Clinical Hypnosis for Pain Control

Clinical Hypnosis for Pain Control

David R. Patterson

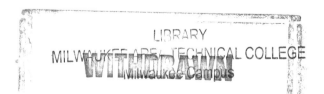
American Psychological Association

Washington, DC

Published by
American Psychological Association
750 First Street, NE
Washington, DC 20002
www.apa.org

To order
APA Order Department
P.O. Box 92984
Washington, DC 20090-2984
Tel: (800) 374-2721; Direct: (202) 336-5510
Fax: (202) 336-5502; TDD/TTY: (202) 336-6123
Online: www.apa.org/books/
E-mail: order@apa.org

In the U.K., Europe, Africa, and the Middle East, copies may be ordered from
American Psychological Association
3 Henrietta Street
Covent Garden, London
WC2E 8LU England

Typeset in Goudy by Circle Graphics, Inc., Columbia, MD

Printer: Edwards Brothers, Ann Arbor, MI
Cover Designer: Minker Design, Sarasota, FL

The opinions and statements published are the responsibility of the authors, and such opinions and statements do not necessarily represent the policies of the American Psychological Association.

Library of Congress Cataloging-in-Publication Data

Patterson, David R.
  Clinical hypnosis for pain control / David R. Patterson. — 1st ed.
    p. cm.
  Includes bibliographical references and index.
  ISBN-13: 978-1-4338-0768-8
  ISBN-10: 1-4338-0768-8
  1. Hypnotism—Therapeutic use. 2. Pain—Treatment. I. Title.

  RC495.P32 2010
  615.8'512—dc22
                                    2009044715

British Library Cataloguing-in-Publication Data

A CIP record is available from the British Library.

Printed in the United States of America
First Edition

CONTENTS

PREFACE

In 1983, I was about four months into my first job, as the psychologist for the rehabilitation medicine unit and the burn unit at the University of Washington Medical School's Harborview Medical Center, when I was given an urgent consult from the patient-care team regarding a 63-year-old man with a large burn injury who was on the intensive care unit. The patient was refusing to return to wound care, which involved a daily regimen of pulling off his bandages (often taking some of the burned skin with them), scrubbing and debriding the wound area, and usually putting a stinging antiseptic on the injury. (I later learned that patients with burn injuries often report that undergoing such wound care is more painful that sustaining the burn injury itself.) Despite high doses of morphine, benzodiazepines, and nitrous oxide, the patient claimed that he would rather die than undergo another dressing change.

I was at a loss as to how I could ask the patient to continue with the excruciatingly painful daily procedure, but I was fortunate enough to have had Bill Fordyce on my faculty at the time. Bill had already established himself as one of the most prominent psychologists ever to work in the area of pain control and one of the architects of the multidisciplinary approach. I called him for a consultation on the patient and was more than taken aback when I heard his brief advice after presenting the case: "Have you tried hypnosis?"

I found a hypnosis induction script in the literature for controlling acute pain and read it to the patient, but I left the room convinced that what I had just done would have little impact on the patient's pain. When I went to check on the patient several hours later, there was a great deal of excitement on the hospital ward. "What did you do to him?" the nurses wanted to know. "We put him in wound care and he fell asleep. He showed no pain at all." The patient underwent the remainder of his dressing changes with little or no pain. Two months later, I saw him in the burn outpatient clinic. I touched the patient on the shoulder as a greeting, and he nearly collapsed in my arms in a seemingly hypnotic state.

It was this experience, as well as several others in the trauma hospital, that led me to become fascinated with hypnosis. I took as many workshops as I could and was lucky enough to meet many of the preeminent names in the field. I also noticed that in the literature hypnosis for pain control had received very little attention, at least in terms of randomized controlled trials with patient populations.

This led me to apply to the National Institutes of Health (NIH) for grant funding, and in 1989 I received funding for my first R01-level study. This was followed by a number of controlled studies and publications in journals such as *Psychological Bulletin*, the *Journal of Consulting and Clinical Psychology*, the *Journal of Abnormal Psychology*, *Pain*, *International Journal of Experimental and Clinical Hypnosis*, and the *American Journal of Clinical Hypnosis*.

In the late 1990s, I began collaborating with Hunter Hoffman on the use of immersive virtual reality in pain control. Hunter was working with the University of Washington Human Interface Technology Laboratory and was interested in creating three-dimensional worlds that are capable of pulling a patient's attention away from pain during medical procedures. Again, with NIH funding, I began applying this technology to hypnosis. Although we will likely never be able to replace the patient relationship and the need to tailor hypnotic suggestions to the needs of patients, virtual reality hypnosis is proving to have tremendous potential for relatively standard applications of hypnosis, such as controlling pain from burn care, trauma, or surgery. My hope is that this technology will make the availability of hypnosis far more widespread, particularly to low-income patients. This technology was reported in two grants submitted to the NIH in 2000 (R01 GM42725-09A1 and 1R21 HD40954-01) and entered the public domain at that point.

Early in my hypnotic training I became fascinated by the work of Milton Erickson and attended several workshops by people who studied with him. However, I was particularly drawn to the work of Steven Gilligan, who had completed a postdoctoral fellowship in Ernest Hilgard's laboratory before studying with Erickson. Thus, although my empirical work was largely structured and relied on scripts to provide standardization, I found that the work of Erickson and Gilligan provided endless creativity and simply made the process of studying hypnosis joyful.

An equally powerful influence on my career and on this book in particular has been Mark Jensen, a colleague on my faculty. Mark has been a prolific pain researcher and became interested in hypnosis over the past few years. Our collaboration led to a review in *Psychological Bulletin* on hypnotic pain control, which has served as a template for the empirically based part of this book. The chapter on chronic pain—one of the more important clinical ones in the book—was written largely by Mark and is primarily driven by his ideas. A book of the quality that I hope the reader will experience would not have been anywhere near possible without Mark's tireless and generous collaboration.

A primary acknowledgment for this book goes to NIH, which funded between 50% and 100% of my salary while I was writing this book and has funded our research in hypnosis since 1989. Scott Sommers has been a wonderful program officer at NIH for over 15 years, and Yvonne Maddox played a significant and early role in encouraging me to stick with my first application. Currently, my research team is funded by NIH under General Medical Sciences (R01 GM42725-09A1) and Arthritis and Musculoskeletal and Skin Diseases (1R01AR054115-01A1).

A number of collaborators at the University of Washington have played a major role in the research that is discussed in this book. I would like to acknowledge Sam Sharar, an anesthesiologist who has lent medical credence to our research on many occasions. Alison Schultz has been my administrative assistant throughout the writing of this book, as well as several years before; she has put countless hours into this book without complaint, and, again, her participation was funded by NIH. Several of my research assistants and nurses, including Maryam Soltani, Gretchen Carrougher, Aubriana Teeley, Sonia Venkatraman, and several others before them, also made valuable contributions. None of this work would have been possible were it not for the long-term support of the surgeons and members of the patient-care team from the University of Washington Burn Center.

Arreed Barabasz and Jeff Borckardt both provided extremely valuable reviews of the first draft of this book. Susan Reynolds, Peter Pavilionis, and Dan Brachtesende from the American Psychological Association have been wonderful in their roles as editors. David Rosengren, Chris Dunn, and Charles Bombardier provided valuable feedback on motivational interviewing, and John Loeser and Judy Turner were very useful in the early chapters.

There are many colleagues in the field of hypnosis who have played a role in my thinking and professional development, and space limitations regretfully prevent me from acknowledging them. Finally, I would like to thank my parents, Roy and Elaine Patterson, whose compassionate careers in health care inspired me to pursue a similar path. My loving wife, Liz, somehow tolerated my partial absence during the years it took to write this, and my boys, Jake, Billy, and Sammy, remain the light of our lives.

Clinical Hypnosis
for Pain Control

INTRODUCTION

It is an exciting time for hypnosis, and its use for pain control represents one of its most compelling and scientific rigorous applications. The number of published experimental theoretical studies and controlled clinical trials in the area of hypnotic pain control has increased significantly over the past 2 decades, and there is a need for a comprehensive treatment of this work. Understanding recent developments in hypnotic analgesia represents one of the best means of advancing the field of hypnosis as a whole.

Unrelieved pain has been increasingly recognized as a serious health problem worldwide but especially in the United States. Over the past 5 decades there have been tremendous advances in both medical and psychological treatments for pain. Yet the field of pain control is also ripe for new developments. Particularly with chronic pain control, medical interventions are known to have limitations and, occasionally, pernicious side effects. Although psychological interventions have provided effective complements—and, occasionally, alternatives—to medical ones, hypnosis offers one of the most promising new clinical approaches for pain control. Although it has been a form of treatment for more than a century, only recently has it been recognized as an empirically supported approach to pain control.

Outside the clinical realm, hypnosis exists in a swirl of popular misconceptions. Even among clinical practitioners, hypnotism finds as many definitions as it does patients. However, for the purposes of this book, Kihlstrom's (2008) definition of *hypnosis* seems appropriate:

> Hypnosis is a process in which one person, designated the hypnotist, offers suggestions to another person, designated the subject, for imaginative experiences entailing alterations in perception, memory, and action. In the classic case, these experiences are associated with a degree of subjective conviction bordering on delusion, and an experienced involuntariness bordering on compulsion. As such, the phenomena of hypnosis reflect alterations in consciousness that take place in the context of a social interaction. (p. 21)

This definition is regarded as being different from training in deep muscle relaxation or guided imagery, both of which are useful psychological approaches for treating pain in themselves.

This book's discussion on hypnosis departs from relaxation and imagery largely by explaining how patients as research subjects can be placed in optimal states to accept suggestions, and in addition, how hypnotic suggestions can be best tailored to reduce suffering from pain. However, there remains a great deal of overlap between hypnosis, relaxation, and imagery, as well as debate over what actually defines hypnosis (Kihlstrom, 1992; Kirsch & Lynn, 1995; Nash, 2001; Patterson & Jensen, 2003). Yet, much like other new, effective clinical innovations that are still acquiring a knowledge base of scientific validity, hypnosis and hypnotic analgesia have already garnered many adherents without such an established base of rigorous scientific validation.

RECENT DEVELOPMENTS IN HYPNOSIS FOR PAIN CONTROL

A number of social and medical trends, and advances in hypnosis itself, have converged in recent years to highlight the utility of hypnotic analgesia in health care. These include the growing importance of nonpharmacological approaches to pain control, societal trends in alternative/complementary medicine, scientific and cost-effectiveness advances in hypnosis, and the potential unique contributions of hypnosis to pain control. Each of these areas is discussed in turn.

The Need for Nonpharmacological Approaches to Pain Control

The importance and value of nonpharmacological approaches to pain control, particularly psychological ones, are increasingly being recognized. Medical and drug therapies have a substantial role in pain control, particularly with acute pain (Loeser, 2001a; Patterson & Sharar, 2001). Without surgeries, medications, anesthetic procedures, and the like, patients would suffer at immensely higher levels (Melzack, 1990). However, overreliance on medical approaches to pain control can have substantial drawbacks. First of all, there are side effects to almost any medications used to treat pain. These can range from gastrointestinal and cognitive effects to, in the case of opioid analgesics, dependence, addiction, and even respiratory arrest (C. Brown, Albrecht, Pettit, McFadden, & Schermer, 2000; Cherny et al., 2001). Surgery for lower back pain is notoriously unreliable. Although 30% of patients improve, 30% remain the same, and 30% actually become worse and experience more pain after back pain surgery (Turk & Okifuji, 1998a, 1998b). Fordyce (1976) was one of the first to point out problems inherent in the medicalization of suffering. When patients pursue solely medical solutions to their pain, the result may be an increase in the chronic nature of their condition and in their suffering (Fordyce, 1976). This is addressed in detail in the discussion on chronic pain conditions, and psychological approaches are also discussed in subsequent chapters.

It would follow that not only is it worthwhile to be conservative in considering drug and surgical options for pain, but it is highly desirable to consider psychological alternatives. Fordyce (1976) has long championed using operant and other psychological approaches to reduce undesirable medical side effects. Hypnosis is increasingly being demonstrated as an approach that can not only supplement medical approaches (Patterson, Everett, Burns, & Marvin, 1992; Patterson & Ptacek, 1997) but also reduce the need for medical interventions (Lang et al., 2000; Montgomery et al., 2007; Ohrbach, Patterson, Carrougher, & Gibran, 1998). There are many ways in which psychological interventions can be used to treat pain, particularly using cognitive–behavioral (Turk, 1978) and operant models (Fordyce, 1976; Patterson, 2005; Turk & Gatchel, 1999). However, what is becoming increasingly clear is that hypnosis provides a new, powerful arena of nonpharmacological approaches that may be able to contribute to pain relief beyond other types of psychological approaches (Kirsch, Montgomery, & Sapirstein, 1995).

Social Trends in Complementary Medicine

Hypnosis should not be categorically labeled as a form of "alternative" or "complementary" medicine. After all, Crasilneck published on the effects of hypnosis in burn injuries in the *Journal of the American Medical Association* in 1955, and the fact that hypnosis was described as a viable treatment for pain in one of the premier medical journals more than 50 years ago should not be neglected. There is nothing "alternative" about the General Medical Sciences section of the National Institutes of Health (NIH) since 1989, which has typically funded bench-level research on hypnotic pain control, yet has also supported clinical studies on hypnotic pain control. Nevertheless, the history of medicine has waxed and waned with regard to alternative approaches to conventional medicine. Often, societal shifts in attitude will occur, sometimes registering frustration with allopathic (conventional) approaches.

A likely source of such frustration is that the amount of time that allo-pathically trained physicians spend with patients has decreased. Because complementary/alternative health care practitioners often spend substantially more time with patients (e.g., consider the time that is typically spent with a massage therapist), patients may respond to frustration with decreased physician time by seeking alternative care. For reasons such as this and concerns about side effects of allopathic medicine, there is a significant trend to pursue complementary treatments (Eisenberg et al., 1993) aggressively. Indeed, there has been an explosion in the use of herbal medications and visits to health care providers who do not fall under the rubric of allopathic. This movement is certain to generate more interest in hypnosis as even "relaxation and imagery" are listed in studies and descriptions of complementary techniques (Eisenberg et al., 1993). The work of Lang and her colleagues (Lang et al., 2000), which is clearly some of the most significant in recent hypnotic analgesia research, was funded by the Complementary and Alternative Medicine branch of the NIH. This is some of the strongest clinical work done in research with hypnosis and demonstrates some potential value to the field if hypnosis is conceptualized as alternative.

The Increased Scientific Basis for Hypnosis

Over the past 2 decades, there has been a welcome increase in scientific support for hypnosis. Whereas randomized controlled studies to test hypnosis in clinical settings were almost nonexistent a few years ago, there is now a body of this literature in support of hypnosis for a number of medical problems, including irritable bowel syndrome (Barabasz & Watkins, 2005; Gonsalkorale, Miller, Afzal, & Whorwell, 2003; Whorwell, Prior, & Faragher, 1984), asthma (Ben-Zvi, Spohn, Young, & Kattan, 1982; Ewer & Stewart, 1986; Isenberg, Lehrer, & Hochron, 1992; Maher-Loughnan, Mason, Macdonald, & Fry, 1962), smoking cessation (Visweswaran & Schmidt, 1992), obesity (Kirsch, 1996), and pain control (Patterson & Jensen, 2003).

From a different source of scientific credibility for hypnosis, investigators are taking advantage of sophisticated methods to investigate brain activity associated with hypnosis (Barabasz et al., 1999; Killeen & Nash, 2003; Rainville & Price, 2004; Ray & Tucker, 2003; Raz, 2005, 2008; Raz, Fan, & Posner, 2005; Raz, Lamar, Buhle, Kane, & Peterson, 2007; Raz & Shapiro, 2002; Woody & Szechtman, 2003). The fact that Rainville published data of this nature in *Science* (Rainville, Duncan, Price, Carrier, & Bushnell, 1997) is testimony to the credibility that hypnosis is gaining validity in the scientific community. Currently, the question with this group of researchers seems not to be, Is there a physiological marker for a hypnotic state? but rather, What is the progression of neurophysiological markers that define hypnosis? Although studies of brain activity during hypnosis do not represent a type of clinical outcome, they certainly add to the theoretical foundation for this type of intervention.

An additional area of research worth discussing is the potential of offsetting health care costs with hypnosis. Lang et al. (2000) published findings in *The Lancet* about the impact that hypnosis has on pain and anxiety associated with perioperative procedures (e.g., insertion of catheters). What was groundbreaking about this research was that a subsequent report (Lang & Rosen, 2002) indicated that hypnosis reduced the cost of care from an average of $635 per patient to $300. Equally important, Montgomery et al. (2007) recently reported that their cost-offset findings were even more impressive in the treatment of breast cancer. Also, there are groups of investigators who are constantly generating and refining sophisticated theories that attempt to explain the mechanisms of hypnosis, and this research activity is common knowledge in the clinical community (Nash & Barnier, 2008). Mike Nash, the former editor of the *International Journal of Clinical Hypnosis*, quipped that without a sound scientific basis, "Hypnosis will go the way of phrenology" (personal communication, October 24, 2007); fortunately, with the trends noted previously, the scientific support for hypnosis is flourishing.

Unique Contributions of Hypnosis to Pain Control

Cognitive–behavioral and behavioral techniques have been receiving attention in the literature for years. Such approaches have a substantial impact on pain control and are well documented (Fordyce, 1976; Turk & Gatchel, 1999; Turk, Meichenbaum, & Genest, 1983; Turk & Okifuji, 1998a, 1998b). Clinicians now have such techniques at their disposal, and some may feel that such operant and cognitive–behavioral techniques have reached their maximum potential for having an impact. To be sure, many psychological approaches to pain control have reached a plateau, and the field is ready for the infusion of new techniques. What is promising in this regard is the potential for hypnosis to offer pain relief above and beyond the levels of other such psychological approaches. In the meta-analysis published by Kirsch et al. (1995), hypnosis was found to produce treatment effects above and beyond the effects of basic psychotherapy approaches. At least with acute pain, hypnosis has been reported to be superior when combined with other treatment approaches (Patterson & Jensen, 2003).

Hypnosis is remarkable for how it can have an impact on some types of pain with some types of patients who do not seem to respond to other approaches (Crasilneck, 1995; Ohrbach et al., 1998). Researchers are only beginning to learn how hypnosis can reduce pain; this area of investigation is in its infancy relative to other types of psychological pain control. Hypnosis has the potential to reduce suffering in patients dramatically, in ways that other approaches do not (Patterson & Jensen, 2003). Conversely, like any approach, hypnosis will have little or no effect on some patients, and in such cases its application should be abandoned in favor of other approaches.

A BRIEF HISTORY OF HYPNOSIS FOR PAIN CONTROL

To the extent that humans have exercised the use of their mind to relieve pain with some sort of ritual that facilitates trancelike states, hypnosis is timeless; the examples across cultures and throughout history are too numerous to even mention here. Whether pain was controlled by a village shaman freeing a patient from evil forces or by a faith healer making use of a person's religious beliefs, throughout time, interpersonal processes have allowed people to reduce or eliminate their pain by relying solely on the mind. There have always been interpersonal and psychological resources that can create profound analgesia; the challenge has been accessing them in a manner that is systematic and routine. It would be presumptuous to attribute all of the amazing examples of "mind over matter" in terms of pain control to hypnosis, yet this approach offers a wonderful porthole to allow us to understand the workings of the human mind.

The history of hypnosis, including early contributions of Franz Anton Mesmer (mesmerism), is reviewed nicely in other texts (see Barabasz & Watkins, 2005; Rainville & Price, 2004). This overview, then, will focus on the history of hypnosis and pain control, which can be traced back largely to the 19th century, when a Scottish physician named James Esdaile reported that he had successfully used hypnosis, or "mesmerism" as he called it, as the sole anesthetic in 345 major operations performed in India. Although Esdaile's success rate has been questioned (Chaves & Dworkin, 1997), he likely did have a profound effect on a large number of patients using the new technique of mesmerism. At about the same time, another Scottish physician, James Braid, cautiously endorsed Esdaile's mesmerism practice but made a departure with his own advance on mesmerism. Braid's technique, which he called "neuro-hypnotism" (or "nervous sleep")—and, later, simply "hypnotism"—involved the first use of eye-fixation induction techniques.

The medical/clinical applications of mesmerism and Braid's hypnosis to pain control were largely dormant for a number of decades. Crasilneck's report in the *Journal of the American Medical Association* in the mid-1950s has already been mentioned. It was also during this time that Milton Erickson began to report his extensive clinical work. Although only a small portion of his work was with pain control, the clinical/therapeutic oeuvre had a huge impact on reviving interest in hypnosis in the psychology and medical communities.

In the 1950s and 1960s, scholars began to turn their attention to the theoretical underpinnings of hypnosis. During this period, pain reduction and analgesia often went hand in hand. A large reason for this is that pain control is a hypnotic phenomenon that is often so clear and capable of measurement that it often was (and still is) used as the dependent variable of perceptual change in laboratory studies. Consequently, many of the investigators during this period were interested in hypnosis as a phenomenon in itself, and pain control was more of an experimental tool than the primary focus of study.

The most salient example in this regard is the work of Ernest Hilgard. In two of Hilgard's greatest contributions to the hypnosis literature, laboratory studies of hypnotic analgesia figured prominently. One such contribution was the trait theory of hypnosis, which held that the ability to be hypnotized is largely an inherent talent. The attempts of Weitzenhoffer and Hilgard (1959, 1962) to measure this variable led to scales of hypnotizability. In turn, pain control in the laboratory setting (e.g., in analog studies, or pain created "artificially"—from a tourniquet, heat, or cold presses) was found to be strongly associated with response to scales measuring hypnotizability. Furthermore, Hilgard's "neo-dissociation" conceptualization of hypnotizability also had its genesis largely in hypnotic analgesia. Hilgard noted that many people who were hypnotized appeared to show simultaneous channels of consciousness, some split off from others (Hilgard & Hilgard, 1975). This allowed a hidden observer to be able to examine the hypnotic phenomena seemingly with other parts of consciousness not being engaged.

To illustrate, Hilgard and colleagues claimed that laboratory subjects often reported a conscious reduction of pain, yet their subject's physiological response to pain remained unchanged (Hilgard & Hilgard, 1975). In other words, under hypnosis human subjects would rate their pain as less, but such indicators as increased heart rate (during the application of pain stimuli) would remain unchanged.

In the 1970s to 1990s (and certainly up to the present), a great number of articles were published on the theoretical underpinnings of hypnosis. Investigators largely fell into two theoretical camps: those who viewed hypnosis as a normal cognitive process that is influenced mainly by social psychological phenomena (Kirsch & Lynn, 1995; Lynn, Kirsch, & Hallquist, 2008) and those who regarded it to be a special cognitive state (Hilgard & Hilgard, 1975; Woody & Sadler, 2008). Once again, pain control was central to many of the studies attempting to demonstrate a particular theoretical point of view in the laboratory. Sociocognitive theorists reported findings, for example, that the process of going through a hypnotic induction is not necessary to create hypnotic analgesia (pain control suggestions will work either way), in support of their approach (Chaves, 1986, 1989, 1993, 1994; Chaves & Barber, 1974, 1976; Chaves & Brown, 1987; Chaves & Dworkin, 1997). In contrast, dissociated-control theorists reported subjects under hypnosis could easily and effortlessly experience pain reduction under an induction, supporting their contention that it worked through facilitating automatic processes (Bowers & Brennenman, 1981; Patterson, Hoffman, Palacios, & Jensen, 2006; Woody & Sadler, 2008). In essence, pain control remained the center of many theoretical studies on hypnosis. Pain reduction was often the dependent variable in studies whose theoretical premises were at the opposite ends of the spectrum.

In the 1990s, there was an increased push for empirical validation of hypnosis and support for its use in clinical interventions in both psychology and medicine. Unfortunately, at that time there were almost no randomized controlled studies for hypnosis and pain control; yet hypnotic analgesia was one of the most scientifically based and time-honored applications of hypnosis. Fortunately, over the next 2 decades there was a steady increase of randomized controlled studies. In 2000, Montgomery et al. reported their meta-analysis on a combination of laboratory and clinical studies and found that hypnosis was able to reduce pain in roughly 75% of the people in a clinical or research setting. A review of such randomized controlled studies in a 2003 *Psychological Bulletin* review found that the majority of such studies reported favorable effects (Patterson & Jensen, 2003). As discussed previously, Elvira Lang and colleagues reported on hypnotic analgesia for periopertative procedures in *The Lancet*— the largest randomized clinical study done on clinical hypnosis at that time. Both Lang and then Montgomery reported (Lang & Rosen, 2002; Montgomery et al., 2007) that hypnotic analgesia can have significant cost-offsetting impacts in surgical procedures and cancer treatment, respectively. Once again, in areas of hypnosis that are important to the literature in general, such as empirically support treatment and cost offsetting, the application of this treatment to pain control has taken a prominent position.

As is increasingly the case in psychology and medicine, the degree to which hypnotic processes can be demonstrated through sophisticated brain imaging studies can be a significant marker for how well such processes are accepted in the scientific community. Over the past few decades, there have been a number of important attempts to demonstrate changes in brain activity associated with various aspects of hypnosis, using such methodologies as skin conductance tests, electroencephalograms, brain positron emission tomography scans, and, more recently, magnetic resonance imaging (Rainville, Hofbauer, et al., 1999). The seminal study in this area was published by Rainville et al. in *Science* in 1997. They reported that not only do suggestions for hypnotic analgesia show related brain activity that can be measured through radiologic techniques but also that the nature and activity of brain activity depend on the nature of hypnotic suggestions given. As such, different hypnotic suggestions for pain will result in different areas of the brain responding. (The theoretical implications of this work is discussed more in Chapter 3.) In terms of historical significance, Rainville's work has a major implication: Pain control was again a central subject area that was prominent in moving the science of hypnosis forward. This time, however, the findings are in one of the most prestigious journals for any area of science, and they advanced the notion that hypnosis has some basic theoretical underpinnings.

Some interesting implications for the future have to do with the application of technology to the delivery of hypnosis, ranging from Borckardt and Nash's (2002) efforts to computerize the delivery of hypnosis and assessment of hypnotizability to the delivery of hypnosis for pain control using immersive virtual reality (Oneal, Patterson, Soltani, Teeley, & Jensen, 2008; Patterson, Tininenko, Schmidt, & Sharar, 2004; Patterson, Wiechman, Jensen, & Sharar, 2006). The latter technique allows patients to go into a compelling visual world for induction purposes with their eyes remaining open, which should be useful to people who are less hypnotizable or who struggle with their imagination. Such innovative techniques may also make hypnosis more widely applicable to clinical situations in which a clinician trained in hypnosis is not available.

In sum, the history of hypnosis has been shaped largely by attempts to control human pain. Pain is a problem that has often driven clinicians to try hypnosis, and it is also a perceptual phenomenon that has been a favorite of many theorists and researchers in the field (based on the ability of scientists to create the perceptual phenomenon of pain). The field has moved from relying on dramatic anecdotal reports to sophisticated studies with randomized controlled designs, to ones that use advanced diagnostic techniques to study brain activity.

OVERVIEW OF THIS BOOK

The recent developments in hypnosis and pain control have moved so quickly that it has been difficult for investigators to compile useful compendiums that keep up with all the advances in knowledge and theory. It is hoped that this volume will be able to present what researchers have discovered from recent developments, but in a way that clinicians will find applicable to their work. More important, however, this book is designed to stimulate both practicality and creativity in applying hypnosis to pain control. Typically, clinicians seem to discuss pain as a general phenomenon, but just as the Inuit (Eskimos) have multiple words for snow, clinicians must know what types and aspects of pain they are dealing with before applying hypnosis. Acute pain and chronic pain are often on opposite ends of the treatment spectrum. The intense pain from predictable procedures usually requires a different approach to treatment than ongoing discomfort that has lasted for months. Ultimately, the goal of this volume is to leave both clinicians and researchers with many clinical tools for understanding and treating pain that are solidly based in science and clinical applications. Equally important, readers should be stimulated to create several new approaches as well.

This book is intended for any health care professional who is interested in hypnosis for pain control. Much of the book is designed to provide practical applications that will be applicable to patients who are suffering from a wide variety of etiologies for pain. Yet the subject matter is also addressed in a manner that, it is hoped, will be of interest to researchers and scientists working in the area of pain control. A number of other agendas were considered in the presentation of the material. Hypnosis as a treatment for pain control has not been adequately recognized either for its rich history of theoretical and laboratory research or for the many randomized controlled clinical trials that provide an empirically supported and evidence-based foundation for using this approach for patients who are experiencing clinical pain. A compilation of such information can be important for professionals promoting hypnosis in most health care systems as well as to make care delivery more efficient and cost-effective.

This book also seeks to provide a synthesis between some of the basic research that has been done on hypnosis and pain control and Ericksonian approaches to hypnosis. In this regard, a central purpose of this volume, again, is to provide the best of scientific analysis and clinical technique that is driven by the pain literature and based on the clinical richness of Milton Erickson's work. However practical the reader finds the clinical presentation, it is also nevertheless intended to generate creative thinking among researchers. The book culminates with ways through which hypnosis can be integrated with brief counseling therapies that are applicable for patients suffering from chronic pain.

Chapters 1, 2, and 3 of this book focus on the scientific foundations of hypnotic analgesia and also provide background on psychological approaches to pain. Chapters 4 and 5 provide an overview of Ericksonian conceptualizations of hypnosis and then describe how Erickson approached pain control specifically. Chapters 6 and 7 discuss in much more detail how to approach acute and chronic pain conditions with hypnosis. Chapter 8 describes how hypnosis can be combined with motivational interviewing, a particularly useful approach for chronic pain; however, this chapter also seeks to provide a culmination of this book—that is, how counseling and practical clinical hypnotic techniques can be combined to provide powerful tools to improve the quality of life in patients suffering from pain.

1

UNDERSTANDING PAIN AND ITS PSYCHOLOGICAL APPROACHES

This chapter is divided into two sections. The first section discusses the nature of pain, emphasizing its attempted reduction using psychological approaches, particularly hypnosis. The second section reviews specific psychological interventions (other than hypnosis) that mental health professionals should be familiar with when treating a patient who presents with pain symptoms. These sections are further subdivided into approaches for acute and chronic pain, consistent with the notion that each type presents a different challenge for aspects of pain control and must be addressed accordingly (Patterson, 2004; Patterson & Jensen, 2003).

PRACTICAL IMPLICATIONS OF PAIN PHYSIOLOGY

The physiology of pain discussed here is from the perspective of its treatment with psychological approaches. More detailed discussions can be found in works by pain experts (Loeser, 2001a, 2001b). My premise is that clinicians will be more effective at controlling pain if they understand its underlying mechanisms, but effective hypnotic analgesia does not require that hypnotic suggestions accurately mirror the physiology of pain. As an example to illustrate this point, there is at least strong anecdotal evidence that hypnosis can reduce blood loss associated with surgical procedures (Bennett, 1993). When hypnotized patients show less blood loss, it is seldom because clinicians have provided hypnotic suggestions that are based on the vascular physiology of reduced blood loss (e.g., "You will find that your capillaries will become constricted in critical regions of your body, thereby reducing internal bleeding in the region of your surgery"). Rather, patients typically receive a more generic hypnotic suggestion that indirectly leads to reduced blood loss (e.g., "You will heal quickly with minimal complication"). Alternatively, hypnotic suggestions for increased relaxation and comfort may reduce the release of catecholamines (i.e., stress hormones) that increase blood pressure, resulting in less physiological arousal and attendant blood loss. Similarly, in the setting of pain, a clinician is less likely to suggest to a patient, "You will be able to activate the descending fibers that travel along your spinal cord in a manner that shuts down the gate in the dorsal horn of your spinal cord." Although this information may be physiologically accurate, the body does not know how to translate this language into corresponding physiological changes. Instead, hypnotic suggestions that are more practical and matched to the patient's educational level are more likely to have clinical benefit. Thus, simply suggesting to patients that they will experience less pain will likely be as effective as describing the mechanisms of gate control theory.

Hypnotic suggestions do not have to mirror pain physiology to have a clinical analgesic effect; however, it is extremely valuable for those using hypnosis to understand the physiological underpinnings of pain. Although hypnotic suggestions seldom have to reflect the neurophysiology of analgesia, understanding the nature of pain will make the clinician more effective in a variety of ways. As a simple example, some types of pain will respond better to topical application of heat, whereas others respond to coolness. Further, for some types of injuries it is more important to use ice early in treatment and heat at a later point. Clinicians using hypnosis obviously will be more effective if they are aware of such medical management strategies.

John Loeser's (1980) "onion model" is helpful for explaining the concepts of pain discussed in this chapter. As shown in Figure 1.1, pain and suffering occur at different levels, with nociception at the core. *Nociception* refers to mechanical, thermal, or chemical energy impinging on specialized peripheral nerve endings, signaling to the central nervous system that adverse events are occurring. Pain is the sensory experience that can arise from nociception. At the next level, *suffering* is the affective or emotional response in the central nervous system, triggered by the experience of pain or by other adverse events. Finally, beyond suffering are *pain behaviors*—that is, what people do to communicate that they are in pain, through interaction with their

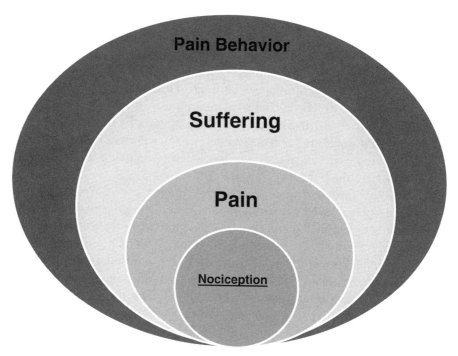

Figure 1.1. The "onion model" for understanding pain. Adapted from "Perspectives on Pain," by J. D. Loeser. In P. Turner (Ed.), *Clinical Pharmacology and Therapeutics,* 1980, pp. 313–316. London, England: Macmillan. Adapted with permission.

environment. Some of these can be obvious, such as limping, grimacing, or groaning. Others are more subtle, such as not going to work with the arrival of disability payments.

The Nature of an Injury Cannot Reliably Predict Pain or Suffering

It is tempting to assume that, based only on the type of injury, lesion, or illness present, one would be able to predict how much pain and suffering a patient will experience. Antiquated models of pain processing would indeed lead us to assume this is the case (Melzack & Wall, 1965). For example, if one stubs a toe, both practical sense and outmoded models would lead one to assume that there is a direct line of the communication between the toe and the brain; the brain registers signals that come from the toe and that the signals are in direct proportion to how hard the toe is stubbed. We know now from the gate control theory and other more sophisticated models that pain signals can potentially be modulated, derailed, enhanced, or suppressed as soon as they enter the dorsal horn and begin their journey to the brain

(Melzack, 1999; Melzack & Wall, 1973). As an example, I might call you on the phone from Chicago when you are in London and tell you that I am calling from Greece. The satellite signals may be carried along a repeater in say, Athens, but at least from the ambient sounds on my end, you have no way of verifying that I am not calling from Chicago. This is the case with pain signals, particularly with chronic pain, nerve injuries, and certain types of disease that cause nerve damage. The pathology may not lie in the body region where the pain is reported but instead may be elsewhere in the nervous system and influence the apparent transmission of nociceptive information from the periphery to the brain.

There are important implications of this complex nature of pain transmission with respect to working with patients. First, a patient's pain complaint should not be questioned merely because the minimal nature of the stimulus (e.g., wound) is such that the clinician determines it could not possibly generate such pain. A typical source of contention in the hospital setting is for a health care professional to observe a minimal wound or injury and conclude that the patient "should not be hurting so much." Current theories and research argue that the patient's perception of his or her own pain should seldom if ever be dismissed (Barabasz & Watkins, 2005; Hilgard & Hilgard, 1975; Melzack, 1999; Patterson & Sharar, 2001; Price & Bushnell, 2004; Ptacek, Patterson, Montgomery, Ordonez, & Heimbach, 1995). Moreover, we now know that there are vast individual differences in the responses to noxious stimuli (Bayer, Coverdale, Chiang, & Bangs, 1998). How one reacts to painful stimuli varies on the basis of age, gender, ethnicity, prior experiences with pain, and a host of other psychosocial factors (R. R. Edwards & Fillingim, 1999; Ellermeier & Westphal, 1995; Woodrow, Friedman, Siegelaub, & Collen, 1972). To use cutaneous burn injuries as an example, it was long assumed that once an injury was healed, there was no reason for patients to feel pain. More recent evidence indicates that burn pain can result in neuropathic damage, so that even if a wound has long been healed, patients may still experience pain of a different, more chronic nature (Schneider, Holavanahalli, Helm, Goldstein, & Kowalske, 2006). Going back to the original points in this section, not only do hypnotic suggestions not need to reflect the exact mechanisms of pain, but in many cases even the most knowledgeable clinician can seldom account accurately for the exact mechanism of pain.

Another practical implication of this poor association between the nociceptive lesion and the actual pain experienced relates to the patients' explanations for why they are hurting. Often, patients with chronic pain will have an *illness conviction,* or an assertion that some type of injury or illness is causing their pain. Consequently, a first step in helping patients cope with their pain is for them to understand that the process underlying their pain may not be what they think it is. A patient may insist that the answer to his or her chronic, severe foot pain problem is to amputate, despite the fact that an amputation would do little to alter the nociceptive input that the patient is experiencing. Again, in terms of the *source* of pain, the "phone call" may actually come from Greece rather than Chicago, and it can be very helpful to educate patients about the difference, particularly when their conceptualization of the pain may lead to aggressive surgical treatments that are unlikely to affect the real source of the problem.

Pain and Suffering Can Become Imprinted Into the Brain

Evidence of nociception is not necessary for the appearance of pain behavior. Patients often complain of pain when there is no evidence of a physical lesion or a disease process that can be clearly linked to that complaint. At the same time, it is extremely rare for pain complaints to arise when there was never any sort of injury or disease process present at the outset. Almost all patients have had some type of anatomic or physiological insult that can explain their initial pain. The clinical problem of chronic pain often arises when pain and suffering persist long (months or years) after the physical source for the problem has disappeared. Several sections in this book address how psychological factors can keep pain behavior and suffering in place long after the source of nociception is gone, as well as how they can be addressed.

With respect to basic theory and research, the concept of *neuroplasticity* helps us understand how the experience of pain can become imprinted into the brain, allowing pain to persist long after the tissue damage has healed. This is described in Ronald Melzack's (1999) article "From the Gate to the Neuromatrix." Over time, humans who have experienced pain can develop neurological responses such that when the proper stimuli are present, the brain will respond as if in pain. Fordyce (1976) described this well in terms of a classical conditioning paradigm. Experiencing pain in the absence of nociception can be no different from salivating at the smell of bread baking in the oven. For a patient with chronic back pain, the idea of picking up a heavy box may be sufficient to recreate the experience of pain. Further, even asking patients with chronic pain about how they are feeling can be a sufficient stimulus to generate internal suffering and external pain behaviors. The presence of a spouse who is solicitous about pain (i.e., reinforces the patient's pain behavior) can also be a factor in increasing pain behavior (Sanders, 1996). In other words, if a spouse responds to pain complaints with compassion and caring (which certainly would not be outside of what might be anticipated in a marriage or partnership), this might actually serve to increase suffering by the patient. Germane to the present discussion is evidence that the mere presence of a spouse is enough to create differences in brain activity (as measured by neurophysiologic brain imaging) in patients with chronic pain. Specifically, brain regions that register pain show increased activity when the patient is in the presence of a spouse (Flor, Kerns, & Turk, 1987).

The concept of neuroplasticity also helps us understand that patients with chronic pain are truly suffering, that the pain is not simply "all in their heads," and that physicians face enormous challenges in attempting to treat chronic pain. While it may seem to be good news when a thorough history and physical examination fail to reveal a physical nociceptive lesion in the patient with chronic pain, the potential bad news is that the patient has become conditioned to respond internally as if pain is being inflicted on him or her, and overcoming such typically longstanding problems can be a formidable task. Certainly one of the greatest challenges in treating chronic pain is not only helping the patient overcome such deep-seated impulses but also helping the patient understand such complex concepts in the first place. Hypnosis represents one of the most promising approaches to address some of the challenges that are presented by neuroplasticity of pain in patients.

Cognitions and the Brain Can Override Pain Signals

The notion that the manner in which one thinks about pain can influence how much suffering one experiences is strongly supported by the gate control theory (Melzack, 1999) and other such theoretical advancements. It was through such empirical and theoretical work that we learned that pain signals are modulated in the spinal cord and the brainstem *before* they reach the brain. Pain is modulated by a complex interaction of ascending and descending neural signals that open or shut the pain gate. However, it is possible for higher cortical function to override modulation of pain signals at the dorsal spinal cord level (i.e., the gate). In other words, the manner in which the brain interprets or attends to pain signals can have a significant impact on the amount of suffering a person ends up experiencing internally.

Melzack (1973), in *The Puzzle of Pain*, described how cultural values can influence the perception of pain. For example, Kosambi (1967) reported on ceremonies practiced in remote villages in India. "Celebrants" are suspended in the air by two metal hooks in the small of their backs. Rather than pain, the celebrants are observed to be in a state of exaltation. Similarly, anthropologists (Kroeber, 1948) have observed the practice of couvades in which women show virtually no distress during childbirth. The authors use this as an illustration of the notion that the context in which pain is experienced can greatly influence how much suffering is experienced. Beecher's (1959) classic work is often cited in this vein. Beecher observed that the wounded soldiers he treated in World War II requested far less morphine for a major injury than did the patients he later cared for in a peacetime setting. He ascertained that the interpretation of the pain was critical in this regard. For the soldiers, the wound and pain meant that they were likely to be released from combat duty and to go home alive. A more recent illustration is the case of a hiker in Utah who was trapped by a large boulder that fell on his arm. He not only performed an amputation of his own arm with a pocketknife to free himself but also intentionally broke his arm in order for the self-performed surgery to occur. In such cases, the option of facing certain death allows individuals to tolerate intense and self-inflicted pain.

There is good anecdotal evidence that in some individuals, hypnosis may act to override the neuroprocessing of pain at the spinal cord level. Most compelling in this respect are the hundreds of surgeries performed by Esdaile (1957) in the 19th century, as well as multiple different types of surgeries performed in modern-day medicine with hypnosis as the only anesthetic (Hilgard & Hilgard, 1975). Major invasive surgery is one of the most challenging types of pain that any human can endure and certainly presents a compelling case that those patients that calmly endure it with only hypnosis might be overriding pain signals in some fashion.

As is discussed throughout this book, hypnosis involves far more than intentionally pulling the patient's attention away from pain. Although attentional processes are certainly involved, with hypnotic analgesia, additional mechanisms are also involved, such as perceptual alterations. Hypnosis is often invoking the effortless perceptual change that seems to bypass the scrutiny of high-level cognitive screening (Price & Bushnell, 2004). Further, even when attentional mechanisms are involved with hypnotic analgesia, they are complex and multilayered. Thus, although hypnotic analgesia partially works through attentional/distraction mechanisms, there is evidence that a number of other cognitive neurophysiological processes play a role in pain relief of this nature (Faymonville et al., 1997; Freeman, Barabasz, Barabasz, & Warner, 2000; Rainville & Price, 2004; J. T. Smith, Barabasz, & Barabasz, 1996).

The important point to be understood is that, in some circumstances, it is possible to override pain signals through higher order cognitive processes. The manner in which such factors as attention and motivation can alter perceptual processes is poorly understood, but hypnosis offers an effective vehicle to allow such changes in pain perception to occur.

Anxiety and Acute Pain

The relationship between anxiety and acute pain is so powerful that it is often not clear clinically which issue is predominant. Certainly, there is a cyclical interaction between acute pain and anxiety; one promotes the other. Undergoing a traumatic procedure that can create acute pain is one of the most unpleasant and threatening events that a human can experience. Such a nociceptive barrage of great intensity can elicit a fight-or-flight response to the current event, as well as a desire to escape further intense episodes of pain in the future. An acute pain episode can create a conditioned anxiety response, whereas the stimulus for a subsequent medical procedure becomes a stimulus for anxiety. As an example, Chapter 6 discusses the "green scrubs" response in children who encountered uniformed medical care personnel. Pediatric patients have been known to demonstrate a fear response to health care professionals wearing hospital attire (green scrubs) because painful procedures are often performed by individuals in such garments. If patients experience pain during one procedure, the resulting anxiety described previously can heighten pain during a subsequent one. Anxiety can create heightened vigilance and arousal. These factors, in turn, can cause a heightened pain response to a procedure (Williams, 1999). With repeated procedures, such as burn wound debridement, cancer treatment, or dental care, both pain and anxiety can increase over time. It is not a matter of the patient becoming less tolerant of the procedures; rather, the cyclical interaction between pain and anxiety makes tolerating such repetitive medical procedures increasingly difficult.

It follows that providing adequate analgesia and sedation for the first of several medical procedures can prevent this unfortunate cycle from beginning. This can be seen in the practice of an effective pediatric dentist who will have young patients merely sit in the dental chair for their first sessions, with the only purpose being to have fun. The dentist is first ensuring that the chair itself does not become a threatening stimulus. Having the patients open their mouth and be exposed to potentially painful dentistry procedure comes later. Unfortunately, in many instances, children (and adults) do not receive adequate analgesia during their first procedure. With children, this creates a "runaway train" clinical problem in which their anxiety as well as need to escape is so powerful that no amount of subsequent analgesia can be sufficient. In addition, there are many instances of acute pain from unexpected trauma and related medical procedures for which appropriate analgesic preparation is not possible. Referrals for reducing pain with hypnosis will often be with patients who have built up such conditioned anxiety.

PSYCHOLOGICAL APPROACHES TO PAIN CONTROL

Practitioners who use hypnosis for pain control must be aware of basic psychological approaches to the conceptualization and management of this clinical challenge. For some patients with chronic pain, an educational focus is most beneficial, whereas for others, the most important intervention will involve increasing activity in a manner that does not overwhelm the patient. A clinician who knows nothing about such interventions will be sorely deficient in patient treatment skills. Along the same lines, the clinician must understand the patient's medical disorder and history. Although medical training cannot be expected in professionals managing the psychological part of care, the patient should have had a through medical work up before this type of care is initiated.

For all psychological interventions, including hypnosis, it is important to distinguish whether a patient's pain is acute or chronic. The sections below describe what psychological approaches are appropriate based on these parameters.

Chronic pain is generally of 3 to 6 months duration, often refractory to medical interventions, and associated with complications such as depression, anxiety, and inactivity. Given that acute and chronic pain are discussed extensively in Chapters 6 and 7, their definitions are touched on only briefly here.

Acute Pain

With acute pain, clinicians are often addressing spikes of pain that are temporary but intense, extremely uncomfortable, and usually related to tissue damage or potential tissue damage. Anxiety is often a challenge in patient care.

Educational Interventions

Pain from medical procedures often comes with warning and anticipation. There are both advantages and disadvantages to this. Most patients who know that they will be going through a painful procedure experience anticipatory anxiety. Such anxiety is unpleasant leading up to the procedure but can also exacerbate pain at the time of the procedure. Particularly with children, treating the anxiety can be a greater challenge than the pain itself. The good news that comes with warning the patient before a medical procedure is that it often affords the clinician the opportunity to prepare the patient. Psychological interventions for patients undergoing acute pain involve, in large part, the provision of information, as reviewed by Everett, Patterson, and Chen (1990).

There are two types of information that can be given to patients to prepare them for procedures. The first is procedural information, which focuses on what will happen during the procedure. A patient undergoing a magnetic resonance imaging (MRI) scan, for example, might be told that she will slide into a cavernous machine and is instructed not to move for 30 minutes. She will be warned about the noise that she will hear during the MRI scan. A number of studies have indicated that providing procedural information can make medical procedures more tolerable (Everett et al., 1990).

Sensory information focuses on what a patient will feel during the procedure. With burn wound debridement, for example, patients might be told that they will feel some of their necrotic skin being pulled off when bandages are pulled away and that they will experience a stinging sensation when an antiseptic is applied. The provision of sensory information has also been reported to help patients to tolerate procedures (Patterson, 1992).

There is an important caveat to consider in providing preparatory information, and this has to do with patients' preferred coping strategies. Although providing procedural or sensory information may benefit some patients, for others it may actually serve to exacerbate their anxiety. The variable to consider here is whether patients cope best with medical threats by mentally removing themselves from the situation or whether they tend to focus on threatening procedures. Patients with avoidant/repressor coping styles typically will not benefit from information. They will not want to hear much about the procedure before it happens, and they find information only makes them more anxious. On the other hand, patients who are sensitizers tend to take a hypervigilant stance toward their procedures. They will actively seek information and will want to know in great detail what will occur to them during the procedure. In summary, providing patients with preparatory information can be very helpful to patients in managing acute pain; however, it is important that this be done with sensitivity to the patient's coping style. If nothing else, just asking the patient how much information he or she would like to have can be useful in this respect.

Discriminative Conditioning

When patients undergo painful procedures, they frequently experience a stress response. In extremes, a painful procedure can even elicit phobic responses or, more rarely, posttraumatic stress disorder. Even in the absence of more disabling or severe responses, the environment in which medical procedures take place may become a cue for anxiety or unpleasant anticipation. The best safeguard against this is for patients not to experience acute pain in the first place. If they are sufficiently treated by pharmacological and/or psychological approaches, then this process of conditioning will be far less likely to occur. In any event, making the environment less threatening can be beneficial. An increasing number of medical and dental offices have fish tanks or waterfalls in the waiting area for this reason. Playrooms for children serve a similar function, as do making pediatric MRI machines appear as "caves in the jungle" or burn hydrotanks as playful tubs with "rubber ducks." While decreasing the threat of the environment is one strategy to prevent or reduce anticipatory anxiety, treating fear of procedures as a type of phobic response can also be a useful approach. Training the patient in deep relaxation and then introducing the threat of the stimulus in a gradual manner might be useful to patients who have a conditioned fear of procedures, as well as anxiety from any source. This is the essence of the hypnotic approach presented in Chapter 6 but the same task can also be addressed through basic psychological approaches.

Distraction

Burn pain and wound treatment procedures often increase patients' anxiety, and such emotional responses exacerbate acute pain (Chapman & Nakamura, 1999; Chapman & Turner, 1986; France, Krishnan, & Houpt, 1988). Distraction can reduce this anxiety. The efficacy of distraction techniques is often explained in the context of a gate control heuristic (Gasma, 1994). Specifically, attention, beliefs about pain, expectations, and attributions are thought to inhibit or modify the nociceptive signals (Turk, Meichenbaum, & Genest, 1983).

At a less theoretical level, regardless of the mechanism, the effectiveness of cognitive interventions involving distraction is empirically supported in the literature. In a meta-analysis of adjunctive treatments for several types of pain, Fernandez and Turk (1989) found that cognitive–behavioral strategies significantly reduced measures of pain in 85% of the 47 studies analyzed, with distraction proving to be among the most effective strategies. A growing number of recent laboratory and field studies from several disciplines are consistent with this conclusion. Pain tolerance to cold pressors increased significantly for subjects viewing humorous or repulsive movies (Weisenberg, Tepper, & Schwarzwald, 1995). Distraction with movies improved pain tolerance to gastrointestinal procedures in 82% of patients in one study (Kozarek et al., 1997). Cartoon distraction paired with coaching reduced children's distress during immunizations (Cohen, Blout, & Panopoulos, 1997), and a program combining behavioral training with a video cartoon/movie distraction technique allowed 9 of the 11 child patients to avoid traditional sedation for daily cancer radiation treatments (Slifer, 1996). Most relevant, A. C. Miller, Hickman, and Lemasters (1992) found that showing scenic movies and playing music during burn wound dressing changes led to significant reductions in pain and anxiety. Further controlled evaluations on pain distraction during burn wound care are needed, and a technology capable of creating a more dramatic reduction in pain than videos might be more widely adopted in hospital practice.

Immersive Virtual Reality

Immersive virtual reality (VR) distraction is the foundation for the VR hypnosis that is discussed in Chapter 3. The following provides some detail on the theory behind this approach.

Investigators have proposed that immersive VR can serve as an unusually powerful psychological pain control technique (Hoffman, Patterson, Carrougher, & Sharar, 2001). Pain requires attention to process (Chapman & Nakamura, 1999; Eccleston & Crombez, 1999), and VR has the exceptional ability to divert attention from the painful procedure and into the computer-generated virtual world. The illusion of entering the 3-D computer-generated world (known as *presence*) is uniquely compelling in immersive VR. Patients who experience a stronger illusion of going into the virtual world will be more distracted by VR and will thus report more pain reduction than those who experience a less compelling illusion of presence in the virtual world (Hoffman, Sharar, et al., 2004).

A number of small studies have investigated the use of immersive VR pain control (Hoffman, 2004; Hoffman, Patterson, et al., 2004). In an early case study, VR distraction reduced pain during staple removal from skin grafts more effectively than a two-dimensional video game (Hoffman, Doctor, Patterson, Carrougher, & Furness, 2000). The two patients in this study reported feeling more present in the computer-generated world during the VR condition than during the video-game condition. When compared with standard of care (no distraction), burn patients consistently report clinically meaningful (i.e., greater than 30%) reductions in pain during wound care and physical therapy sessions while in VR (Das, Grimmer, Sparnon, McRae, & Thomas, 2005; Hoffman, Doctor, et al., 2000; Hoffman, Patterson, & Carrougher, 2000; Hoffman, Patterson, Carrougher, & Sharar, 2001). Furthermore, although larger studies with longer treatment durations are needed, preliminary results indicate that VR does not decline in analgesic effectiveness when used on multiple occasions (Hoffman, Patterson, Carrougher, Nakamura, et al., 2001).

On the one hand, Slater and Wilbur (1997) reported that VR presence is a subjective illusion created in the user's mind, (i.e., a psychological state of consciousness). On the other hand, immersion is an objective, measurable description of the sensory input that a particular VR system delivers to a participant. Although presence and immersion are distinct concepts, increasing the immersiveness of a VR system is predicted to increase the illusion of presence in virtual reality, and this relationship is often found. As an example, increasing the size of the eyepieces in the VR helmet, thus increasing the field of view (Prothero & Hoffman, 1995), and adding or improving the quality of sound in VR (Hendrix & Barfield, 1995) have both been shown to increase participants' subjective illusion of presence inside the virtual world. Further, tracking the orientation of the patient's head such that what the patient sees in VR changes as the patient moves his or her head around can also enhance presence (Hendrix & Barfield, 1995), as can tactile augmentation (adding tactile feedback to virtual objects; Hoffman, Garcia-Palacios, Carlin, Furness, & Botella-Arbona, 2003). One of Hoffman and colleagues' studies demonstrated that a low-tech VR system (no head tracking, low-quality helmet, and no sound effects) led to a less compelling illusion of presence and less pain reduction than a high-tech VR system with head tracking, high-resolution video, and stereophonic sound (Hoffman, Sharar, et al., 2004).

It is of interest to determine how VR distraction and hypnosis interact with each other. In a 2006 article published in the *Journal of Abnormal Psychology*

(Patterson, Hoffman, Palacios, & Jensen, 2006), my colleagues and I attempted to combine VR distraction and hypnosis in the laboratory. In a 2 × 2 design, normal participants were subjected to experimentally induced thermal pain with four possible interventions: (a) VR distraction, (b) audiotape hypnosis with posthypnotic suggestions for pain relief, (c) combined VR distraction and audiotaped hypnotic suggestions, or (d) a control condition with none of the treatments. Participants who received VR distraction showed the largest amount of pain reduction. The participants who showed reduced pain levels with either hypnosis or combined hypnosis and VR distraction were ones who, on average, scored higher on a scale of hypnotizability (Stanford Clinical Hypnosis Scale). In this study, the combination of VR distraction and hypnosis did not appear to create a large advantageous effect, but the two interventions were not designed to facilitate one another. Our current research is focusing on whether hypnotic suggestions designed to facilitate VR distraction will facilitate the magnitude of pain reduction. It should be noted that this line of research is different from the use of VR technology as a means to actually induce hypnosis; this is discussed in Chapter 3.

In summary, distraction for acute pain can be as simple as watching TV or engaging the patient in conversation. VR offers an ability to capture the patient's attention in a highly efficient, practical manner.

Self-Coping Statements

For acute as well as chronic pain, self-coping statements can be useful. It is useful to determine first any negative cognitions that patients have about their acute pain. Then, based on the patients' individual characteristics, they can repeatedly make adaptive statements to themselves. Examples might include, "This will go away in a while," "This is not causing any damage," "I can breathe slowly and regularly," or "Tomorrow I will be playing golf."

Chronic Pain

Chronic pain has been defined as pain that has persisted beyond normal healing time; typically, noncancer pain that has persisted for longer than about three months is considered chronic. Chronic pain is almost by definition is refractory to medical interventions. Often, it is associated with complications such as depression, anxiety, and inactivity. This section focuses on psychological interventions for patients with chronic pain. These include education and behavioral and cognitive–behavioral therapies. A number of additional approaches should be considered that are not covered here; these include biofeedback, group therapy, and family therapy (especially when the patient is a child) and are reviewed by Gatchel and Turk (1996). One type of approach that is not covered in detail here but does require some mention is the psychodynamic.

Some experts view many chronic pain problems as an expression of inner conflict and unresolved emotional issues. Patients with histories of physical and/or emotional abuse as children may be more vulnerable to chronic pain. Grzesiak, Ury, and Dworkin (1996) pointed out a number of psychodynamic themes that can be associated with chronic pain, including early experiences with pain and illness, anger, helplessness, depression, loss, punishment, and interpersonal conflict. This is a difficult area to study with rigorous design, and consequently there is little empirical basis to support psychodynamic approaches to chronic pain. However, some report that effectively treating patients' psychodynamic conflicts will have a positive impact on their chronic pain (Baker & Nash, 2008).

Operant Behavioral Approaches

From an operant behavioral perspective, a patient's pain behaviors (e.g., guarding the painful part of the body, limping, grimacing, moaning) function like any other behavior. Like any behavior, pain behaviors are under the control of the environment, are learned, and may change under new learning conditions. The focus of the intervention is on targeting maladaptive pain behaviors for change, and the target of the intervention is not on changing the patient's experience of pain. For some professionals and patients, the notion that changing pain behaviors can reduce pain and suffering may seem nonsensical. Further, applying principles such as extinction may seem like a callous disregard of a patient's suffering. Fordyce (1976) advanced this understanding by explaining how, when the proper stimuli are in place, pain will be elicited in the absence of nociception. When eliciting stimuli and environmental reinforcers are in place, people will experience pain, much as a classically conditioned dog will salivate at the sound of a bell. If a patient is experiencing chronic pain and the response of family members is to start off conversations asking about that pain, this response can stimulate suffering in the patient. A number of useful principles that fall under operant techniques, including reinforcement, extinction, discriminative stimulus control, and operant conditioning (Sanders, 1996), can help address this issue.

Educational Approaches

One of the more critical variables to address in assessing and treating patients in chronic pain is determining the model that the patient uses to explain his or her pain. It is important to ask patients what they think may be causing their pain. Most patients, understandably, hold a biomedical/biomechanical model of their pain. For example, many patients with chronic low back pain believe they must have a problem with their disks or spine and thus look to an intervention such as a spine operation that will make a mechanical change to resolve the cause of the pain. Many patients with chronic pain have seen multiple specialists in the search to find the right one to solve their problem. Certainly almost every one of these patients indeed had an injury or disease process that was likely at the original core of the problem. However, a pain problem that was once driven by tissue damage is now maintained by variables such as central nervous system changes, environmental factors, deconditioning, and emotional sequelae. The challenge is to identify these maintaining factors and to help the patient move to a view of his or her pain as influenced importantly by these factors. A related challenge is to move the patient (and health care provider) from an acute care model to a chronic disease management model.

Education is a primary treatment modality in moving a patient from a biomedical acute care model to a biopsychosocial chronic care model. It is critical with educational approaches to meet patients "where they are." It is also important for nonmedical providers to work with credible medical providers in explaining patients' pain problems to them. When a patient insists that there is something wrong with his back and a surgeon needs to go in and fix it, it is important that a credible medical provider educate the patient about his specific condition in the context of current scientific understanding of chronic pain. It is often helpful to schedule a session involving the medical provider, the mental health provider, and the patient, to review back anatomy and discuss the structures in the back and in the central nervous system that may be involved in the patient's pain, as well as the various options for treatment, including potential risks and benefits of each. It is further extremely helpful to educate patients regarding the importance of the central nervous system in maintaining a pain problem that may have begun peripherally and to emphasize that inactivity will result in a gradual worsening over time, whereas a program of gradually and systematically increasing activity may at first increase pain but will be essential in the long run to the patient's recovery. Along these lines, information that "hurt does not equal harm" is important.

Once the clinician is working within the patient's frame of reference, education can be provided on a number of fronts. Again, one important concept is neuroplasticity, which can help patients understand why they continue to suffer in the absence of any identifiable source of nociception. As described earlier, chronic pain can be imprinted into the central nervous system (brain and spinal cord) so that patients continue to experience pain long past healing of the peripheral injury. For example, if a patient sustains an injury through a certain activity, the thought of facing that activity can be enough to reactivate the experience of the pain itself. Another important concept is the role of stress. Stress activates the autonomic nervous system and results in increased muscle tension, which in turn can increase pain. Patients experiencing considerable psychosocial stress are likely to experience more pain and have diminished resources for coping effectively with pain. Helping patients to recognize stress and to apply stress management strategies can result in patients feeling much better able to manage their pain.

Reinforcement

According to learning principles, a behavior is likely to increase when it is followed by consequences that are reinforcing. Reinforcers may be positive (e.g., for some patients, attention and sympathy from a spouse are such positive reinforcers) or negative (e.g., removal of aversive conditions). A simplistic example would be a man who is currently unable to work as a result of back pain sustained from an on-the-job injury. He spends most of his days in a recliner watching TV, because his back pain increases with physical activity. Occasionally, he gets up and attempts to do a household chore such as mowing the lawn (which he has always disliked doing). However, when he does this, he limps and grimaces. Occasionally, he stops and clutches his back. His wife responds by expressing concern and urging him to let her take over mowing the lawn, and recommends he take pain medication and lie down.

In an operant model, there are at least two reinforcers for this man's pain behaviors (limping, grimacing, clutching his back). The first is the solicitous response from his wife. Several studies have demonstrated that pain behavior increases when the response of a spouse is solicitous or reinforcing to that behavior (Flor, Turk, & Rudy, 1989). In fact, brain imaging studies have even demonstrated that when a patient is experiencing pain, the presence of a spouse can even heighten the manner in which the pain is registered in the brain. The second reinforcer is a negative one: the removal from the unpleasant chore of mowing the lawn.

Although beyond the scope of this book, it is also important to recognize that patient involvement in a workers' compensation system is likely to heighten the risk of poor outcomes with any pain therapy. Especially when a patient has been out of work for many months or even years, loss of disability payments and medical benefits if a patient improves may serve as a powerful disincentive for improvement. Many patients are understandably concerned about how they will support themselves and their families if they lose their workers' compensation benefits and are not able to return to a job that paid as well as their last job. If a patient has been out of work for some time, his or her former job may no longer be available.

It important to understand that these behavioral principles can, and often do, operate without the patient's awareness. In terms of overall base rates of chronic pain presentation, malingering is quite rare, and it is important to assume the patient is genuinely suffering and wants to get better.

Extinction

If operant reinforcers play an important role in maintaining a behavior, then extinction is the most effective means to decrease that behavior. It is important to understand that, in extinguishing pain behaviors, one is ignoring the patient's behaviors rather than the patient himself or herself. Further, nonsickness behaviors are reinforced rather than extinguished; it is as important to reinforce wellness behavior as it is to extinguish pain behavior. It is interesting that, in work with families of patients with chronic pain, the families are often relieved when this concept is brought up. Families of patients experiencing extended periods of chronic pain are often exhausted and seem to have arrived at this conclusion themselves. In explaining this to the patient, the clinician can put it in terms of distraction:

> We will do everything we can from a medical and pharmacological approach to control your pain. Beyond that however, we have learned that the more people talk about and focus on pain, the more suffering they experience. Talking about pain becomes a constant reminder of it and it makes patients feel worse. We are going to encourage you and your family to focus as much as possible on something other than pain. In fact, we are going to encourage your family not even to discuss your pain with your anymore.

Although the focus of this chapter is not on hypnosis, it is important to note that when pain behaviors are importantly influenced by such operant factors, using hypnosis for pain relief may only serve as a reinforcer for pain behaviors that, in term of the patient's best interest, should ideally be extinguished. This is one of many reasons a clinician using hypnosis for pain relief should be familiar with broad-based psychological approaches as a prerequisite.

Discriminative Stimuli Control

Pain behaviors are not only under the control of the consequences that follow but may also be under the control of the stimuli that precede them. Classical and operant approaches have led to the understanding that many patients with chronic pain can develop a fear of movement that borders on the phobic. Patients learn at some point that movement exacerbates pain, and they stop moving as a protective mechanism. The movement that is so critical to a functional lifestyle becomes a source of fear for the patient. Treatment involves very gradually allowing the patient to move at a rate that their conditioned anxiety allows (Fordyce, 1976; Sanders, 1996).

Application of Operant Conditioning Principles to Therapy

Behavioral principles can be used to build functional behaviors as well as to extinguish unwanted pain behaviors. Perhaps no area is as important as that of increasing activity and exercise, particularly in patients who are deconditioned (many patients with chronic pain spend much of their days lying down or sitting) and in those with "pacing problems" (i.e., the tendency of patients to let pain guide their activity in a way that they end up overdoing activity on some days, "paying for it" with increased pain, and subsequently resting and moving very little). What occurs is this: Patients with chronic pain have a "good day," without much pain, and their reaction is to overextend themselves in activities. The next day, they find themselves in pain and limit their activity. Over the course of several days, their activity decreases and their pain increases. Often they have complaints of constant pain, but there is very little movement. They may even have developed the fear of movement described earlier. Enabling the patient to move in a manner that it does not result in another surge of pain and downward cycle is a challenge to the clinician. On the basis of operant conditioning principles, Fordyce (1976) proposed the *quota system* as an approach to such pacing problems. The quota system involves a behavioral analysis and treatment that uses rest as a reinforcer for activity.

To illustrate, take a patient who is trying to walk after long-term neuropathic pain in his legs. If he walks too far, his pain is incapacitating and he cannot get out of bed for 2 days. The quota system prescribes that a patient work to pain for fatigue for three baseline periods, taking 80% of the average of those three sessions as a starting point, and then increasing activity by 5% each session. To put "working to fatigue" in another way, the patient is instructed to walk or do some other exercise until the pain level or sense of being tired becomes uncomfortable. For this particular patient, the therapist walks him for as far as he is comfortable for three therapy sessions. In the first session, he walks 150 feet, the second for 50 feet, and the third for 100 feet. The average of those three sessions is 100 feet, and 80% of that is 80 feet; 80 feet thus becomes the starting point. For the next session, the patient is instructed to walk 80 feet and 80 feet only, even if he feels good and desires to walk more. This amount is increased by 5% each session (5 feet is close enough), so he will go 85, 90, 95, and 100 feet over the next few sessions. If the patient fails to meet the quota in a given session, then the therapist goes back to the last successful quota that he reached. By using this formula, patients should show a steady improvement in activity that does not overwhelm them.

Cognitive–Behavioral Approaches

Cognitive–behavioral approaches followed the popularity that behavioral approaches enjoyed in the 1960s and 1970s, stemming from the belief of proponents that patient cognitions, in addition to behaviors, played important roles in psychological problems (e.g., in depression and anxiety). Using this approach, therapies were designed for treating anxiety and depression (Holzman, Turk, & Kerns, 1986). This progression of paradigms was paralleled in the chronic pain treatment literature. Operant behavioral approaches somewhat revolutionized approaches to treating chronic pain. A natural next stage was to apply cognitive–behavioral approaches to chronic pain (e.g., see Turk et al., 1983).

Cognitive–behavioral approaches have been an emphasis in the pain literature for the past 2 to 3 decades. They work by helping patients learn to identify and modify cognitions related to emotional and behavioral responses to pain. Beck, a pioneer of cognitive therapy, discussed identifying the automatic thoughts that people with depression experience: "I will always be depressed. I am worthless. Life is not worth living." The cognitive therapist works with patients to recognize such cognitions and to challenge them. As patients learn to effectively challenge overly negative thoughts, they learn to generate alternatives such as, "I may be depressed now but it will not last forever. I feel inadequate in some, but not all areas of my life. Life is a series of ups and downs." Substantial evidence has established the efficacy of cognitive and cognitive–behavioral therapies for depression, anxiety, pain, and other disorders (Beck, 1976, 1979; Turk et al., 1983).

Catastrophizing. One of the more robust findings to come out of recent research related to the psychological aspects of pain is the importance of catastrophizing. This was likely first discussed in Albert Ellis's work on cognitive–behavioral approaches in general psychotherapy (A. Ellis, 1961, 1980, 1995; J. A. Ellis & Spanos, 1994) and has been generally defined as an exaggerated negative mental set brought to bear during painful experiences (Sullivan et al., 2001). There is growing evidence that a tendency to catastrophize during experiments with clinical pain situations leads to more intense pain and more emotional distress (Sullivan & D'Eon, 1990; Sullivan, Stanish, Waite, Sullivan, & Tripp, 1998; Sullivan et al., 2001). Catastrophizing thoughts may have to do with the perceived duration of the pain ("This will never get better"), the meaning of pain ("This means I have cancer and I will die"), the affective quality of pain ("This is horrible"), or the ability to tolerate it ("I can't stand the pain"). Catastrophizing thoughts of this nature have an impact on patients' ability to tolerate both acute and chronic pain. It is not hard for a clinician to realize that if patients are attempting to face pain with any one of these cognitions driving their schemas, they are going to have more difficulty. Moreover, if they are able to counter such negative thoughts with more adaptive appraisals, it is certainly easy to see how this will have a positive effect on the patient's ability to cope.

Hurt Versus Harm. A central issue to both acute and chronic pain is whether the patient perceives pain as being a signal of bodily harm. The point is that with "hurt versus harm," the patient may perceive the pain only to hurt. Hurt is regarded as something that, although undesirable, is generally something that the patient can tolerate. Harm is a completely different matter. If patients believe that what they are experiencing is harmful to them, they will likely invoke a series of self-protective actions and do what they can to cease the pain. Self-protective actions fly in the face of most types of psychological approaches for pain control, and the concept of fear avoidance is useful here (Patterson, 2005). Many patients with back pain, for example, avoid activities both because they believe the activity will cause increased pain and because they worry the activity could cause further damage to their back. At one level, patients are being asked to accept and tolerate their pain. If patients are operating under the assumption that such tolerance or acceptance is likely to cause them damage, such approaches are likely to fail.

Enabling patients to shift their perspective from harm to hurt understanding is an important part of educational and cognitive–behavioral approaches. Usually, a thorough medical workup will be required to provide the assurance that the patient needs. Patients are able to gain an intellectual understanding that their pain is not harming them, but, emotionally, they continue to struggle with the concept. One of the greatest clinical challenges can be overcoming the tremendous conditioned anxiety that patients can build up regarding pain. Cognitive–behavioral, relaxation, and hypnotic techniques all can be useful in this regard.

Beyond these aforementioned categories, a number of other cognitions can affect pain control. The cognitions that keep pain in place for patients may be subtle and require several sessions of treatment to identify and modify. Typically, cognitive–behavioral therapies for pain are provided over a number of sessions and include a variety of behavioral techniques, such as training in imagery or relaxation (Bradley, 1996).

Relaxation Approaches

There is certainly a great deal of overlap between relaxation techniques and hypnosis. However, in a discussion of psychological approaches, relaxation techniques deserve a discussion in their own right. One important point to consider is that some patients will not respond to hypnosis, so relaxation training is an important option for this group. Arena and Blanchard (1996) defined *relaxation therapy* as a "systematic approach to teaching people to gain awareness of their psychological responses and achieve both a cognitive and physiological sense of tranquility without the use of the machinery employed in biofeedback" (p. 180). The authors listed the major forms of relaxation therapy as progressive muscle relaxation (E. Jacobson, 1938), meditation (Lichstein, 1988), autogenic training (Luthe, 1969–1973), and guided imagery (Bellack, 1973).

There are a number of reasons why deep relaxation will be of benefit to a patient in chronic pain. An important group of patients to consider for relaxation training are those with headaches. A review of the literature (Patterson & Jensen, 2003) indicates that hypnosis and relaxation tend to be of equivalent efficacy for this patient population. Most patients with chronic pain hold a great deal of tension in their bodies, and muscular spasms are common. Muscular tension has a cyclical relationship with pain and nociception. In the case of headaches, particularly tension headaches, tension plays a key role in the genesis and maintenance of pain. Deep relaxation offers one of the most effective means to offer relief to patients.

Autogenic training is often discussed in the literature as being effective for chronic pain and is one of the easier approaches to teach to the patient. To provide an example of an autogenic approach, clinicians would have patients repeat each of the following statements to themselves:

My right hand is heavy.
My right hand is warm.
My right hand is feeling relaxed.
My right arm is heavy.
My right arm is warm.
My right arm is feeling relaxed.

This sequence is repeated for the right shoulder, left hand, left arm, left shoulder, right foot, right calf, right thigh, left foot, left calf, left thigh, top of the head, forehead, checks, mouth, jaw, neck, chest, and stomach.

The clinician continues with:

My entire body is heavy.
My entire body is warm.
My entire body is feeling relaxed.
My entire body is heavy.
My entire body is warm.
My entire body is feeling relaxed.

Finally, the clinician can make autogenic statements that have to do with general well-being or pain control. At this stage, the distinction between autogenic statements and hypnosis becomes blurry. Statements such as "I am totally at peace," "I am in control of the sensations in my body," or "Nothing seems to bother me" are examples of autogenic statements linked to pain control.

Imagery

Imagery can be useful for both acute and chronic pain management. A. Richardson (1969) defined *imagery* as "quasi-sensory or quasi-perceptual experiences of which we are self-consciously aware and which exist for us in the absence of those stimulus conditions that are known to produce their genuine sensory or perceptual counterparts" (p. 35). Hypnosis incorporates imagery but extends far beyond it, in terms of engaging attentional processes, deliberately creating dissociation, and the elaborate nature of suggestions. Because there is still a great deal of overlap between hypnosis and imagery, however, this approach is not discussed at length. Pincus and Sheikh (2009) recently published a book on imagery for pain relief that includes numerous examples of imagery scripts that are useful for chronic pain.

Acceptance Therapy and Mindfulness

Acceptance and commitment therapy (ACT) and mindfulness to chronic pain represent relatively new and exciting approaches to chronic (far less to acute) pain management. ACT departs from many conventional approaches to chronic pain because its approach with patients is not necessarily to cope with or control pain, rather acceptance of chronic pain includes an active willingness to have pain present, along with associated thoughts and feelings (McCracken, Carson, Eccleston, & Keefe, 2004; McCracken, Vowles, & Eccleston, 2004). Such acceptance involves responding to pain-related experiences without attempts at control or avoidance.

Other relatively unique features of ACT are its emphasis on the context in which chronic behavior occurs as well as the use of patient values in directing treatment. These concepts are intertwined in ACT as the context of treatment is largely based on the patient's value. *Values* are defined as verbally constructed, global, desired, and chosen life directions (Dahl, Wilson, Luciano, & Hayes, 2005). Another unique feature is the emphasis of this approach on functional analysis. Rather than trying to change dysfunctional thoughts, therapists using the ACT approach teach clients to treat thoughts as thoughts and to examine their function rather than contents (Dahl et al., 2005).

Much of the empirical research on acceptance of chronic pain has been done by McCracken and colleagues (McCracken & Eccleston, 2003, 2005; McCracken, Vowles, & Eccleston, 2004). Using ACT concepts, patients with chronic pain have reported greater willingness to have pain and engagement in activities (McCracken & Eccleston, 2005) and fewer sick days and medical visits associated with pain (Dahl, Wilson, & Nilsson, 2004). ACT and mindfulness show promise for the treatment of not only chronic pain but also anxiety (McMain, Korman, & Dimeff, 2001), depression (Dougher, 2002), and even borderline personality disorder (Linehan, 1993).

The concepts of ACT are complex, and their applications to chronic pain are worthy of an entire chapter or book in themselves (e.g., Dahl et al., 2005). The juxtaposition of hypnosis with such approaches is yet an entirely different discussion. Many of the clinical hypnotic approaches described in the latter part of this book are based on my interest in ACT and mindfulness. For example, a repeated message is that people with chronic pain may benefit the most with suggestions that are not focused on pain reduction itself. Hypnotic approaches that emphasize the transient nature of thoughts rather than eliminating them are discussed. Also discussed is the motivational interviewing concept of using a patient's core values and integrating them into hypnotic suggestions. Fordyce (1988) decried the medicalization of suffering, a concept discussed by ACT therapists. Finally, many of the principles discussed in ACT were embodied by Erickson (and Gilligan), as discussed in Chapters 4 and 5. The principle of utilization, which is central to Erickson's approach, encourages therapists to use patient symptoms to their benefit rather than to try to make them go away. These are only a few of the many parallels between the clinical hypnotic approaches described in this book and the concepts of ACT and mindfulness.

SUMMARY

This chapter summarized how basic physiologic knowledge can be translated into psychological approaches. Although the clinician does not need to know the complex intricacies of pain that usually only neurophysiologists can understand, appreciating the basic nature of pain can help guide both hypnosis and psychological approaches in general.

A clinician working with hypnosis for pain control should also be well versed in psychological approaches to this issue. First, psychological approaches in general often apply a guide for how hypnotic suggestions are applied to pain, particularly chronic pain. Second, hypnosis has definite limitations, particularly with some patients. Often, it will be necessary to use educational, operant, or cognitive–behavioral techniques prior to—or instead of—hypnosis.

2

THE SCIENTIFIC BASIS OF HYPNOTIC ANALGESIA AND PAIN CONTROL

Two decades ago, if a clinician suggested hypnosis in a medical setting, this form of treatment would have most likely been greeted with skepticism. Today, this is still the case in many medical settings. The difference is that 2 decades ago, much of the reluctance to accept hypnotic analgesia on a scientific basis was at least partially justified The good news is that over the past 20 years, a significant body of scientific research has grown to support hypnosis for the treatment of pain, and in general, skepticism from a scientific standpoint is no longer warranted (Barabasz, Olness, Boland, & Kahn, 2006). The science behind hypnotic analgesia can be divided into studies that represent more basic science and are laboratory or theoretically based and clinical trials with patient populations. This chapter addresses laboratory studies of hypnotic analgesia, physiological correlates of hypnosis, and the more recent research that has been done on virtual reality hypnosis. The next chapter discusses clinical trials.

LABORATORY STUDIES OF HYPNOTIC PAIN CONTROL

There is a rich history of laboratory analog studies on hypnosis for pain control. Typical paradigms involve administering pain stimuli through means such as swirling ice water, heat, or pressure and then measuring pain reduction after hypnosis; usually, hypnotizability is measured as a covariate—highs and lows are compared—on this variable. It is interesting that many or most of these studies have not been done with testing hypnotic analgesia in mind; rather, they have used the phenomenon of hypnotic analgesia to test the mechanisms that underlie hypnosis itself. In other words, analgesia is used to test theories of hypnosis. A parsimonious means of discussing this body of literature will be to categorize it by the hypnotic theory tested.

At times, the boundary between hypnotic theory and mechanisms of analgesia becomes indistinguishable. In other cases, there are theories as to how hypnosis works that seem to have little bearing on how they relate to analgesia. In terms of tight, controlled studies as to how hypnosis works, theoretical views differ widely, and vigorous debates at national symposiums and journals abound. Clinicians often disregard such debates and either ignore theory or use paradigms that seem more suitable to clinical practice.

One purpose of this chapter is to demonstrate that most of what has been produced about hypnosis from a scientific standpoint can be useful to the clinician. George Kelly argued that every scientific theory has a "range of convenience" (Patterson & Sechrest, 1983). Even when operating in a domain of science as basic as physics, this concept is applicable. In scientifically explaining light, for example, the particle theory accounts for some phenomena, whereas wave theory seems preferable for others. It is remarkable at times that theorists in hypnosis are not more tolerant of multiple theories, for the science behind hypnosis is infinitely more ambiguous and softer than that of physics.

Clinicians will be more effective with hypnosis if they are able to use Kelly's range of convenience and apply that to clinical interventions. Hypnosis does not work for every patient, and any clinician or scientist who claims that it does is being misleading at best. However, if a clinician is approaching a patient using one theory of hypnosis without success, using an alternative paradigm might very well produce results. Further, when clinicians can operate using elements from several theories, they are likely enhancing their overall efficacy with a given patient. There are elements of any theoretical approach that are bound to be helpful to a patient. One example of this is *expectancy*, which is often reported to have at least a moderate effect related to outcome in hypnosis, as well as virtually any type of clinical intervention. Clinicians can usually enhance expectancy in their patients regardless of the treatment approach they are using.

With the notion in mind that any well-established line of analog research can have useful clinical implications, it is useful to discuss some of the theoretical approaches to understanding hypnosis that will have some utility.

Trait Theory

While perhaps not best described as a trait theory, the idea that hypnotizability is largely hard-wired into an individual's makeup is important to pain control. Conceptualizing hypnotizability as a trait has a number of important implications for clinical practice: Some patients are going to respond to this approach better than others; some will not respond at all. Researchers and clinicians are limited in what can be done to change responsiveness, and the capacity to respond to hypnotic suggestion is largely related to brain structure and information-processing capacity, which is independent of learning and the environment.

The concept that hypnosis has traitlike features stems largely from attempts to measure hypnotizability. Beginning with the Stanford Hypnotic Susceptibility Scale (Weitzenhoffer & Hilgard, 1959, 1962), a number of scales have been developed to measure hypnosis (Spiegel & Spiegel, 1978). One of the strongest arguments that hypnotizability is at least partially a trait is that scores such as those on the Stanford scale are reliable even after 10 years (Morgan, Johnson, & Hilgard, 1974; Stern, Spiegel, & Nee, 1979). Further, hypnotizability appears to have a genetic component (Morgan et al., 1974). Hypnotizability has even been found to be more powerful than the treatment effect in some studies (Frischholz, Blumstein, & Spiegel, 1982).

It is interesting to note that hypnotic pain control was the perceptual change favored in many of the early studies that investigated hypnotizability. The purpose of these studies, in other words, was more to delve into the properties of hypnosis than to investigate pain control. Hilgard and Hilgard (1975) divided normal subjects into high, medium, and low "hypnotizables" according to Stanford Clinical Hypnotizability Scale scores and found a close association between reduction of cold pressor pain and hypnotizability; several others replicated this finding (Freeman, Barabasz, Barabasz, & Warner, 2000; Hilgard, 1969; W. R. Miller & Rollnick, 1991). Ischemic muscle pain perception has also been found to be related to hypnotizability (Hilgard & Morgan, 1975; Knox, Morgan, & Hilgard, 1974).

McGlashan, Evans, and Orne (1969) reported a seminal study in which low hypnotizables showed the same minimal response to hypnosis as they did to placebo. Unlike the low hypnotizables, the high hypnotizables showed an analgesic response to hypnosis but minimal response to placebo. It is hard to understand how various writers have argued that hypnosis is "all placebo" when such evidence was reported more than 40 years ago. Finally, Montgomery, DuHamel, and Redd (2000) reported a meta-analysis on the effects of hypnotic analgesia. In their review of a number of studies, subjects who showed higher levels of hypnotizability generally reported greater reductions in pain.

What are the practical applications of hypnotizability trait theory for the clinician? First, even if a clinician or theorist rejects the notion of a bell-shaped curve of hypnotizability, it is difficult to throw out the concept that there are individual differences in response to a standard induction. For some clinicians, this may mean providing a hypnotizability scale, and if the patient scores low, then hypnosis is rejected for another psychological treatment. For other models, the failure of a patient to respond to conventional hypnotic interventions could suggest a shift in approach to hypnosis. Barabasz (1982; Barabasz & Barabasz, 1989) suggested interventions to increase hypnotizability, and Holroyd (1996) indicated that improving hypnotizability can relate directly to pain treatment. Much of the later part of this book will be focusing on Ericksonian approaches, many of which appear to be useful when more traditional induction techniques fail.

Sociocognitive Approaches

Sociocognitive views represent a notable contrast to trait theories. Within the framework of sociocognitive theory, hypnotic talent, altered states, or even hypnotic inductions are not necessary for hypnotic function. Some of the early thinking behind this approach came out of laboratory studies demonstrating that responses of hypnotic simulators (those pretending to be hypnotized) could not be distinguished from those subjects who had undergone an actual hypnotic induction. Rather than the subject entering a special state then, theorists contended that hypnosis is a product of social interaction, and hypnotic response is a product of the subject's response to cues from the social environment. Some of these sociocognitive processes include expectancy, contextual cues in the social environment, demand characteristics, and role enactment (Kirsch & Lynn, 1995). In the case of expectancy, the success of a hypnotic induction is influenced by what subjects anticipate will occur through the process. However, clearly there is more to hypnotic induction than expectancy.

One of the most important studies in this regard was reported by Benham, Woody, Wilson, and Nash (2006). Milling, Shores, Coursen, Menario, and Farris (2007) reported that response expectancies are an important mechanism of hypnotic and cognitive–behavioral pain treatments, and hypnotizability is a trait variable that predicts hypnotic responding across situations. The authors reported that even ideal levels of expectancy could not overcome such variables as hypnotizability. In terms of contextual cues, hypnosis is regarded as an ambiguous social reaction to suggestions or cues from the hypnotist, however subtle they may be (Lynn, Kirsch, & Hallquist, 2008). Role enactment follows similar principles, in that a subject undergoing a hypnotic induction is fulfilling a role. This is particularly the case in stage hypnosis, in which the social pressure of "going along with the act" is thought to account for the often outlandish response to hypnotic suggestions. There are a variety of manners in which sociocognitive theorists conceptualize how social cues and normal cognitive processes account for hypnotic processes; regardless, hypnosis is viewed not as a special state or function of unusual talents but as everyday cognitions in the context of social interactions.

It follows that interventions for pain control in a sociocognitive framework involve working with everyday cognition. Hypnotic suggestions from a sociocognitive standpoint differ little from the cognitive–behavioral interventions that have become a fixture for the treatment of chronic pain over the past 25 years (Bradley, 1996; Holzman, Turk, & Kerns, 1986). Using such interventions, maladaptive thoughts about pain are modified, and patients are trained to replace them with thoughts that facilitate pain control. A particularly salient example of this is catastrophizing thoughts (e.g., "My pain will never get better," "I can't stand the pain"). Chaves (1989) pointed out that subjects who catastrophize tend to amplify the negative effects of pain. It is interesting that Chaves, a leading proponent for a sociocognitive approach to hypnosis for pain control, reported that a hypnotic induction is not necessary for pain control (Chaves, 1993). As such, it is not clear how hypnosis for pain control from a sociocognitive framework differs from standard cognitive–behavioral interventions.

Turning to the range of convenience for clinical applications of sociocognitive theory, there are a number of practical implications from this theory. As mentioned before, increasing patient expectancy for any type of medical treatment is likely to improve outcome. Thus, whatever the clinician can do within ethical boundaries (e.g., flagrant exaggeration of treatment potential should be considered unethical) to increase patient expectations for hypnotic pain treatment will likely be of benefit. Interestingly, there is evidence that the clinician's expectation is equally or more important than that of the patient (Galer, Schwartz, & Turner, 1997).

A clinician who is aware of the influence of role enactment might define the clinical intervention in a way in which the patient will respond positively to hypnotic suggestion. This might be in terms of defining the therapist–patient relationship, or it may manifest itself in rituals of induction. For some patients, perhaps watching a swinging watch may help them play the role. Another consideration is for a patient who is struggling with conventional hypnosis. It may be that having a patient simulate or role-play hypnosis will facilitate the induction.

Dissociation Theories of Hypnosis

Woody and Sadler (2008) discussed dissociation theory in terms of some of Hilgard's easy observations about hypnotic pain control. Specifically, Hilgard and Hilgard (1975) observed that, "For the highly hypnotizable subject within hypnosis, pain reduction is essentially effortless" (p. 156). However, for subjects who are not naturally highly hypnotizable, they must use "considerable effort, initiative and ingenuity to achieve success" (p. 181). Dissociation theories of hypnosis such as the neodissociation (Hilgard, 1992) and the neodissociation reformulation (Bowers, 1990, 1992; Bowers & Davidson, 1991) stress the increased effortlessness or decreased self-awareness of effort associated with responding to suggestions (Woody & Sadler, 2008).

Bowers and colleagues argued that subsystems of control can be activated directly rather than through higher level executive control. Along these lines, Hargadon, Bowers, and Woody (1995) reported that consciously evoking pain strategies was not necessary for subjects to experience a reduction in laboratory-induced pain. In addition, Eastwood, Gaskovski, and Bowers (1998) reported achieving analgesia in laboratory pain through cognitive mechanisms that were effortlessly engaged. In a number of studies, subjects have been reported to reduce pain automatically, without any type of conscious, thought-out strategy (Barabasz, 1982; Barabasz & Barabasz, 1989; Bowers, 1992; Freeman et al., 2000; M. F. Miller, Barabasz, & Barabasz, 1991; J. T. Smith, Barabasz, & Barabasz, 1996). In addition, a series of studies by DePascali and colleagues (De Pascalis, Bellusci, Gallo, Magurano, & Chen, 2004; De Pascalis, Cacace, & Massicolle, 2004) have indicated that dissociated models of pain control are supported in studies using psychophysiological monitoring (e.g., event-related potentials).

Neodissociation theory has a number of practical implications for clinical pain. An obvious one is that highly hypnotizable patients often will respond differently to pain control strategies compared with those with less hypnotic talent. The studies reviewed above suggest that highly hypnotizable patients might often respond well to simple, self-generated strategies for pain control (Patterson, 2001). In contrast, lower hypnotizable patients might require some of the detailed cognitive–behavioral strategies discussed above under sociocognitive theory. This line of research would imply that enabling patients to dissociate through hypnosis might serve as a useful approach to pain control. In addition, when patients are placed in situations that engender acute stress disorder and the tendency to dissociate, such as trauma hospitalization, patients might be more receptive hypnotic subjects (Patterson, Adcock, & Bombardier,

1997). Suggestions designed to elicit dissociative responses will be discussed frequently in the clinically applied chapters of this book.

PHYSIOLOGICAL CORRELATES
OF LABORATORY PAIN REDUCTION

For many years hypnosis researchers sought after specific physiological indicators of a hypnotic state. As discussed previously, there has been an ongoing debate in the field as to whether hypnosis represents a special state of consciousness. It was thought that unique physiological indicators would support special state conceptualizations (Dixon & Laurence, 1992). The physiological studies that have been done have seemed to be most definitive in saying what hypnosis is *not* rather than what it is. For example, cortical activity during hypnosis is not the same as during sleep (Dynes, 1947). To date, no specific markers have been tied to a hypnotic state. However, Pierre Rainville, one of the most prolific investigators in this area, believes that asking what the markers of a hypnotic state are is asking the wrong question. Hypnosis actually demonstrates a series of physiological changes, and those can indeed be monitored by brain activity (Rainville, 2004). Further, Arreed Barabasz was arriving at similar conclusions using cortical event-related potentials in his laboratories (Barabasz et al., 1999; S. M. Jensen, Barabasz, Barabasz, & Warner, 2001). It is really the progression of brain activity that interests brain hypnosis research than what occurs at a given time. What should be of more interest to the reader of this particular chapter is the relationship between physiological changes and hypnotically induced analgesia. There has been a notable amount of research done with physiological markers of hypnotic analgesia, and, again, interpreting the literature depends largely on the question being asked.

Physiological responses to hypnotic analgesia that have been the subject of studies include sympathetic responses (e.g., heart rate and blood pressure), electrocortical activity (i.e., assessment of brain wave and cortical stimulation evoked potentials at various sites), endogenous endorphin release, and regional blood flow. Much of the following review of these types of responses was reported in Patterson and Jensen (2003); all of the studies involve laboratory pain paradigms rather than clinical subjects.

Sympathetic Responding

The autonomic nervous system, which is part of the peripheral nervous system, is made up of two types of nerves: sympathetic and parasympathetic. The sympathetic and parasympathetic input that the organs within the autonomic nervous system receive are opposing. The sympathetic nerves are responsible for organizing, stimulating, and mobilizing energy to respond to threatening situations, such as fighting an intruder or escaping from a fire. Parasympathetic nerves, conversely, are responsible for conserving energy, generally during a state of rest, or reregulating the body after a threatening situation has passed. Generally speaking, sympathetic activity is indicative of both physiological and psychological arousal, whereas parasympathetic activity is indicative of physiological and psychological relaxation. Much of the early hypnotic pain research focused on autonomic responses such as changes in heart rate and galvanic skin response. Some decreases in heart rate and blood pressure have been reported with hypnotic analgesia (Casiglia et al., 2007; De Pascalis & Perrone, 1996; Hilgard & Morgan, 1975; Lenox, 1970); however, there are an equal number of findings that autonomic activity is not altered by hypnosis (T. X. Barber & Hahn, 1962; Hilgard, 1967, 1969; Shor, 1962; Sutcliffe, 1961).

To complicate matters further, Rainville, Carrier, Hofbauer, Bushnell, and Duncan (1999) reported a selective link between heart rate and pain unpleasantness. The finding that nonvoluntary physiological parameters may be less influenced by hypnosis than self-report may be used to argue that this form of analgesia is more focused on subjects' willingness to report pain. However, as Hilgard and Hilgard (1975) long ago pointed out, these data only reflect subjects' response to a subset of physiological responses; they do not reflect the overall experience of pain. Moreover, we are learning more and more that what occurs in some part of the body may not translate into suffering at higher cortical levels. To illustrate, patients may undergo an invasive medical procedure with the amnesic drug midazolam (Versed). This drug has no analgesic properties; however, patients who take it will have no recall of the painful event in many cases. If the residual effects of the pain are later controlled upon their awaking, the patients will respond largely as if they never experienced pain in the first place.

Endogenous Opioids

It has long been known that humans are able to modulate internally their pain experience through the use of endogenous opioids (Melzack & Wall, 1973). Specifically, it is well known that humans produce endorphins that have pain-reducing qualities (Chance, 1980).

A natural question would be whether hypnotic analgesia operates partly by generating endogenous opioids. The manner in which this has been studied has been to induce hypnosis with suggestions for analgesia for experimental pain and then administer opioid receptor antagonists such as naloxone. Theoretically, if hypnosis is creating analgesia by generating production of endorphins, the administration of an agent that blocks these receptors will reduce the analgesia and patients will begin to feel more pain. In the studies that have attempted this, naloxone has failed to reverse the effects of hypnotic analgesia (J. Barber & Mayer, 1977; Goldstein & Hilgard, 1975). As clever as these studies were, they should not be used to dismiss the notion that hypnosis can stimulate endogenous opioid production or release. First, what studies that have been done have been indirect tests that did not actually measure the presence of endorphins, but, rather told us only if opioid antagonists are reducing analgesia. Second, this research is done with laboratory-induced pain from which subjects know they can escape. Little is known about what happens physiologically when hypnosis is administered for clinical pain. Acute clinical pain results in a number of physiological changes, including the release of stress hormones. Mechanisms for reducing this and experimental pain may be very different in physiological terms.

Evoked Potential Studies

Brain function may be assessed by measuring the electrical activity that the brain produces when it is functioning. Electroencephalography (EEG) measures the electrical activity of the cerebral cortex, the part of the brain responsible for higher order functions, including sensation, movement, and thought processes, whereas evoked potentials are specific, discrete electrical measurements of sensory function, such as sight, feeling, and hearing. Evoked potential studies were the earliest type of methodology used to try to get at what occurred in the brain during hypnosis, particularly during pain control. Late evoked potentials have been found to be associated with the level of pain intensity perceived and are influenced by attention (Chen, Chapman, & Harkins, 1979; Stowell, 1984). The methodology commonly used is to determine somatosensory potentials in response to baseline pain stimulation and then to measure them under hypnotic analgesia. A number of studies have shown reductions in such evoked potentials after hypnosis (Arendt-Nielsen, Zachariae, & Bjerring, 1990; Barabasz & Lonsdale, 1983; Crawford et al., 1998; Danziger et al., 1998; De Pascalis, Magurano, & Bellusci, 1999; Halliday & Mason, 1964; Meier, Klucken, Soyka, & Bromm, 1993; Meszaros, Banyai, & Greguss, 1980; Spiegel, Bierre, & Rootenberg, 1989; Zachariae & Bjerring, 1994).

There is substantial support for reduced evoked potential amplitude with hypnotic analgesia. This body of research demonstrates that subjects show a decreased physiological response that is associated with a lessening of pain activity. It also suggests that hypnotic analgesia can result in physiological changes that are not under conscious control. This line of research is somewhat in contrast to the studies on autonomic response discussed previously. Also see De Pascalis, Cacace, and Massicolle (2008) for a study on somatosensory evoked potentials in high, low, and medium experimental subjects.

Surface EEG Recordings

General surface EEG measures have also been applied to studies of hypnotic analgesia. Crawford (1990) studied EEG response to cold pressor pain in high and low hypnotizable subjects. Subjects with high hypnotizability scores showed significantly greater theta-wave activity during hypnotic analgesia than did subjects with low hypnotizability scores during the hypnotic analgesia condition, particularly in the anterior temporal region. In terms of laterality in brain function, the low hypnotizable subjects showed little hemispheric difference during the two experimental conditions. In contrast, the high hypnotizable subjects showed relatively greater left hemisphere activity during pain stimulation and then a reversal in hemispheric dominance during hypnotic analgesia (see also De Pascalis & Perrone, 1996). These results and others led Crawford (1994) to argue that subjects who rank higher in hypnotizability scores demonstrate a greater ability to shift from left to right brain functioning than those who score lower in this area.

Further, Crawford maintained that hypnotic analgesia may operate through attention filtering and that the frontolimbic system is central to this process. De Pascalis and colleagues (De Pascalis, Magurano, Bellusci, & Chen, 2001) have reported, however, that hypnotic suggestions for focused analgesia are as effective or more so than those for dissociative imagery to reduce pain. Such findings, in addition to those of Rainville, Duncan, Price, Carrier, and Bushnell (1997), argue against an explanation of hypnotic analgesia that operates solely through attention-filtering mechanisms. It appears that the type of pain reduction that occurs through hypnosis at least partly depends on the type of hypnotic suggestion given. While attentional processes are an important part of the equation, it seems that the brain also responds with specificity to the type of suffering; thus hypnosis includes but goes beyond filtering of attention.

Brain Imaging Studies

Somatosensory and EEG studies provide a measure of brain functioning associated with hypnosis based on electrical activity; however, they do not provide information about the specific neuroanatomical sites at which the modulation of pain experience occurs (Price & Barrell, 2000). Brain imaging studies can provide a different type of information regarding possible physiological substrates. In the 1990s, the most available technology included positron emission tomography (PET) scans, a technique designed for physiological imaging based on some metabolic component (in contrast to the kind of anatomical outlines one sees with an X-ray or computed tomography [CT] scan).

Rainville, Hofbauer, et al. (1999) studied PET scans of brain activity before, during, and after subjects' exposure to hypnotic analgesia while experiencing thermal pain (i.e., hot water). The focus of hypnotic suggestions was for unpleasantness, but not intensity, of the noxious stimulus. The investigators found that when the focus of hypnotic suggestions was on unpleasantness, brain function changes centered on the anterior cingulate gyrus rather than the primary somatosensory cortex.

The limbic system is the part of the brain that is more likely to register emotion, as opposed to the somatosensory cortex, which is more likely to register physical sensation. In a second study, again using PET scans, Hofbauer, Rainville, Duncan, and Bushnell (2001) found that hypnotic suggestions for sensory reductions resulted in more activity in the somatosensory cortex. Price and Barrell (2000) concluded that hypnotic analgesia can produce an inhibition of signals that arrive at the somatosensory cortex (pain intensity) and can also modulate pain processing in the limbic system (pain unpleasantness, suffering). As Rainville et al. (1997) made clear in an important paper in *Science*, the nature of the hypnotic suggestions makes a big difference in how the brain responds to pain control. To a degree, clinicians "get what they ask for" when they give a patient a hypnotic suggestion for pain relief. Also see Sharav and Tal (2006) for an experimental study on focused hypnotic analgesia.

Faymonville, Boly, and Laureys (2006) used PET methodology to describe the distribution of cerebral blood flow during the hypnotic state. They reported that hypnosis-induced reduction of affective and sensory responses of experimentally induced thermal pain was modulated by activity in the midcingulate cortex (area 24a). They also reported that the hypnotic state significantly enhanced the functional modulation between midcingulate cortex and a large neural network. This network was involved in sensory affective cognitive and behavioral aspects of nociception.

M. P. Jensen (2008) published an award-winning article titled "The Neurophysiology of Pain Perception and Hypnotic Analgesia: Implications for Clinical Practice" that provides an excellent, thorough review of the issues discussed here and also discusses clinical applications. Table 2.1 lists the areas of the brain that process pain and what type of hypnotic suggestions might be tailored to each, according to Jensen's review.

Neuroprocessing at the Spinal Cord Level

Because of the work of Melzack and Wall (1965) and others, we have long known that pain is modulated through an interaction of inhibitory and excitatory signals that operate in the dorsal roots of the spinal cord. Pain can

TABLE 2.1
Pain-Processing Areas of the Brain and Corresponding Hypnotic Suggestions

Neurophysiological site problem	Goals of suggestion
Diffuse cortical activation	Generalized calm
	The experience of being in a calming "safe place"
Periphery	Experience peripheral analgesia
	Produce the experience of decreased nociceptor responsivity
Spinothalamic tract (STT; dorsal horn and thalamus)	Experience or produce activities that reflect descending STT cell inhibition, such as warm or cool sensations
	Metaphors and images related to the inhibition of flow
Somatosensory cortex	Decrease pain intensity
	Alter the pain site
	Alter pain extent
	Alter pain quality
	Metaphors that alter the sensory aspect of pain
Insula	Experience comfortable bodily sensations (e.g., relaxation, warmth, lightness)
	Age regression to the experience of physical sensations incompatible with pain
Anterior cingulate cortex	Experience a feeling of "not caring" about the pain, a feeling of not having to do anything about it
	Amnesia for pain to reduce recall of distress and dread of future pain
Prefrontal cortex	Alter the meaning of pain
	Focus on valued goals other than pain reduction
	Focus on physical activity and fitness
	Age regression to experience memories of comfort
	Age progression
Cortical connectivity	Experience oneself as distant from one's body
	Disconnect sensations from an emotional response
Plasticity	Experience the painful area as able to move comfortably and easily
	Posthypnotic suggestions to make any benefits permanent

be decreased when inhibitory nerves fire at the "gate," and an interesting premise is that hypnosis might reduce pain through this mechanism. Studies have demonstrated hypnotically induced reductions in arm skin reflex (Hernandez-Peon, Dittborn, Borlone, & Davidovich, 1960), ankle muscle response (Holroyd, 1996), and nerve response in the jaw (Sharav & Tal, 1989).

Keirnan and colleagues also demonstrated a hypnotically induced muscle response in the ankle (Kiernan, Dane, Phillips, & Price, 1995), but their study received particular attention because they demonstrated that hypnotic suggestions for analgesia were correlated with spinal nociceptive (R-III) reflex. The R-III reflex has little to do with higher order central nervous system processing and would suggest that pain reduction is occurring, at least partially, through the inhibitory processes discussed above. Danziger et al. (1998) used a similar methodology to report that two distinct patterns of R-III reflex appear to be associated with hypnotic analgesia. Specifically, 11 of their subjects showed strong inhibition of the R-III reflex, whereas seven showed a strong facilitation. Rather than try to read too much into these findings, one may conclude that suggestible subjects can show a marked change in R-III reflex processing with hypnotic analgesic suggestions. Hypnotic effects on nervous system inhibition have also been demonstrated by alterations in galvanic skin response (Gruzelier, Allison, & Conway, 1988; West, Niell, & Hardy, 1952). All of the studies discussed in this section are subject to the limitations of many psychophysiological studies of hypnosis, in that they do not include control groups of nonhypnotized subjects. However, they do provide compelling preliminary data that hypnotic analgesia has physiological correlates and that those mechanisms may extend beyond higher cortical processing.

Sensory Versus Affective Pain Effects

As the thinking about the nature of pain has become more sophisticated, the notion that pain can be understood as simple unilateral phenomenon has been abandoned. In other words, understanding pain is not simply a matter of "how much it hurts," and this notion has been reflected in advancements in conceptualization and measurement. Specifically, it is useful to look not only at how strong the pain is (pain intensity) but also at how much it bothers the patient. This is what is known as the *sensory* versus *affective* components of pain. Sensory pain is thought to be more related to nociceptive (e.g., tissue damage) components of pain, whereas affective pain is linked more to cognitive-evaluative dimensions.

A number of studies have attempted to discern which of these pain dimensions are more affected by hypnosis. In an early study, Price, Harkins, and Baker (1987) reported that affective components of pain showed a greater reduction with hypnosis than did sensory ones. The same finding was demonstrated more recently with a sample of patients undergoing burn wound care (Wiechman Askay, Patterson, Jensen, & Sharar, 2007). However, a study by Price and Barber (1987) showed that both components of pain were affected by hypnosis and that it was largely a matter of how the suggestions were put. This certainly appeared to be the case in the brain activity studies by Rainville and colleagues (Rainville, Carrier, et al., 1999), described above. They reported that different parts of the brain show activity based on whether hypnotic suggestions are focused on sensory or affective pain components. Also see Feldman (2009) for a clinically oriented discussion of this topic. A more recent understanding (Wiechman Askay et al., 2007) is that when generic hypnotic suggestions for pain control are made, people seem to show more reduction on affective dimensions; clearly, however, appropriately targeted hypnotic suggestions can have an impact on both sensory and affective domains.

VIRTUAL REALITY HYPNOSIS

Virtual reality (VR) hypnosis involves the use of immersive VR technology as a medium to deliver hypnotic inductions and suggestions. The use of immersive VR as a distraction for pain is discussed in detail in Chapter 1. It may be useful to describe briefly here how the technology for immersive VR evolved. In the late 1990s, work by Hoffman and colleagues at the University of Washington began on the application of immersive VR to pain control, particularly that from acute procedures such as burn wound debridement. The experimental approach involved placing patients in a computer-generated three-dimensional environment in which they interacted with a simulated world around them. The operative cognitive processes involved distraction and, specifically, pulling attentional resources away from processing pain (Hoffman, Patterson, & Carrougher, 2000). In 2000, my colleagues and I developed an immersive VR world in which hypnosis could be delivered. Our hope was that this technology would allow the application hypnosis to patients without the presence of a trained clinician.

Currently, we have two ongoing randomized controlled trials on the use of VR hypnosis for burn and trauma pain. The following sections will review our findings to date on the studies that we have published, and also to discuss some of the theoretical and methodological issues that have been generated as we have attempted to deliver hypnosis through this new technological medium.

Scientific Evidence for Virtual Reality Hypnosis

Our first case study using VR technology to administer hypnosis was published in 2004 (Patterson, Tininenko, Schmidt, & Sharar, 2004). A 37-year-old man who was admitted to the burn center with full-thickness burns to 55% of his body, including his arms, legs, and hands, was the first to try this new technology. Upon admission to the intensive care unit, he was heavily medicated with opioid analgesic (analgesic and benzodiazepine agents) and was minimally responsive during this phase. The patient began to have panic attacks and intense anxiety in anticipation of his twice-daily painful wound debridements as he became more alert. His records indicated that he was receiving more than 15 times the dose of opioid analgesics typically given on the burn unit for wound care and was still reporting excruciating procedural pain.

The patient consented to participate in this study and reported that he had never received any type of hypnosis and also had no prior mental health history. His score on the Stanford Hypnotic Clinical Scale (SHCS) was 3 out of 5, indicating medium hypnotizability, and he scored 18 out of 34 on the Tellegen Absorption Scale, indicating a moderate ability for absorption. Pain was measured through a series of 10-point Graphic Rating Scales (Karoly & Jensen, 1987) used to determine the worst pain and the average pain experienced and the time spent thinking about pain. The Burn Specific Anxiety Scale (Taal & Faber, 1997) was used to measure anxiety. Baseline measures were taken on Day 1 of the study (wound care with medication but no hypnosis). The patient received VR hypnosis 2 hours prior to the wound care on Day 2 of the study.

The intervention relied on the posthypnotic suggestions given for pain control prior to wound care rather than intervention during the actual wound care. The patient listened to an audiotape-only hypnotic induction based on the audio of the VR intervention on Day 3. He was instructed to imagine himself going into the virtual world as he was guided through the hypnotic induction. The effect size of the intervention for this patient was encouraging: a 40% reduction in pain ratings from baseline to Day 2, another 60% reduction in pain after the audiotape alone on Day 3, a 50% reduction in anxiety from Baseline to Day 2, and a 60% reduction after Day 3. The patient further reported a positive, subjective experience with the VR technology. Although this was only an initial case study, the findings suggested the value of conducting a larger case series.

The same VR technology and a similar study design were used to study 13 patients on the same burn unit (Patterson, Wiechman, Jensen, & Sharar, 2006). Patients requiring a minimum of 3 days of hospitalization and daily wound debridements were enrolled consecutively from ongoing admissions. Baseline measures were again taken on Day 1, using the same measures as previously mentioned. On Day 2, patients received VR hypnosis prior to their wound care, and outcome measures were repeated just following their wound care. However, on Day 3 of the study, patients were given VR hypnosis again, instead of an audio-only hypnotic intervention. Nurses were instructed to medicate patients for wound care and background pain as usual and were not aware of the patients' condition assignment. Data were analyzed for eight patients as five were dropped from the study because of unexpected changes in the initial burn management plan, (e.g., unanticipated surgery or early discharge).

On average, patients in this study scored in the moderate range for absorption and the medium range for hypnotizability, using the SHCS and Tellegen scales. Results indicated an average 20% drop in worst pain scores from baseline to Day 3, a 29% drop in the time that patients spent thinking about their pain, and a 29% drop in anxiety scores. There was an unanticipated 50% reduction in the amount of opioids (calculated opioid equivalents) that patients required before, during, and immediately after wound care, providing further evidence of the analgesic efficacy of this technique. Because the intervention was done prior to wound care, there was no added time required to complete wound care for patients in the study. More studies are currently being conducted on the use of VR hypnosis for acute pain procedures and address some of the methodological issues and limitations raised in this case series, including the use of both a control group and randomized treatment allocation.

More recently, Patterson, Jensen, Wiechman Askay, and Sharar (in press) used VR hypnosis to control the ongoing pain of patients hospitalized in a Level I, regional trauma hospital for long bone fractures or internal injuries from trauma. Twenty-one patients were randomly assigned to conditions in which they received either VR hypnosis with suggestions for pain relief and improved sleep or a control condition (either standard care or VR distraction that was not linked to pain control). VR hypnosis patients reported less pain intensity and unpleasantness relative to control patients.

The only published report of the application of VR hypnosis to chronic pain recently appeared in the *International Journal of Clinical and Experimental Hypnosis* (Oneal, Patterson, Soltani, Teeley, & Jensen, 2008). This was a single-subject design study with a 36-year-old woman with a 5-year history of a high-level spinal cord injury (C4 tetraplegia) who suffered from bilateral upper extremity neuropathic pain. She described her pain as a constant burning sensation along her shoulders, arms, and forearms. She reported being unable to wear clothes with sleeves or to be outdoors in the heat or wind. The pain also reportedly interfered with her sleep and quality of life. No prior psychiatric history was reported by the patient. Numerous pain management treatments had been attempted over the years for this pain, including various medications, physical therapy, massage therapy, meditation, acupuncture, and standard hypnosis, all with no relief.

With respect to the intervention, the patient received 33 sessions of VR hypnosis over a 6-month period. The technology was similar to the studies described previously; however, modifications in hypnotic suggestions were made for chronic pain, including posthypnotic suggestions aimed at overall comfort. Between sessions, the patient was encouraged to practice self-hypnosis at home and was given an audiotape version of the VR hypnosis induction. The patient kept a pain diary of ongoing pain that included Graphic Rating Scales of pain intensity, pain unpleasantness, and amount of time the patient experienced a reduction or absence of pain between treatment sessions. In order that an ABA (treatment, no treatment, treatment) design could be established, she was also asked to take a 1-month hiatus from treatment (both the VR hypnosis and audiotapes). The patient's rating of pain intensity and pain unpleasantness declined by an average of 36% and 33%, respectively, over the course of the treatment. She also reported no pain for an average (over the 33 sessions) of 3.86 hours after treatment and a reduction in pain for 12 hours after treatment. Although the effects of the intervention did not persist over a longer time (1 month), the duration of the treatment effects and the relief provided were superior to other methods that she had tried. She also indicated that she persisted with the treatment because even having 3 hours free of pain was enough relief to improve her quality of life. What was particularly interesting is that the patient returned for 33 sessions of treatment; traveling to the hospital was a cumbersome task that required the assistance of an attendant. Apparently the patient did not tire of the technology after 33 sessions and reported that she found the induction presented through the immersive VR technology to be preferable to the audio-only (for which she could have stayed home). These results are also promising and indicate the potential viability of the use of VR hypnosis for chronic pain problems.

Methodological Issues With Virtual Reality Hypnosis

The aforementioned studies have led to the identification of methodological issues that need to be addressed to advance this technology and our understanding of the processes involved. First, there is a clear need for randomized controlled trials of VR hypnosis for both acute and chronic pain problems. Without randomized controlled trials, clinicians will not be able to isolate conditions in the environment and within patients that can have an impact on results, particularly when the intervention is conducted in clinical settings. Second, the importance of an audio-only control group to establish the efficacy of VR technology over standard hypnosis, or simply attention from a therapist, is apparent. The treatment effect sizes in the studies discussed above are equivalent to what has been achieved in studies that used a clinician. However, it is important that VR hypnosis be compared with audio-only hypnosis in a controlled trial. The technology used in VR hypnosis is far more expensive than that of a simple audiotape, and distinct advantages of VR hypnosis would have to be demonstrated in a direct comparison to establish a rationale for the increased equipment costs.

One advantage of VR hypnosis is that it is completely standardized and does not depend on the skill or availability of a trained therapist. This standardization is appealing in conducting more research and understanding more fully the underlying physiological mechanisms involved in hypnosis. In many studies of clinical hypnosis, even if the exact same wording is used, clinicians can vary substantially in their delivery of the hypnosis. With VR hypnosis, this issue of consistency is no longer subject to question.

The role of hypnotizability and the impact of clinical (as well as laboratory) effects of hypnosis are important variables in any experimental study of this type. With VR hypnosis, there have been some efforts to assess user hypnotizability. Unfortunately, this has been measured with the SHCS, which is only a five-item scale. The SHCS lacks the range and psychometric properties of superior scales such as the Stanford A or C (Hilgard & Hilgard, 1975). As such, the role of hypnotizability and response in VR hypnosis is not fully understood. In the aforementioned studies, as is the case in most studies, the majority of participants score in the medium range of hypnotizability. Future studies with larger subject numbers may want to separate out those with high versus low hypnotizability scores in their analyses to see if there is a differential analgesic effect in these two patient populations.

Theoretical Issues With Virtual Reality Hypnosis

The studies discussed above have generated several questions and theoretical issues that warrant further investigation. First, can VR hypnosis enhance hypnotic response in those with low hypnotizability scores? Hypnotizability was first described by Hilgard and Hilgard (1975) as a trait measure that assesses a person's ability to be hypnotized. As mentioned previously, assessing a person's hypnotizability is important in these studies. It has been theorized that VR hypnosis may capture attention in those who have trouble with imagination and absorption. The concept of presence, described earlier, is believed to be central to the efficacy of VR hypnosis. The sensation of "going into" the virtual world enhances a patient's presence in the environment and draws attention away from the pain. Attentional processes are regarded as central to hypnotic analgesia as well. Attention is an important step in a hypnotic induction (Crawford, 1994). With attentional mechanisms as a common denominator, the potential for a synergistic effect between the attention-captivating qualities of VR and the suggestion inherent in hypnosis is significant for several reasons. First, hypnotic suggestion may help inhibited patients relax and immerse themselves in a virtual world. Further, hypnotic suggestion can be used to deepen a patient's sense of presence in the virtual world. As mentioned before, however, the critical question is whether VR plays a role in facilitating hypnotic suggestion.

A second theoretical issue is the potential for this technology to expand the application of hypnosis as an analgesic treatment modality. VR hypnosis could potentially eliminate the need for the physical presence of a clinician at most such interventions. With less dependence on the skill of a trained hypnotist, such technology may increase the capacity to reach a greater number of patients who could benefit from hypnotic analgesia. The initial acquisition cost of this technology may be expensive now but is certain to come down in price, with improved electronic technologies. With the move toward telemedicine and providing more services to patients in rural areas and underserved regions, this is an exciting concept to explore. At its extreme, this question becomes whether VR hypnosis can completely replace live hypnosis. The answer is clearly that it cannot. For complex clinical problems there will always be the need to individualize hypnotic interventions to identifiable patient characteristics. However, at this point, there are many diverse clinical settings, such as pain control from medical procedures or smoking cessation, that are amenable to the more generic type of hypnosis afforded by VR hypnosis. This technology also holds great promise for those patients with hearing impairments as written hypnotic suggestions can be incorporated into the program.

A third theoretical issue is the question of what constitutes optimal VR hypnosis. We have only scratched the surface in exploring the potential application of this modality both in the laboratory and in the clinical situation. What can be offered now with respect to VR hypnosis technology is only an early prototype. There are countless variables to be investigated, such as the nature of the virtual environment, the role of auditory stimulation, the ideal duration of treatment, and whether patients should have their eyes closed and rely on imagination for some of the time in VR or keep their eyes open the entire time.

Another question is whether we can ever provide computer-generated stimuli that are more compelling than human imagination. At this point we are not at a point where we can consider rivaling human imagination with computer technology, and it is questionable whether this could ever be the case. Ultimately, the optimal use of VR hypnosis may be in the form of an interaction between patients and technology. Some patients may generally prefer imagination, whereas others may show a proclivity toward passively experiencing computer-generated stimuli, especially in situations in which cognitive functioning is compromised and the need for cognitive effort is minimized. These are all questions yet to be explored. With society's increasing reliance on technology, however, the application of VR to a spectrum of medical issues, including pain relief, is an exciting prospect that could potentially benefit millions of people.

SUMMARY

Far more than other areas of psychology, the results for analog studies in hypnosis can help guide clinical work. The body of literature on hypnosis with laboratory pain is simply useful. It provides a foundation of carefully controlled scientific work on which to base clinical applications of hypnosis. It further provides ideas on how to improve clinical interventions. The concepts of hypnotizability, expectancy, and dissociated control that have grown out of experimental work have proved applicable to clinical pain. The growing number of psychophysiological studies on hypnosis and pain has only served to enhance the scientific legitimacy of hypnosis. Hypnotic analgesia created in the laboratory is reflected in a number of measurable psychophysiological phenomena. This body of research puts to rest the argument that hypnosis is solely a placebo effect. Moreover, although there are no discrete markers for whether subjects are or are not in trance states, there are physiological correlates of hypnosis that vary by the nature of suggestion. The main question now has to do more with what progression of changes occur in the brain and other systems, and how they vary by the nature of hypnotic suggestion. Finally, a promising area for future scientific and theoretical work is the application of immersive VR to the delivery hypnosis. It is hoped that the use of this, as well as other types of technologies, will not only improve the impact of hypnosis but also greatly enhance its dissemination to patient populations in need of pain relief.

3

CLINICAL RESEARCH AND HYPNOSIS AS AN EVIDENCE-BASED PRACTICE

Like other forms of psychological and medical treatment, hypnosis is under increased demand to show empirical support for its clinical application. This push has come not only from the basic tenets of the scientist–practitioner perspective but also from the fact that health care is increasingly shaped by pressures from funding sources such as insurance coverage and payer mix. Chapter 2 laid out what should be a compelling body of laboratory and psychophysiological research supporting hypnotic analgesia. However, as impressive as that support is, it is not sufficient for hypnosis to be accepted as an actual clinical treatment. Twenty years ago, there were almost no randomized clinical trials investigating hypnosis for pain. For that matter, there were almost no trials of this nature examining hypnosis for any type of medical or psychological problem. The purpose of this chapter is to examine the scientific evidence for using hypnosis to treat clinical pain in patient populations.

ANECDOTAL AND CLINICAL REPORTS

For most of the history of hypnosis and perhaps up to 2 decades ago, the sole scientific evidence for clinical hypnotic analgesia was in the form of anecdotal or case report studies. Often such reports lacked any form of objective measurement. Most commonly the reports were a matter of investigators stating that the patient's pain improved. However, it is useful to review this body of research from clinical reports for a number of reasons. First, it is important to determine the range of pain conditions that have been successfully addressed by hypnosis. Second, there are a number of highly creative approaches that are reported in such anecdotal reports. Controlled studies really do nothing to replace the creativity that might go into an intervention in a case report.

The most famous of case reports was the series of 345 operations that Scottish surgeon James Esdaile reported as performed with mesmerism as the sole anesthetic (Esdaile, 1957). As early as 1975, Hilgard and Hilgard reported 14 different types of surgeries that have been published by different investigators in which hypnosis was the only form of anesthesia. Examples of such surgeries include hysterectomies, tumor excisions, gastrostomies, and appendectomies. Victor Rausch, a dentist who advocated using hypnosis in his field, reported undergoing a cholecystectomy with self-hypnosis, remaining awake and walking back to his room immediately after the procedure (Rausch, 1980).

Burn injuries have been one of the most popular applications of hypnosis reported in the literature. Crasilneck, Stirman, and Wilson (1955) reported on eight patients hospitalized for burn care. One of the cases involved giving a patient the hypnotic suggestion that he "will eat everything on his tray." This suggestion had to be revised after the patient was observed attempting to eat his milk carton and paper plate (Crasilneck et al., 1955). There are a number of other case reports indicating successful burn pain control with hypnosis (Gilboa, Borenstein, Seidman, & Tsur, 1990; Patterson, Questad, & Boltwood, 1987). Of particular significance, Finer and Nylen (1961) reported on a burn patient undergoing excision and grafting using hypnosis rather than chemical anesthesia. See Hammond (2008) for a review of hypnosis as a sole anesthetic for major surgeries.

In the anecdotal literature in general, what it is remarkable is the breadth of pain disorders that have been treated with hypnosis. This list includes pain associated with dental work (J. Barber, 1977; J. Barber & Mayer, 1977; Hartland, 1971; Hilgard & LeBaron, 1984), reflex sympathetic dystrophy (Gainer, 1992), acquired amputation (Chaves, 1986; Siegel, 1979), childbirth (Haanen et al., 1991), spinal cord injury (M. P. Jensen & Barber, 2000), sickle cell anemia (Dinges et al., 1997), arthritis (Appel, 1992; Crasilneck, 1995), temporomandibular joint disorder (Crasilneck, 1995; Simon & Lewis, 2000), multiple sclerosis (Dane, 1996; Sutcher, 1997), causalgia (Finer &

Graf, 1968), lupus erythematosus (S. J. Smith & Balaban, 1983), postsurgical pain (Mauer, Burnett, Ouellette, Ironson, & Dandes, 1999), and unanesthetized fracture reduction (Iserson, 1999). Other types of pain problems reported to respond to hypnotic analgesia include low back pain (Crasilneck, 1979, 1995), headaches (Crasilneck, 1995; Spinhoven, 1988), and mixed chronic pain (Evans, 1989; Jack, 1999; Sacerdote, 1978). Despite the extensive nature of this list, it is certainly not exhaustive. There are very few pain problems for which hypnosis has not been reported to be successful, and I am not aware of any pain issue for which hypnosis cannot at least be considered.

CONTROLLED CLINICAL STUDIES

Both hypnosis in general and its use for pain control suffered for years in terms of scientific support. Hypnosis has always been regarded with a certain amount of skepticism in the scientific community, and the influence of stage hypnosis, as well as "lay hypnotists" attempting to treat health problems, has not been of any help in this regard. Before the 1980s, few randomized controlled studies could be identified for clinical hypnotic analgesia. Now pain control has become somewhat of a standard for the field. The body of literature that has developed in this area is respectable.

A basic problem in the hypnotic pain literature up, at least, until recently, is that often no distinction is made between whether the type of pain being treated is acute or chronic. In fact, regarding acute and chronic as the same treatment identity is akin to saying that the treatments for anxiety and depression or for obesity and sleep disorders are similar. In many ways, the treatments for these two types of pain are on opposite ends of the spectrum. Acute pain is generally a response to tissue damage (Melzack & Wall, 1973; Williams, 1999). Hypnosis can usually focus directly on reducing acute pain; with chronic pain, treatment is often more complex. The following sections represent an update on the 2003 *Psychological Bulletin* (Patterson & Jensen, 2003) review of hypnotic pain control and are divided into the categories of acute and chronic pain. These sections are accompanied by tables (originally appearing in the *Psychological Bulletin* article) summarizing controlled studies on the respective types of pain.

Acute Pain

As is discussed several times in this volume, acute pain is different from chronic pain in that it is usually intense, short-lived, and frequently caused by some sort of medical procedure. Table 3.1 describes the controlled hypnosis studies done with acute pain. The sections that follow are divided according to

TABLE 3.1
Controlled Studies in Acute Pain Hypnotic Treatment

Study (type of acute pain)	Hypnotizability assessed?	N	Randomized?	Control condition(s)	Adult or child?	Outcome dimensions	Findings
Zeltzer and LeBaron (1982); bone marrow aspiration pain	No	33	Yes	Deep breathing and distraction (DBD)	Child (age range = 6–17 years)	Patient-rated pain intensity Patient-rated anxiety Observer-rated pain intensity Observer-rated anxiety	H > DBD H > DBD H > DBD H > DBD
Katz et al. (1987); bone marrow aspiration pain	No	36	Yes	Nondirected play (NDP)	Child (age range = 6–11 years)	Observed distress (PBRS) Nurse-rated anxiety Patient-rated fear Patient-rated pain Therapist-rated rapport Therapist-rated response to hypnosis	H = NDP H = NDP H = NDP H = NDP H = NDP H = NDP
Kuttner (1988); bone marrow aspiration pain	No	25	Yes	Standard care (SC) Distraction (D)	Child (age range = 3–6 years)	Observed distress (PBRS-R) Observer-rated pain Observer-rated anxiety Patient-rated pain Patient-rated anxiety	H > SC (.91), H > D (.64) H > SC, H > D H > SC, H > D H = SC = D H = SC = D
Liossi and Hatira (1999); bone marrow aspiration pain	Yes (Stanford Hypnotic Clinical Scale for Children)	30	Yes	Cognitive–behavioral therapy (CBT) Standard care (SC)	Child (age range = 5–15 years)	Observed distress (PBCL) Patient-rated pain intensity Patient-rated anxiety	H > CBT > SC (H = CBT) > SC H > CBT > SC

Study		n		Control condition	Age	Outcome measure	Result
Wakeman and Kaplan (1978); burn wound dressing change and debridement pain	No	42	No	Attention control (AC)	Both (age range = 7–70 years)	Percentage of allowable medication use during study participation	H > AC
Patterson et al. (1989); burn wound dressing change and debridement pain	No	13	No	Standard care (SC)	Adult	Patient-rated pain intensity	H > SC
Patterson et al. (1992); dressing change and debridement pain among burn patients	No	30	Yes	Standard care (SC) Attention control (AC)	Adult	Morphine equivalents for administered pain medications Patient-reported pain Nurse-rated pain	H = SC = AC H > (SC = AC) H > (SC = AC)
Everett et al. (1994); burn wound dressing change and debridement pain	No	32	Yes	Attention control (AC) Lorazepam (L)	Adult	Patient-rated pain intensity Patient-rated anxiety Nurse-rated patient pain intensity Nurse-rated patient anxiety	(H+L) = (H) = (AC+L) = (L) (H+L) = (H) = (AC+L) = (L) (H+L) = (H) = (AC+L) = (L) (H+L) = (H) = (AC+L) = (L)
Patterson and Ptacek (1997); burn wound dressing change and. debridement pain	No	61	Yes	Attention control (AC)	Adult	Self-reported worst pain intensity Nurse-reported worst patient pain intensity Patient-rated effectiveness of hypnosis Opioid Intake	H = AC (among subjects with high pain, H > AC) H > AC H = AC H = AC

(continues)

TABLE 3.1

Controlled Studies in Acute Pain Hypnotic Treatment   (Continued)

Study (type of acute pain)	Hypnotizability assessed?	N	Randomized?	Control condition(s)	Adult or child?	Outcome dimensions	Findings
Wright and Drummond (2000); burn wound dressing change and debridement pain	No	30	Yes	Standard care (SC)	Adult and child (age range = 16–48 years)	Medication consumption	H > SC
						During procedure pain intensity	H > SC
						During procedure pain unpleasantness	H > SC
						Postprocedure pain intensity	H > SC
						Postprocedure pain unpleasantness	H > SC
						Pre-post procedure change in patient-rated relaxation	H > SC
Davidson (1962); labor pain	No	210	No	Standard care (SC) Relaxation training (RT)	Adult	Duration of labor	H > (RT = SC)
						Patient-rated pain in the first stage	H > (RT = SC)
						Patient-rated pain in the second stage	H > (RT = SC)
						Analgesia intake	H > (RT = SC)
						Patient-rated pleasantness of labor	H > (RT = SC)
Freeman et al. (1986); labor pain	Yes (Stanford Hypnotic Clinical Scale)	65	Yes	Standard care (SC)	Adult	Duration of pregnancy	H longer than SC by .06 weeks
						Duration of labor	H longer than SC by 2.7 hours
						Analgesic intake	H = SC
						Mode of delivery	H = SC
						Pain relief	H = SC
						Satisfaction with labor	H > SC (p = .08)

Study	Hypnotizability measured	N	Randomized	Comparison condition	Age	Outcome measure	Results
Harmon et al. (1990); labor pain	Yes (Harvard Group Scale of Hypnotic Suscep-tibility, Form A)	60	Yes	Breathing and relaxation exercises (BR)	Adult	Length of stage 1 labor	H > BR
						Length of stage 2 labor	H = BR
						Newborn Apgar, 1-min	H > BR
						Newborn Apgar, 5-min	H > BR
						Spontaneous delivery (%)	H > BR
						Percentage given medications	H > BR
						MMPI Depression (scale 2) scale score	H = BR (among highs, H > BR)
						Pain intensity (MPQ)	H > BR
						Sensory pain (MPQ)	H > BR
						Affective pain (MPQ)	H > BR
						Evaluative pain (MPQ)	H > BR
						Miscellaneous pain (MPQ)	H > BR
Weinstein and Au (1991); pain during angioplasty	No	32	Yes	Standard care (SC)	Adult	Pulse	H = SC
						Systolic BP	H = SC
						Diastolic BP	H = SC
						Total time of balloon inflation during procedure	H = SC
						Requests for additional medicine	H > SC
Syrjala et al. (1992); pain following chemotherapy for cancer	No	45	Yes	Cognitive—behavioral therapy (CBT) Attention control (AC) Standard care (SC)	Adult	Catecholamine levels	H > SC
						Oral pain	H > (AC = CBT)
						Nausea	H = AC = CBT = SC
						Presence of emesis	H = AC = CBT
						Opioid intake	H = AC = CBT

(continues)

TABLE 3.1
Controlled Studies in Acute Pain Hypnotic Treatment   *(Continued)*

Study (type of acute pain)	Hypnotizability assessed?	N	Randomized?	Control condition(s)	Adult or child?	Outcome dimensions	Findings
Lang et al. (1996); mixed invasive medical procedures—primarily diagnostic arteriograms	Yes (Hypnotic Induction Profile)	30	Yes	Standard care (SC)	Adult	Self-administration of analgesics	H > SC
						Blood pressure increase	H = SC
						Heart rate increase	H = SC
						Oxygen desaturation during procedure	H > SC
						Procedural interruptions due to hemodynamic instability	H > SC
						Patient-rated pain intensity	H = SC
						Patient-rated maximal pain	H > SC
						Patient-rated anxiety (BAI)	H = SC
Faymonville et al. (1997); elective plastic surgery	No	56	Yes	Emotional support (ES)	Adult	Analgesic requirements	H > ES
						Perioperative patient-rated anxiety	H > ES
						Patient-rated pain intensity	H > ES
						Patient-rated level of control	H > ES
						Observed complaints during surgery	H > ES
						Diastolic BP	H > ES
						Maximum decrease in SpO2	H > ES

Study; procedures	Randomized	N	Population	Control group(s)	Outcome measure	Result
Lambert (1996); variety of surgical procedures	No	52	Child (age range = 7–19 years)	Attention control (AC)	Maximum increase in heart rate	H > ES
					Maximum increase in respiratory rate	H > ES
					Maximum increase in systolic BP	H > ES
					Maximum increase in cutaneous temperature	H = ES
					Patient-rated surgery satisfaction	H > ES
					Observer-rated surgical comfort	H > ES
					Postoperative nausea and vomiting	H > ES
					Surgeon's satisfaction	H > ES
					Patient-rated pain	H > AC
					Patient-rated postoperative anxiety (SSAIC)	H = AC
					Length of surgery	H = AC
					Length of hospital stay	H > AC
					Length of anesthesia	H = AC
					Time in postanesthesia care unit	H = AC
					Medication consumption	H = AC
Lang et al. (2000); variety of surgical procedures including arterial and venous surgery and nephrostomy	No	241	Adult	Standard care (SC) Attention control (AC)	Patient-rated pain intensity	H > (AC = SC)
					Patient-rated anxiety	H > SC; H = AC; AC = SC
					Medication use	(H = AC) > SC
					Time needed for procedure	H > SC; H = AC; AC = SC
					Hemodynamic stability	H > (AC = SC)

(continues)

TABLE 3.1
Controlled Studies in Acute Pain Hypnotic Treatment *(Continued)*

Study (type of acute pain)	Hypnotizability assessed?	N	Randomized?	Control condition(s)	Adult or child?	Outcome dimensions	Findings
Wiechman Askay et al. (2007); burn wound care pain	Yes	46	Yes	Attention plus relaxation (AR)	Adult	Patient-rated pain intensity	H > AR
						Patient rated average pain intensity	H > AR
						Patient rated worst pain intensity	H > AR
						Patient rated anxiety	H > AR
Lang et al. (2006); large core needle biopsies of breast	No	236	Yes	Standard care (SC) Empathy (E)	Adult	Patient rated pain	H > SC; H = E; E > SC
						Patient rated anxiety	H > SC; H > E; E > SC

Note. H = hypnosis alone; PBRS-R = Procedural Behavioral Rating Scale—Revised; PBCL = Procedural Behavior Checklist; MMPI = Minnesota Multiphasic Personality Inventory; MPQ = McGill Pain Questionnaire; BAI = Beck Anxiety Inventory; BP = blood pressure; SpO2 = oxygen saturation; STAIC = State–Trait Anxiety Inventory for Children. Adapted from "Hypnosis and Clinical Pain Control," by D. R. Patterson and M. Jensen, 2003, *Psychological Bulletin, 129,* 501–503. Copyright 2003 American Psychological Association.

some of the causes of acute pain, including invasive medical procedures, burn injuries, labor, bone marrow aspirations, and women's health procedures.

Pain From Invasive Medical Procedures

Angioplasty is an invasive and potentially frightening procedure that involves insertion of a catheter that runs into the heart. In a study that compared 16 patients who received the procedure with 16 control patients, E. J. Weinstein and Au (1991) used a modification of J. Barber's (1977) rapid induction analgesia (RIA) procedure. The outcome measures included the amount of time the patients allowed the doctor to keep the balloon catheter inflated; this was increased by 25% in the hypnosis group but was statistically insignificant. In addition, the group that received hypnosis demonstrated a significantly reduced use of opioid analgesics as well as catecholamine levels in blood samples. However, the hypnosis group did not show differences in other physiological variables measured including blood pressure or pulse.

Intervention radiology involves procedures that are similar to angioplasty. Lang and her colleagues reported two studies using hypnosis for such procedures. Sixteen patients who received hypnosis (relaxation and guided imagery) for procedures that primarily involved diagnostic anteriograms were compared with a control group that received standard care (Lang, Joyce, Spiegel, Hamilton, & Lee, 1996). The hypnosis group reported less maximal pain, used less pain medication, and showed more physiological stability. However, there were no differences between treatment groups in anxiety ratings, blood pressure, or heart rate increases. In addition, scores on a scale of hypnotizability did not correlate with differences. Treating clinicians were not blinded to the study condition.

Their second study was one of the largest and best designed of any clinical hypnosis study to date. Lang et al. (2000) studied patients undergoing cutaneous vascular and renal procedures, also in the realm of interventional radiology. A total of 241 patients were randomly assigned to groups that received self-hypnotic relaxation ($n = 82$), structured attention control ($n = 80$), or standard care ($n = 79$). A particular strength of this study, in addition to the large sample size, was that both the hypnosis and the structured attention control group received a manualized type of treatment. The attention control group had eight key components; the hypnosis group had these same components plus hypnotic suggestions (having patients imagine themselves in a safe and pleasant place during the procedure). Unlike most studies in the field, it would be relatively easy to replicate the hypnosis and control group treatment based on these requirements. Further, the fidelity of treatment was established through videotaped coding. The hypnosis group showed less procedure room time, more hemodynamic stability, and less use of analgesic/sedating medications. Repeated measures of pain and anxiety were also reduced for the hypnosis group. The investigators used measures that allowed them to perform a cost analysis of experimental versus control. In a follow-up study, they were able to demonstrate that the hypnosis treatment cut costs in half (mainly by reducing operating room time and anesthetic agents), even when the time of training clinicians was taken into account. More recently, Lang et al. (2008) reported reduced pain and anxiety with hypnosis in 201 patients undergoing percutaneous tumor treatments. Ratings were lower by patients receiving hypnosis than those randomly assigned to empathic listening or standard treatment control groups.

Surgery is certainly an area that could be considered an invasive medical procedure, perhaps the most extreme, on this continuum. Lambert (1996) compared children ($n = 52$) who received hypnosis and guided imagery with a control group of those who spent an equal amount of time discussing both the surgery and topics that were of interest to them. The hypnosis treatment involved a single 30-minute session that occurred approximately a week before surgery (the hypnosis clinician was not present during surgery). Children were given hypnotic suggestions for relaxation, minimal pain, and positive surgical outcome based on images that they selected. The children randomly assigned to the hypnosis group reported lower levels of pain as well as shorter hospital stays than did those in the control group. The experimental group showed less anxiety, but this finding was not significant. The groups did not differ on length of surgery, anesthesia care, or postanesthesia care. Related to this, Saadat et al. (2006) reported that hypnosis reduced preoperative anxiety in patients randomized to a hypnosis group rather than attentive listening and support or standard care.

Plastic surgery is the area in which Faymonville and colleagues (Faymonville et al., 1997) have reported some of the most dramatic results for hypnosis and invasive medical procedures. Thirty-one patients received hypnosis, and 25 received what was described as a stress-reducing technique. For the hypnosis group, a hypnotic state was induced using eye fixation, muscle relaxation, and permissive and indirect hypnotic suggestions. The exact words and details of the induction technique depended on the anesthesiologist's observation of patient behavior. The stress-reducing group received a number of strategies including deep breathing and relaxation, positive emotional induction, and cognitive coping strategies (imaginative transformation of sensation or imaginative inattention). In terms of results, patients in the hypnosis group received significantly less analgesic and sedation drugs. Further, the hypnosis group reported significantly less pain and anxiety, higher levels of satisfaction, greater perceived control, lower (improved) physiological rates (blood pressure, heart rate, and respiratory rate), and less nausea and vomiting. Surgeons of the patients in the hypnosis group reported higher levels of satisfaction in those patients than did those for the stress reduction group. This study was compelling because, for the patients in the hypnosis group, what they received was never actually defined as hypnosis. This approach to the study raises an interesting argument: Can patients receive an actual hypnotic intervention without the term *hypnosis* ever being used? The experimental design was somewhat limited in that the treating anesthesiologist provided both of the treatments and was certainly aware of which patients were in the two conditions. Nevertheless, the findings of this study were compelling, and it would be interesting to see if they are replicated.

Bone marrow transplants are one of the most painful types of treatments included in cancer care. Harvesting the marrow is certainly painful in itself. Further, patients undergo supralethal does of irradiation that can cause nausea, vomiting, and mucositis for days or even weeks. Syrjala, Cummings, and Donaldson (1992) compared hypnosis with cognitive–behavioral and attention control conditions in patients with cancer undergoing this difficult procedure and 20 days of chemotherapy and irradiation. Hypnosis included relaxation and suggestions for pain control that were tailored to the needs of the patient and then provided on audiotapes. Patients were instructed to listen to the tapes daily for the 20 days of treatment. The cognitive–behavioral intervention involved information, cognitive restructuring, information, goal development, and exploring the meaning of the disease. Patients in the hypnosis group reported significantly less pain than did the cognitive–behavioral or attention control groups. However, no differences between the groups were reported on nausea, emesis, or pain medication use.

Burn Pain

Burn wound debridement is known to be one of the worst among acute pain procedures. It is interesting that psychopathology has long been overemphasized after severe burn injuries (Pattterson, Everett, et al., 1993), which can have dire ethical implications (Patterson, Miller-Perrin, McCormick, & Hudson, 1993), and pain control has often been neglected (Melzack, 1990). Pain control issues after burn injuries are not necessarily a problem of the initial burn injury itself as much as with the treatment that ensues. Standard care requires that many burn injuries be debrided and cleaned once or twice a day; such care commonly causes more pain than does the initial trauma itself. Opioid analgesics (i.e., morphine and its derivatives) are generally the treatment of choice for burn pain (Patterson & Sharar, 1997, 2001); however, it is well established that such interventions will often not control all of the pain (Patterson, Ptacek & Esselman, 1997). Several patients respond poorly to such agents or have adverse reactions to them. Moreover, patients can develop tolerance to opioid analgesic; large dosing can lead to withdrawal symptoms and lengthen hospital stays. Hypnosis for burn pain is one of the most frequently cited applications of this treatment approach. This is not surprising because it often can have a dramatic impact on pain levels, even when other modalities are not working well.

As has been mentioned, Crasilneck et al. (1955) published some of the earliest work in this area in the *Journal of the American Medical Association,* which won the research some attention from the medical community. Ewin (1983, 1984, 1986) has also produced some work of historical merit in this area. In a series of clinical reports, Ewin, a surgeon, reported that the early application of hypnosis (within 4 hours after meeting a patient) had the effect of not only controlling pain but also retarding the progression of the thermal injury. By having patients "go to a special place" and placing cool towels on their injuries, patients who sustained injuries that would have progressed to full thickness levels (third degree, requiring skin grafts) witnessed wounds healing with no surgical intervention. Ewin's results were dramatic and compelling and, if replicated in controlled trials, would represent one of the more significant applications of hypnosis.

Wakeman and Kaplan (1978) randomly assigned patients with burn injuries to groups that received hypnosis or attention control from the psychologist. Treatment included live and audiotaped hypnosis with suggestions for analgesia, anesthesia, dissociation, and reduction of anxiety and fear. The treatment outcome was the amount of required medication, and a huge effect was found in this study. Most recently, Wiechman Askay, Patterson, Jensen, and Sharar (2007) reported that RIA appeared to have a greater input on affective as opposed to sensory ratings of burn pain.

My colleagues and I have conducted a number of studies on hypnosis for burn care with funding from the National Institutes of Health in the General Medical Sciences. Our first study involved a quasi-research design, using a convenience sample of patients with burn injuries as a control (Patterson, Questad, & DeLateur, 1989). Patients with high levels of baseline pain received a hypnotic induction; posthypnotic cues were provided by the nurses performing wound debridement. Visual Analog Scale (VAS) scores for pain dropped significantly.

We attempted to compensate for the nonrandomized design in our next study (Patterson, Everett, Burns, & Marvin, 1992). We randomized 30 patients to treatment conditions in which they received active hypnosis, attention-placebo, or standard treatment control (medication only). The attention-placebo condition involved the equivalent amount of time as hypnosis. Patients were visited by the psychologist and engaged in a discussion about their burn injury and the nature of their pain. Strategies for pain control were discussed. Toward the end of the session, the patients were instructed to count from 1 to 20 and put themselves in a relaxing place; they were instructed to also do that during their upcoming dressing changes. The patients' ratings of their expectations for treatment did not differ between the hypnosis and attention-placebo groups. In terms of results, the VAS pain scores dropped significantly for the hypnosis group but not for the attention-placebo or standard treatment groups (Patterson et al., 1992). In a subsequent study (Everett, Patterson, Burns, Montgomery, & Heimbach, 1994), we used a similar design but had one group receive the tranquilizer lorazepam. In this study, we did not find a treatment effect for any of the groups, including hypnosis.

With the assumption that our sample sizes were inadequate, we attempted to replicate our initial findings using a large cohort of patients with burn injuries (Patterson, Ptacek, Carrougher, & Sharar, 1997). The patients in the hypnosis, attention-placebo, and standard treatment groups did not show a difference in their pain ratings. However, when we looked specifically at patients with high initial pain scores, we found an interaction effect, suggesting that such patients showed a significant drop in pain ratings (Patterson, Ptacek, et al., 1997).

Other studies with hypnosis for burn pain have shown analgesic effects independent of initial levels of pain (Wright & Drummond, 2000). However, from our findings, we regarded initial levels of pain to be at least somewhat of a factor. Our interpretations of these findings is that patients with higher levels of pain will be more motivated to escape it and try techniques that might be foreign to them, such as hypnosis (Patterson, Adcock, & Bombardier, 1997). We also postulated a number of other factors that might make inpatients with burn pain better candidates for hypnosis. Many of them might be undergoing the dissociation that accompanies acute stress disorder (ASD), and patients with burn injuries commonly demonstrate ASD (Difede et al., 2002; McKibben, Bresnick, Wiechman Askay, & Fauerbach, 2008). Because elements of hypnosis often involve dissociation (Spiegel & Spiegel, 1978), an effective clinician can use these tendencies to the patient's advantage. As a side note, Shakibaei, Harandi, Gholamrezaei, Samoei, and Salehi (2008) reported that hypnosis reduced pain and reexperiencing trauma in their sample of burn patients. Another factor is the functional dependence that comes with trauma hospitalization. Often a trauma patient's survival depends on complying with the directives of health care workers. Patients are routinely asked to disrobe, provide stool samples, or undergo exams or procedures. In many respects, a hypnotic suggestion to relax and enter some sort of dissociative state pales in comparison with the level of demands patients undergo on a daily basis (Patterson, Adcock, & Bombardier, 1997; Sharar, Patterson, & Wiechman Askay, 2007). Unfortunately, most of the studies done with burn pain have not included research to determine if trauma hospitalization alters hypnotizability or at least receptivity to try hypnosis.

Labor Pain

Although labor pain may not be classified as the result of a medical procedure, it is unquestionably a source of acute pain. Women are increasingly opting for epidural-routed analgesia/anesthesia to manage delivery pain. Even with such effective pain control techniques, labor can be a painful event, and there is a potential role for hypnosis independent of whether epidurals are used (McCarthy, 2001). Early reports on the potential benefits were anecdotal or quasi-experimental designs (Flowers, Littlejohn, & Wells, 1960; Moya & James, 1960). Davidson (1962) actually published a controlled trial of hypnosis for labor pain, although this study did not include randomized assignment. After six sessions of hypnosis with posthypnotic suggestions, mothers reported shorter Stage I labor, more effective analgesia, less labor pain, and a more pleasant birth experience.

A subsequent study by Freeman, MacCaulay, Eve, Chamberlain, and Bhat (1986) compared 29 women who received hypnosis before labor with 36 who received standard care. The suggestions in hypnosis involved relaxation and transferring pain relief from the hand to the abdomen. Hypnosis did not seem to make a difference in this study; analgesic intake, reported pain relief, and mode of delivery did not differ between groups. In fact, the hypnosis group actually had longer delivery times. Patients were administered the Stanford Hypnotic Clinical Scale for Adults (Morgan & Hilgard, 1978/1979). Patients with good to moderate hypnotic suggestibility reported that hypnosis reduced their anxiety and helped them cope with labor. Again, however, the overall study did not demonstrate differences.

Despite this study, the preponderance of evidence for hypnosis with labor and delivery pain is positive. Harmon, Hynan, and Tyre (1990) divided 60 pregnant women into two groups on the basis of high or low hypnotizability scores. Half of the women were randomly assigned to a group that received hypnosis. The hypnosis group received a number of suggestions for relaxation and analgesia and were also provided with an audiotape of the induction for home use. In a particularly interesting twist, the women were given the opportunity to practice hypnotic skills on controlling ischemic pain during the sessions leading up to delivery. Parenthetically, women with higher hypnotizability scores reported lower ischemic pain scores that those with lower hypnotizability scores.

The women who received hypnosis were compared with a control group of women who listened to a commercial prebirth relaxation tape (which likely had some hypnotic suggestions in itself). In terms of results, the women assigned to the hypnosis group showed benefits across several variables; they had shorter Stage I labor, gave birth to children with higher Apgar scores, used less pain medication, and had a higher rate of spontaneous deliveries than did the control group of women. Ratings for labor pain on the McGill Pain Questionnaire (Melzack & Perry, 1975) were less than controls. Further, women with high hypnotizability scores showed less depression scores after birth than those with low scores. In general, all of the women randomized to the hypnosis group seemed to show some benefit, but those with high hypnotizability scores seemed to benefit relatively more.

With respect to anecdotal evidence as a supplement to the afore-mentioned trials, it might be useful to mention Patrick McCarthy's work. As a physician practicing in New Zealand, he reports using a hypnotic procedure for childbirth with over 600 women. His protocol is discussed in Barabasz and Watkins (2005). Further, a recent review by D. C. Brown and Hammond (2007) reiterated the benefits of hypnosis in preterm labor and delivery at term. However, they also reported risk factors, including prolonged pregnancy. Further, a meta-analysis performed by Cyna, McAuliffe, and Andrew (2004) showed less use of analgesia with hypnosis but also indicated a need for better designed trials.

Bone Marrow Aspiration Pain

Bone marrow aspiration involves the insertion of thick gauge needles into the lumbar section of the spinal cord to harvest marrow. In our review (Patterson & Jensen, 2003), we were able to find several studies that have shown positive findings of hypnosis with such procedures (Katz, Kellerman, & Ellenberg, 1987; Kuttner, 1988; Liossi & Hatira, 1999; Syrjala et al., 1992; Zeltzer & LeBaron, 1982). In one of the earlier studies, Zeltzer and LeBaron (1982) compared children receiving hypnosis with a control condition that included deep breathing and distraction. Thirty-three children ages 6 to 17 years were randomly assigned to one of these two conditions. The hypnosis interventions were unique to each child and involved such approaches as storytelling, fantasy, imagery, and deep breathing. Although both groups reported a reduction in pain, lower pain was reported in the hypnosis group, and those patients reported an anxiety reduction not seen in the controls. See Neron and Stephenson (2007) for a general review of hypnosis with cancer pain, emesis, and anxiety.

Katz et al. (1987) studied 36 children (ages 6 to 11 years) who required bone marrow aspirations for lymphoblastic leukemia. The patients were randomly assigned to a hypnosis group (imagery and suggestions for pain control and distraction) or a control group consisting of nondirected play for the time equivalent of hypnosis. Both groups showed decreases in ratings of pain and fear, and hypnosis was not found to be superior to the play control group.

Kuttner (1988) studied 25 children who also required bone marrow aspirations for the treatment of leukemia. Children ages 3 to 6 years were randomly assigned to groups that received standard care (information, reassurance, and support; $n = 8$), a distraction treatment (popup books, bubbles; $n = 8$), or a hypnotic intervention ($n = 9$). The hypnotic intervention used the child's favorite story to create imaginative involvement. The therapist was present to provide the two experimental treatments (hypnosis and distraction). A behavioral checklist completed by observers indicated that the hypnotic intervention had an impact on observed distress, pain, and anxiety; however, the effect was not found in self-reports from the children.

Liossi and Hatira (1999) investigated hypnosis with 30 children (ages 5 to 15 years) undergoing bone marrow aspirations. The researchers randomized children to groups that received hypnosis, cognitive–behavioral skills training, or standard treatment (lidocaine injections alone). Relative to baseline, children in the hypnosis and cognitive–behavioral skills group reported less pain and anxiety. The authors concluded that both treatments are effective, though children in the cognitive–behavioral group reported more anxiety and showed more behavioral distress than the hypnosis group. Hypnotizability measured by the Stanford Hypnotic Clinical Scale for Children (Morgan & Hilgard, 1978/1979) showed a strong association with outcome in the hypnosis group. Liossi, White, and Hatira (2009) obtained similar findings in a more recent, larger study comparing the efficacy of analgesic cream. What's more, they have also reported the effectiveness of a brief hypnosis intervention to control venepuncture-related pain in pediatric cancer patients (Liossi et al., 2009). Richardson and colleagues (J. Richardson, Smith, McCall, & Pilkington, 2006) provided a review for hypnosis for procedure-related pain and distress in pediatric cancer patients.

Invasive Procedures for Women's Health

Lang et al. (2006) conducted another prospective randomized trial to determine the impact of hypnosis on large core needle biopsies of the breast. Patients ($N = 236$) were assigned to groups that received hypnosis, standard empathic attention, or standard care. Hypnosis consisted of an induction with suggestions for sensory substitution for pain and, if needed, anxiety management. VAS ratings were taken every 10 minutes from pain and anxiety. As expected, pain ratings increased for all three groups as the procedure was initiated. However, scores increased more slowly for the hypnosis and empathic listening group. There was no difference between the hypnosis and empathic listening group.

Marc et al. (2008) investigated hypnosis for women undergoing voluntary termination of pregnancy. The authors randomized 30 women to groups receiving hypnosis or standard care. Hypnosis included suggestions for relaxation, comforting imagery, pain reduction, and abdominal numbness. The induction was provided prior to the procedure, and then patients were walked into the operating room, where suggestions for deepening the hypnotic state were again provided by the clinician performing hypnosis. Patients were given the option to request anything that would make them more comfortable, and such requests became the dependent (outcome) variable. Significantly fewer patients in the hypnosis group (36%) requested nitrous oxide than did the control group (87%). However, the two groups did not show a difference on self-reported pain intensity or unpleasantness.

Montgomery et al. (2007) performed a randomized study of patients who were scheduled to undergo excisional breast biopsy or lumpectomy. The study population consisted of 200 patients who were randomly assigned to either receive a 15-minute presurgery hypnosis session conducted or nondirective empathetic listening (attention control), both conducted by a psychologist. The results of this study showed that patients in treatment (hypnosis) group required less intraoperative anesthesia (propofol and lidocaine) than did patients in the control group. In addition to requiring less intraoperative anesthesia, patients in the hypnosis group also reported less pain intensity, pain unpleasantness, nausea, fatigue, discomfort, and emotional upset compared with those in the control group. A cost analysis also showed that patients in the hypnosis group cost the institution $772.71 less than patients in the control group, on average per patient. In a more recent study, Schnur et al. (2008) reported that hypnosis was also a good technique for controlled presurgical distress in women awaiting excisional breast biopsies. In short, the data support use of hypnosis with breast cancer surgery patients from both clinical and cost-effectiveness perspectives.

This group of investigators (Montgomery et al., in press) also examined the mediators of hypnotic benefits among breast surgery patients. This study revealed that hypnotic effects on postsurgical pain were partially mediated by pain expectancy but not by emotional distress. These data highlight the importance of expectancies as a mediator of hypnoanalgesic effects within clinical settings.

Montgomery, David, Winkel, Silverstein, and Bovbjerg's (2002) meta-analysis of published studies that used hypnosis with surgical patients should also be mentioned at this point. Their results indicated that patients in hypnosis treatment groups had better clinical outcomes than 89% of patients in control groups. Significant beneficial effects of hypnosis were demonstrated for pain, negative affect, pain medication use, physiological indicators, recovery from surgery, and treatment time. These data strongly support the use of hypnosis with a wide variety of surgical patient populations.

Chronic Pain Studies

In contrast to acute pain, chronic pain persists beyond the time needed for the lesion to heal or is associated with an ongoing degenerative or disease process. Chronic pain is often defined as having a 3- to 6-month duration (Chapman, Nakamura, & Flores, 1999). The location, pattern, and description of acute pain often reveals what is known about its cause (Gatchel & Epker, 1999), but chronic pain communicates little about the underlying disease process. Further, a number of factors that have little to do with the initial pain play a role in keeping it in place, such as patient cognitions, coping styles, and social and financial disincentives (Fordyce, 1976; Turk & Flor, 1999). Treatments that are known to be effective for acute pain, such as rest or opioid analgesics, may exacerbate rather than improve chronic pain (Fordyce, 1976).

Such distinctions between acute and chronic pain have important implications not only for how hypnosis is administered but also in terms of how outcome is measured in research. With acute pain, the intervention can focus on reducing or eliminating symptoms, and measurement can reflect how much pain reduction occurs during a given period. Chronic pain is a far more nebulous problem. Typically, chronic pain has been in place for so long that it is ingrained in the patient's perceptual experience; it is usually constantly present, but it can vary widely in intensity over a 24-hour period. Further, a number of complex factors can keep chronic pain in place beyond actual tissue damage. It is interesting that the outcome of success in chronic pain treatment may not even involve reductions of pain. A patient may return to work, increase functional activities, and report a greater satisfaction with life without reporting reductions in pain (Turk & Flor, 1999). Thus, in terms of treatment and conducting research, chronic pain is a different clinical entity.

Given these factors, it is not surprising that hypnosis has not fared as well in outcome with chronic pain as compared with acute pain. Indeed, early reviews on this topic were dismal with respect to outcome. Turner and Chapman (1982) rated the clinical research as "appallingly poor" at that time. Six years later, Malone and Strube (1988) performed a meta-analysis of nonmedical approaches to pain reduction. Out of 14 studies that used hypnosis, only one had enough information to be included in the meta-analysis. The mean pain reduction in this study was only 13%, which was far less than the average improvement rate reported by other nonmedical studies reviewed by Malone and Strube.

Fortunately, this situation has improved dramatically over the past 20 years. A review by Patterson and Jensen (2003) found 12 studies on hypnosis that used solid randomized controlled designs, and there have been a few additional studies reported since that time (see Table 3.2). The types of pain that have been reported in the literature include that from headaches, cancer, fibromyalgia, spinal cord injuries, and mixed etiologies.

Headaches

In terms of chronic pain, there are far more studies on the application of hypnosis on headaches than any other etiologies. In many of these studies, hypnosis is compared with relaxation, biofeedback, or autogenic training condition. Andreychuck and Skriver (1975) compared hypnosis with biofeedback training in 33 patients with migraine headaches. Biofeedback training lasted 10 weeks and included alpha enhancement and hand warming. Hypnosis

TABLE 3.2
Controlled Studies in Chronic Pain Hypnotic Treatment

Study (type of chronic pain problem)	Hypnotizability assessed?	N	Randomized?	Control condition(s)	Adult or child?	Follow-up	Outcome dimensions	Findings
Spiegel and Bloom (1983); cancer-related pain	No	54	Yes	Standard care (SC) Support group without hypnosis (SG)	Adult	None	Patient-rated pain intensity	H > SG > SC
Haanen et al. (1991); fibromyalgia (FM) pain	No	40	Yes	Physical therapy (PT)	Adult	3 months	Morning stiffness	H = PT
							Muscle pain	H > PT
							Fatigue	H > PT
							Sleep disturbance	H > PT
							Self-reported global assessment of outcome	H > PT
							Physician reported global assessment of outcome	H = PT
							FM point tenderness	H = PT
							Symptoms (HSCL-90)	H > PT
Anderson et al. (1975); headache	No	47	Yes	Meds (Prochlorperazine) (M)	Adult	None	Number of headaches	H > M
							Number of Grade 4 headaches	H > M
							Frequency of being headache free	H > M
Andreychuk and Skriver (1975); headache	Yes (Hypnotic Induction Profile)	33	Yes	Hand temp biofeedback (HTB) Alpha enhancement biofeedback (AEB)	Adult	None	Headache Index (product of headache duration × headache severity)	H = HTB = AEB

(continues)

TABLE 3.2

Controlled Studies in Chronic Pain Hypnotic Treatment *(Continued)*

Study (type of chronic pain problem)	Hypnotiz-ability assessed?	N	Randomized?	Control condition(s)	Adult or child?	Follow-up	Outcome dimensions	Findings
Schlutter et al. (1980); headache	No	48	Yes	Biofeedback (BF) Biofeedback + relaxation (BFR)	Adult	10–14 weeks	Number of headache hours per week Pain intensity Pain intensity during submaximum effort tourniquet technique	H = BF = BFR H = BF = BFR H = BF = BFR
Friedman and Taub (1984); headache	Yes (Stanford Hypnotic Susceptibility Scale, Form A)	66	No	Hypnosis without thermal suggestion (H) Hypnosis with thermal suggestion (HT) Biofeedback (BF) Relaxation (R) Wait-list (WL)	Adult	1 year	Highest headache intensity Number of headaches Medication use	(H = HT = BF = R) > WL (H = HT = BF = R) > WL (H = HT = BF => WL
Melis et al. (1991); headache	Yes, but used for descriptive purposes only (Stanford Hypnotic Clinical Scale)	26	Yes	Wait-list (WL)	Adult	4 weeks	Number of headache days per week Number of headache hours per week Headache intensity	H > WL H > WL H > WL

Study; pain type	Hypnotizability assessed	N	Randomized	Conditions	Age	Follow-up	Outcome measures	Results
Spinhoven et al. (1992); headache	Yes, but only used for description purposes (Stanford Hypnotic Clinical Scale)	56	Yes	Autogenic training (AT) / Baseline control (BC)	Adult	6 months	Headache intensity / Psychological distress (CSQ) / Headache relief	(H = AT) > BC / (H = AT) > BC / (H = AT) > BC
Zitman et al. (1992); headache	No	79	Yes	Autogenic training (AT) / Hypnosis not presented as hypnosis (HN)	Adult	6 months	Headache intensity / Headache relief / Medication use / Anxiety (STAI) / Depression (SDS)	H > AT, H = HN, HN = AT / H = HN = AT / H = HN = AT / H = HN = AT / H = HN = AT
ter Kuile et al. (1994); headache	Yes (Stanford Hypnotic Clinical Scale)	146	Yes	Wait-list (WL) / Autogenic training (AT)	Adult	6 months	Headache index (intensity and duration) / Medicine use / Psychological distress (SCL-90)	(H=AT) > WL / H = AT = WL / H = AT = WL
Melzack and Perry (1975); various chronic pain problems including back, nerve injury, cancer-related, and arthritis pain	No	24	Yes	Alpha feedback alone (A) / Hypnosis alone (H) / Hypnosis + alpha feedback (HA)	Adult	4–6 months	Sensory pain (MPQ) / Affective pain (MPQ) / Pain severity (MPQ)	HA > (H = A) / HA > (H = A) / HA > (H = A)
Edelson and Fitzpatrick (1989); various chronic pain problems	No	27	No	Cognitive–behavioral therapy (CBT) / Attention control (AC)	Adult	1 month	Walking / Sitting / Reclining / Pain intensity (MPQ) / Pain severity (MPQ)	CBT > (H = AC) / CBT > (H = AC) / H = CBT = AC / H = CBT = AC / H > AC, H = CBT, CBT = AC

(continues)

TABLE 3.2
Controlled Studies in Chronic Pain Hypnotic Treatment *(Continued)*

Study (type of chronic pain problem)	Hypnotiz-ability assessed?	N	Randomized?	Control condition(s)	Adult or child?	Follow-up	Outcome dimensions	Findings
M. P. Jensen et al (2005); chronic pain from disability	Yes	33	Yes		Adult	3 months	Average pain intensity	Decreased with H ($p <$ .05), maintained at 3 months
							Pain unpleasantness	Decreased with H ($p <$ .05), maintained at 3 months
							Pain interference	Decreased with H ($p <$ .01), maintained at 3 months
							Depressive symptoms	No change
							Perceived control over pain	Decreased with H ($p <$ .05), maintained at 3 months

Study; disorder		N		Control	Population	Follow-up	Outcome measure	Results
Roberts et al. (2006); irritable bowel syndrome (IBS)	No	81	Yes	Standard care (SC)	Adult	3, 6, 12 months	IBS specific quality of life	H > SC at 6 months H = SC at 3 and 12 months
							IBS symptom score	H > SC for improvement of pain, diarrhea, at 3 months H = SC at 6 and 12 months
							Self-reported resource utilization	H > SC for decreased use of prescription drugs over 12 months

Note. H = hypnosis alone; HCL-90 = Hopkins Symptom Checklist–90; CSQ = Coping Strategy Questionnaire; STAI = State–Trait Anxiety Inventory; SDS = Self-Rating Depression Scale; SCL-90 = Symptom Checklist–90; MPQ = McGill Pain Questionnaire. Adapted from "Hypnosis and Clinical Pain Control," by D. R. Patterson and M. Jensen, 2003, *Psychological Bulletin, 129,* 508–509. Copyright 2003 American Psychological Association.

included suggestions, visual imagery, verbal reinforcers, and suggestions for relaxation and pain reduction. Hypnosis was provided on audiotapes, and patients were asked to listen to them twice daily. Patients in the biofeedback condition were also instructed to listen to relaxation tapes twice daily. Outcome was measured by the Headache Index (daily headache duration and severity). The Hypnotic Induction Profile (Spiegel & Bridger, 1970) was used. Both groups (all patients) showed reductions in headache pain; however, patients with higher hypnotizability scores showed greater pain reduction than those with low scores. It is interesting to note that this was independent of treatment condition.

Anderson, Basker, and Dalton (1975) compared hypnosis with medications (prochlorperazine) in another randomized trial for migraine headache pain. The hypnosis condition involved six or more sessions over the course of a year. Patients were asked to practice audio-hypnosis daily. Hypnosis included suggestions for relaxations, ego strengthening, decreased tension, and aversion of migraine attacks. Compared with the group that received medication, patients in the hypnotherapy group showed fewer headaches per month, fewer Grade 4 headaches, and a higher reported frequency of remission.

In a study by Schlutter, Golden, and Blume (1980), the comparison group conditions were electromyography (EMG), biofeedback alone, or EMG plus progressive relaxation. Forty-eight patients were randomly assigned to one of these conditions or hypnosis. Hypnosis treatment consisted of four 1-hour sessions over 4 weeks and included an eye-fixation induction and hypnotic suggestions for relaxation, analgesia, or numbness and visualization of an enjoyable experience (Greene & Reyher, 1972). Outcome was measured by the number of headache hours per week and average headache pain. Patients in all three conditions showed reductions in headaches, but there were no differences between groups.

As is the case with several studies on hypnotic treatment of headache pain, Friedman and Taub (1984) also failed to find differences between hypnosis and other treatment approaches in a study of 66 patients with migraines. In their study, they compared hypnosis with a thermal biofeedback condition, relaxation training, and hypnosis with thermal imagining. Again, all groups showed improvement, this time as measured by headache ratings and medication use, relative to wait-list controls. Hypnotizability was measured by the Stanford Hypnotic Susceptibility Scale, Form A (Weitzenhoffer & Hilgard, 1959). In a similar finding to Andreychuk and Skriver (1975), patients with high scores, compared with those with low scores, showed meaningful decrements on outcome variables (at 1-year follow-up) independent of treatment conditions.

Melis, Rooimans, Spierings, and Hoogduin (1991) did 4 weeks of baseline on 26 patients with chronic headaches. They then randomly assigned them either to four weekly hypnosis sessions or a wait-list control group. The hypnotic suggestion involved having patients express and change headaches as a visual image, as well as imagining the pain moving to a different area of the body. The treatment group reported significantly more improvement as measured by number and duration of headaches. The Stanford Hypnotic Clinical Scale failed to demonstrate that hypnotizability played any role in outcome.

Spinhoven and his colleagues are perhaps the most active team studying hypnosis for headaches. In one of their earlier studies (Spinhoven, Linssen, Van Dyck, & Zitman, 1992), they examined 56 patients in a within-subject, randomized design that compared hypnosis with autogenic training. The hypnosis conditions used suggestions for hand heaviness and warming and coolness on the forehead. Both hypnosis and autogenic training were reported to diminish average pain intensity, decrease psychological distress, and improve headache relief in comparison with a wait-list control group (Spinhoven et al., 1992). Ter Kuile et al. (1994) obtained similar findings in a larger study with 146 patients; hypnosis and autogenic training decreased both headache duration and intensity compared with a wait-list control. Hypnotizability was measured by the Stanford Hypnotic Clinical Scale for Adults. Similar to two of the other studies mentioned, patients with high hypnotizability scores showed greater effects at posttreatment and follow-up compared with low scorers, independent of treatment condition.

One of the more interesting studies by Zitman, Van Dyck, Spinhoven, and Linssen (1992) randomly assigned 79 patients to either autogenic training or future-oriented hypnotic imagery (FI). FI was not labeled as hypnosis, a practice that always engenders definitional problems in the research. In any case, the FI condition had patients imagine themselves in a future scenario where pain had been largely eliminated. Six months later, all patients who received autogenic training or FI in the first phase were offered FI hypnosis again, only this time it was "openly presented as hypnotic technique" (Zitman et al., 1992, p. 221). In terms of reducing Headache Index scores, all approaches appeared to be equally effective. However, at 6-month follow-up, the group that had FI labeled as hypnosis showed statistically greater pain relief than did the attention control groups. It was not clear whether patients in this group showed improvement because they received twice as many sessions or whether it was a matter of treatment being labeled as hypnosis.

Spinhoven provided an early review in 1988 and concluded that hypnotic treatments for headache do not differ significantly from autogenic training or relaxation training. The studies that his group subsequently performed certainly appeared consistent with this premise. Holroyd and Penzien (1990) reached similar conclusions, and Holroyd has also done extensive research in this area. There are a number of factors to consider about such conclusions. First, headaches are one of the tougher etiologies of pain to treat. They have a fairly consistent nociceptive element, and although stress and tension certainly play a role, there is much less of an operant component to headaches. Such pain is often refractory to any type of treatment. Any type of psychological intervention will likely require discipline and practice; the potential for a few sessions of any psychological interventions eliminating headaches is rare. Second, this literature brings to the fore that the distinction between hypnosis and deep relaxation can often become blurred. Hypnosis often includes elements of deep relaxation, and it is never clear whether at least some of the statements in deep relaxation constitute hypnotic suggestion.

One of the interesting findings that have come out of the hypnosis-headache research is that hypnotizability predicts outcome regardless of treatment condition. This was the case in at least three of the studies reviewed (Andreychuk & Skriver, 1975; Friedman & Taub, 1984; ter Kuile et al., 1994). In Hilgard's early work (Hilgard & Hilgard, 1975), there was a clear interaction between hypnotizability and treatment; those who score high appear to benefit from hypnosis, whereas those who score low do not. Patterson and colleagues (Patterson, Hoffman, Palacios, & Jensen, 2006) have demonstrated similar findings with hypnosis and virtual reality; all subjects seemed to benefit from virtual reality distraction, whereas only subjects high in hypnotizability seemed to benefit from hypnosis (or combined treatments). This line of research on hypnotizability suggests that if patients with high hypnotizability scores respond well to both autogenic training for relaxation and hypnosis, then there is indeed a hypnotic component to such treatments. As mentioned, some (e.g., Edmonston, 1991) have argued that there is no difference between hypnosis and deep relaxation. In general, Hammond (2007) reviewed the efficacy of clinical hypnosis with headaches and reported it to be a well-established and efficacious treatment, virtually free of side effects or adverse reactions.

Cancer

Spiegel and Bloom (1983) studied 54 women with chronic pain from breast cancer, which can have an acute element related to invasive procedures or spikes in pain. The women were assigned to a usual treatment condition ($n = 24$) or to a group that also received weekly group therapy for 12 months ($n = 30$). The women who received group therapy, in turn, were assigned to groups that received or did not receive 5 to 10 minutes of self-hypnosis at the end of sessions. The hypnotic treatment was based on that published by Spiegel and Spiegel (1978). Although the women in both support groups showed improvements over controls, those who received hypnosis showed greater improvement over those who did not.

Elkins, Marcus, Palamara, and Stearns (2004) also studied chronic pain from cancer. The investigators conducted a prospective randomized study of 39 advanced-stage (III or IV) patients with malignant bone cancer. The hypnosis consisted of at least four weekly sessions and included suggestions for relaxation, comfort, mental imagery, dissociation, and pain control. The hypnosis followed a transcript, and patients were provided with an audiotape and were instructed in home practice. The control group received weekly sessions of supportive attention. The hypnosis group showed an overall significant decrease in pain, and the mean-rated effectiveness of the self-hypnosis practices was 6.5 on a 10-point scale.

Fibromyalgia

Fibromyalgia is a syndrome that involves chronic pain as well as a series of other symptoms, usually ongoing fatigue. Haanen et al. (1991) randomly assigned patients with refractory fibromyalgia to either eight sessions of hypnotherapy or 12 to 24 sessions of physical therapy that included massage and muscle relaxation training. The hypnotherapy group received 1-hour sessions, supplemented by audiotapes, over a 3-month period. Patients who received hypnosis showed improvements compared with the physical therapy group on measures of muscle pain, fatigue, sleep quality, and overall outcome and distress scores. Such differences were maintained at follow-up assessment. Although the time spent in the two treatment conditions was different and the study did not include a no-treatment control group, this study was significant for a number of reasons. This was the first randomized controlled trial on fibromyalgia, a complex type of chronic pain to treat that is growing in prevalence (Goldenberg, Burckhardt, & Crofford, 2004). Further, physical therapy is a compelling form of treatment, and it is notable that hypnosis actually showed greater improvement compared with what would likely be the treatment of choice. It would be interesting to see a study on the combined effects of hypnosis and physical therapy for a variety of chronic pain conditions, including from fibromyalgia.

In a second study with fibromyalgia, Castel, Perez, Sala, Padrol, and Rull (2007) randomly assigned 45 patients to one of three groups. One group received hypnosis with suggestions for analgesia, and the intervention was labeled as hypnosis. The other two groups received relaxation interventions; however, in one of the groups, the intervention was labeled as hypnosis, and the other was presented as relaxation training. As such, the authors were interested on whether the label of hypnosis had an impact on pain reduction. Pain was assessed using the Spanish adaptation (Lazaro, Bosch, Torrubia, & Banos, 1994) of the McGill Pain Questionnaire (MPQ; Melzack, 1975) as well as the VAS.

Treatment consisted of one 20-minute session. Hypnotic suggestions included imagining a blue analgesic stream fill into the painful area, and relaxation suggestions involved visualizing a pleasant beach. The authors used only the Pain Rating Index Summary and the Pain Rating Index Affective from the MPQ to determine if the treatment interventions would differentially influence sensory and affective components of pain. Patients who received hypnotic suggestions for pain reduction showed greater reductions in pain intensity and sensory components than did either of the other two (relaxation) groups. Whether patients showed relaxation labeled as hypnosis or relaxation alone did not appear to have a significant reduction in pain. No differences were found among the three groups on affective dimensions of pain. It should be pointed out that with a clinical problem like fibromyalgia, a 20-minute intervention should be considered more as an experimental manipulation than a form of treatment.

Mixed Chronic Pain

Melzack and Perry (1975) examined hypnosis and alpha biofeedback in 24 patients with a variety of chronic pain problems (back pain, peripheral nerve injury, arthritis, amputation, and "head" pain). Patients were randomly assigned to one of three groups. The first received 6 to 12 sessions of hypnosis plus alpha training ($n = 12$), the second received hypnosis alone ($n = 6$), and the final group received alpha training alone ($n = 6$). Alpha training alone did not seem to reduce pain. Hypnosis had a nonsignificant impact. However, the combination of hypnosis and alpha training had a significant impact on pain reduction as measured by the MPQ (Melzack & Perry, 1975). For example, 58% of the patients reported pain reductions of 33% or greater. As the authors acknowledged, the study design suffered from the lack of no-treatment and placebo-control groups. At the same time, it is remarkable that there have not been more investigations of the compelling combination of hypnosis and biofeedback.

In another study on mixed chronic pain, Edelson and Fitzpatrick (1989) randomly assigned 27 patients to four 1-hour sessions of hypnosis, cognitive–behavioral treatment, or attention control (supportive, non-directive discussions). Back pain was the most frequent type of pain in the patient sample, although there were mixed etiologies. The hypnosis group showed improvements in subjective pain ratings as measured by the MPQ, whereas the cognitive–behavioral group showed increases in walking and decreases in sitting time.

Low Back Pain

McCauley and colleagues (McCauley, Thelen, Frank, Willard, & Callen, 1983) assigned outpatients to either self-hypnosis ($n = 9$) or relaxation ($n = 8$). After a 1-week baseline period, patients experienced 8 weeks of weekly treatment with one of the two conditions. They were assessed 1 week and then 3 months after treatment. Significant reductions in both groups on the MPQ were reported by both groups. Although the hypnosis group reported 25% to 30% improvement on the pain measures at 3-month follow-up, both interventions seemed to reduce pain, with neither superior to the other.

Spinhoven and Linssen (1989) used a crossover study design to compare self-hypnosis with an education program for 45 patients with chronic low back pain. Patients were assigned to one of the two treatments for 2 months, followed by 2 months of no treatment. They received the other treatment (crossover) and then another 2 months of no-treatment follow-up. Outcome was measured by a diary that included pain intensity, "up" time, and use of pain medication. The Symptom Checklist–90 was used to assess distress and depression. The hypnosis treatment included suggestions for relaxation, imaginative inattention, future-oriented imagery, and pain displacement. Patients were instructed in self-hypnosis and given an audiotape at the fifth session. The education condition included lectures and facilitated discussion designed to enhance pain control. Twenty-four patients completed the entire study protocol (several dropped out). Patients, independent of treatment condition, showed improvement from pretreatment to 2-month follow-up, except for pain intensity. This seemingly surprising finding is actually consistent with some reviews in the chronic pain literature; patients do not necessarily have to report less pain for treatment to be a success. If patients are able to report improved function and quality of life, then whether or not they report less pain may not be important (Turk, 1996; Turk & Flor, 1999; Turk & Okifuji, 1998a, 1998b).

Arthritis

Gay, Philippot, and Luminet (2002) randomly assigned 36 patients with osteoarthritis pain to hypnosis, relaxation training, or a no-treatment/standard-care control condition. Hypnosis treatment consisted of eight weekly sessions and included standard relaxation, with suggestions for positive imagery as well as childhood memories of good joint mobility. Standard control patients were asked to provide assessment and then were offered the hypnosis treatment. The patients in the hypnosis group showed significant pain reduction at 4 weeks, compared with no-treatment controls, and this was maintained at 3- and 6-month follow-up. However, similar to many of the studies with headache pain, the scores of the hypnosis and relaxation group patients did not differ statistically.

Temporomandibular Pain

Simon and Lewis (2000) conducted a noncontrolled clinical trial on hypnosis for temporomandibular pain in 28 patients. Pain intensity, duration, and frequency were measured during wait-list, before treatment, after treatment, and at 6-month follow-up. The intervention included education about hypnosis, an eye closure induction, metaphors and suggestions for relaxation, analgesia, and anesthesia. Patients were provided audiotapes and were instructed to practice self-hypnosis daily. Hypnosis resulted in significant reductions of pain frequency and duration, as well as increases in daily function. The authors reported that treatment gains were maintained at 6-month follow-ups.

Winocur and colleagues (Winocur, Gavish, Emodi-Perlman, Halachmi, & Eli, 2002) treated patients with temporomandibular pain with what they referred to as "hypnorelaxation" (presumably hypnosis). They randomly assigned 40 patients to groups that received hypnosis ($n = 15$) or education/advice ($n = 10$). The hypnosis intervention emphasized progressive relaxation in general and suggestions for relaxation of facial muscles. Patients in the education/advice condition were provided with information about how best to manage their pain. VAS scores of current and worst pain were taken before and after treatment. Hypnosis and occlusion appliances were both more effective than the education/advice condition in alleviating sensitivity to palpitation. Only hypnosis patients, however, reported significantly greater decreases in current and worst pain.

Sickle Cell Disease

The various reviews have been able to find only one study on the use of hypnosis for sickle cell disease (SCD). Although this study did not use a randomized controlled design, it did use a careful pre/post design. Dinges et al. (1997) conducted a 2-year study of 37 adults and children who were experiencing vaso-occlusive pain from SCD. Patients were asked to complete daily pain diaries for 4 months of baseline and then 18 months of treatment. Treatment was a cognitive–behavioral intervention that centered on self-hypnosis. Hypnosis included ideomotor suggestions (hands moving together or rising), development of metaphors, and self-suggestions for pain management. The investigators reported that hypnosis resulted in a significant decrease of pain days. Significant baseline versus treatment phase differences were also reported on the percentage of days for which pain was characterized as non-SCD pain, as well as "bad sleep nights." However, such medication or sleep differences were not reported for SCD pain days. The authors contended that hypnosis was particularly helpful in reducing less severe episodes of pain.

Disability-Related Pain

M. P. Jensen et al. (2005) investigated the effects of hypnosis on chronic pain from disability in a case series. Thirty-three patients received 10 sessions of standardized (script-driven) hypnotic analgesia, pain intensity, and unpleasantness, depression, and perceived control over pain. Measurement was taken before and after a baseline period, after treatment, and at 3-month follow-up. Hypnosis included suggestions for alteration of pain, including relaxation, imagined analgesia, reduced pain unpleasantness, and replacement with nonpainful sensations. Although suggestions were given for self-practice, patients were not given audiotapes prior to the 3-month follow-up. Results indicated posttreatment improvement in pain intensity, unpleasantness, and perceived control relative to baseline. Improvements were not observed in depression ratings. Improvement was maintained at 3-month follow-up. Neither hypnotizability nor treatment concentration was associated with outcome. Cognitive expectancies assessed after the first session showed a moderate association with pain reduction.

In another study of disability-related pain, M. P. Jensen, Barber, Romano, Hanley, et al. (2009) randomized 22 patients with multiple sclerosis to either 10 sessions of self-hypnosis training or progressive muscle relaxation (PMR). The hypnosis intervention was a modified version of the protocol reported by M. P. Jensen et al. (2005). The intervention consisted largely of inviting patients to be in a "special place" of their choosing, experiencing classic (nonanalgesic) phenomena such as ideomotor movement, and altering the number and content of analgesic suggestions. In terms of hypnotic analgesic suggestions, patients experienced five types of these over the first two sessions. The clinician then used two of these suggestions for the remaining eight sessions of "live" hypnosis. Patients were given CDs of the first two sessions and were encouraged to listen to them daily for the remainder of the study period.

The PMR condition was designed after what M. P. Jensen and Patterson (2005) described as a minimally effective control condition. In other words, the PMR patients received a treatment that controlled for therapist time, attention, and patient expectancy. Further, this intervention came as close to actual hypnosis as possible without having all of the components of hypnosis (e.g., suggestions for pain control). Patients in the hypnosis group reported significant pre/post ratings of pain intensity as well as pain interference (Pain Interference Scale from the Brief Pain Inventory; Cleeland & Ryan, 1994; Daut, Cleeland, & Flanery, 1983) relative to the PMR controls. These gains were maintained at 3-month follow-up. Hypnotizability was not related to outcome. However, while treatment expectancy did not differ between two groups, it was related to outcome in the hypnosis group.

As a brief final note about hypnosis for disability pain, a recent publication by Slack et al. (2009) might be mentioned. EMG is a common procedure to test nerve conduction in patients experiencing neurological and other disability-related medical disorders. In a small, randomized study, the authors were able to find some minor success in reducing pain and anxiety among adults undergoing needle EMG. This suggests a potential application of hypnosis for patients with disability undergoing rehabilitation medical care.

Irritable Bowel Syndrome and Abdominal Pain

Many excellent studies have been done on hypnosis for irritable bowel syndrome, or IBS (Covino, 2008; Gholamrezaei, Ardestani, & Emami, 2006; Palsson, Turner, Johnson, Burnelt, & Whitehead, 2002; Whorwell, Prior, & Colgan, 1987; Whorwell, Prior, & Faragher, 1984). The following two studies are included as examples of ones that included pain as an outcome.

Simren, Ringstrom, Bjornsson, and Abrahamsson (2004) studied 28 patients who were described as being refractory to standard treatment for IBS. Patients were randomized to conditions in which they received either 12 one-hour sessions of "gut-directed" hypnosis or a wait-list control condition. The control group received supportive therapy from a dietician, a physical therapist, a gastroenterologist, and a study nurse who made telephone support available. Hypnosis involved progressive relaxation and suggestions aimed at restoring normal gastrointestinal (GI) function. For example, patients might receive imagery of a blocked river that is cleared by the patient and then flows smoothly. GI response was measured through a barostat procedure. A balloon on a flexible scope was expanded to provide readings at baseline and postadministration of a lipid solution. The hypnosis group, after administration of the lipid solution, demonstrated increased tolerance for gas and discomfort, but not pain. The control group demonstrated a decreased threshold for all three variables. The hypnosis treatment group also showed decrease colonic tone response compared with controls during lipid infusion.

Roberts and colleagues (Roberts, Wilson, Singh, Roalfe, & Greenfield, 2006) used a randomized controlled design to compare hypnosis with standard care for the treatment of IBS. Eighty-one patients were randomized to a condition in which they received five sessions of "gut-directed" hypnosis in addition to standard care or received standard care alone. Hypnosis consisted of 30-minute sessions with a standard induction and deepening. Suggestions were tailored to each patient's difficulties with IBS, such as constipation or pain. Hypnosis patients were given a CD at the first session and were encouraged to practice. Patient ratings of pain, constipation, diarrhea, and quality of life were taken at baseline and 3, 6, and 12 months postrandomization. At 3 months, the hypnosis group showed lower ratings of pain than the control group. However, both groups showed significant decreases in pain at 12 months. Patients in the hypnosis group reported that they were significantly less likely to require medication at 12 months.

Noncardiac Chest Pain

Jones and colleagues (Jones, Cooper, Miller, Brooks, & Whorwell, 2006) randomly assigned 15 patients to receive 12 sessions of hypnosis and 13 patients to receive 12 sessions of supportive therapy and placebo medication, both over a 17-week period. Hypnosis involved standard eye closure, progressive relaxation, and deepening techniques. Patients were given hypnotic suggestions for pain reduction, health improvement, and what the authors described as "chest-focused" suggestions. Daily practice was encouraged with a CD that was provided. The hypnosis group showed an 80% improvement in global chest pain, as compared with 23% in the control group, a large effect that was statistically significant. However, ratings of pain severity, while less in the hypnosis group, did not differ significantly between the two groups. Patients in the hypnosis group decreased their use of pain medications, whereas this actually increased in the control group.

CLINICAL AND RESEARCH IMPLICATIONS

Several conclusions can be drawn from this body of research with respect to clinical treatment as well as future research in the area. In general, it is clear that a large number of studies reported in this chapter—most of them randomized clinical trials—are encouraging about the potential for treating clinical pain with hypnosis. In over 40 studies, hypnosis has been shown to have treatment effects superior to standard treatment, placebo, or some type of minimal treatment control. Further, in the majority of studies in which hypnosis is compared against another form of treatment for acute pain, hypnotic interventions have demonstrated superior effects. Despite this encouraging trend of results, there are a number of shortcomings to almost all of the controlled trials, and it is worthwhile to discuss how such research can be improved. In addition, it will be helpful to discuss some of the common findings that can apply to clinical practice.

Hypnotizability and Pain Control

The association between hypnotizability as measured by scales and reduction of laboratory pain in relation to this variable has been long established (Freeman, Barabasz, Barabasz, & Warner, 2000; Hilgard, 1969; Hilgard & Hilgard, 1975; Hilgard & Morgan, 1975; Knox, Morgan, & Hilgard, 1974; M. F. Miller, Barabasz, & Barabasz, 1991). This is one of the more frequently reported findings in the experimental literature, although it is not a universal finding among all of those completed. Subjects with high hypnotizability scores generally report less pain from such sources as tourniquet, electrical stimulation, thermal, or ice water. The role of hypnotizability in pain control is one of the more convincing lines of evidence that hypnosis is far more than a placebo effect (Frischholz, 2007).

Until recently, there was not the same clarity of findings with respect to the relationship between hypnotizability and clinical pain (Patterson & Ptacek, 1997). Gillett and Coe (1984) reported no differences between response to pain in dental patients based on their hypnotizability. In the review of randomized controlled studies presented earlier, eight studies examined the association between hypnotizability and clinical pain relief in samples of patients. The majority of these studies have demonstrated a positive association between hypnotizability and at least one outcome measure of pain (Andreychuk & Skriver, 1975; Freeman et al., 1986; Friedman & Taub, 1984; Harmon et al., 1990; Lang et al., 1996; Liossi & Hatira, 1999; ter Kuile et al., 1994). The preponderance of current evidence is that hypnotizability is an influential variable in clinical as well as experimental pain reduction.

An interesting associated finding is that patients in nonhypnotic treatment groups for pain often report greater pain reduction when they show higher hypnotizability scores (Andreychuk & Skriver, 1975; Friedman & Taub, 1984; ter Kuile et al., 1994). It is difficult to determine whether this suggests that patients with high hypnotizability scores may be more receptive to psychological interventions for pain, or whether some of the "nonhypnotic" treatments actually have components of hypnosis. This is certainly the case with relaxation training; no investigator can clearly establish that relaxation training does not contain at lease some components of hypnosis. However, none of this diminishes the strong association between hypnotic treatments themselves and hypnotizability. Along these lines, Appel and Bleiberg (2005) reported that hypnotizability is related to pain reduction but not relaxation (Milling, 2008).

This is not to suggest that patients with high levels of hypnotizability are the only ones who can benefit from hypnotic interventions. Montgomery, DuHamel, and Redd (2000) demonstrated that although patients with high scores show the greatest benefit from hypnosis, the majority of individuals studied (a reported 75%) will show some benefit. Milling (2008) provided a review on the relationship of hypnotizability to pain relief; patients with moderated levels also show clinical improvement. The findings might be better interpreted as suggesting that patients with very low hypnotizability scores may not benefit from hypnosis, at least initially. There are two ways to consider this relationship.

First, if a patient is very low on measured hypnotizability, it might be the most parsimonious use of the clinician's and patient's time to pursue a treatment other than hypnosis. Hypnosis is not for every patient, and this can provide some useful guidance for who may not be a good treatment candidate. However, if one takes the view that there are multiple theories of hypnosis, and each that can apply to different patient circumstances, then it may be useful to consider whether more can be done with low hypnotizable patients. More specifically, in both sociocognitive and Ericksonian approaches, the role of hypnotizability is considered much less important. This is not to suggest that it will be easy to perform a hypnotic intervention on a low hypnotizable patient if an Ericksonian approach is used. However, the Ericksonian approach does provide a model of approaching patient care in which the interaction between the clinician and patient may be able mitigate such trait characteristics of the patient (see Chapter 4, this volume).

The second main consideration with patients with low hypnotizability is that there is some evidence that hypnotizability can be improved with training (Holroyd, 1996). Barabasz (1982) reported that restricted environmental simulation (REST) can increase both hypnotizability scores and experimental pain stimulation. Further, Barabasz and Barabasz (1989) reported that a sample of people with chronic pain were able to increase their scores on the Stanford Hypnotic Susceptibility Scale, as well as tolerance to ischemic pain, following REST.

The Challenge of Control Groups

A substantial challenge in clinical studies of any nature is to control for nonspecific effects. Often the literature discusses the placebo effect as accounting for improvement that can be attributed directly to the treatment. A more specific variable that has been championed by Kirsch and Lynn (1995) is expectancy. There are actually a number of effects that can potentially account for improvement in patients after hypnosis or psychotherapy in general. Kazdin (1979) recommended the term *nonspecific effects* to capture those effects that are common to all treatments but not specific to the treatment being examined. With hypnosis, it is particularly challenging to control for all of the potential nonspecific effects.

One vexing problem in this respect is that there is not universal agreement on how hypnosis should be defined. For example, an immediate assumption may be that hypnosis involves relaxation, and some argue that hypnosis is essentially deep relaxation (see Lynn & Rhue, 1991). However, Wark (1996, 2006) and others (e.g., Banyai & Hilgard, 1976) have long taught the concept of *alert hypnosis* that is performed with the subject's eyes opened in an awake state. Similarly, there is the question of the need for an induction. Chaves (1993) and others have argued that an induction is not necessary for suggestions to be effective for pain reduction. In other words, several have argued that all that is needed for hypnosis to be effective are the suggestions.

Further, hypnosis is often described and even defined as being an inter-personal process. Yet we know that subjects can be hypnotized by listening to an audiotape. In any case, it is difficult to determine the elements that should be controlled. Barnier and Nash (2008) provided an excellent discussion of the issues associated with defining hypnosis.

Even more potentially problematic is that elements of the control group might be hypnotic in nature. The most obvious illustration of this is deep relaxation. When subjects receive deep relaxation, it becomes impossible to establish that they are not hypnotized. This might be why studies that compare hypnosis and deep relaxation for headaches do not generally differ in their effects, and why patients with high hypnotizability show better pain reduction with relaxation training than those who score low on this variable. M. P. Jensen and Patterson (2006) offered the concept of minimally effective control groups to address this issue. Examples might include providing biofeedback without actually offering suggestions for relaxation or providing hypnotic inductions without suggestions for comfort or analgesia. The authors pointed out that the minimal-treatment control groups have the potential ethical issue of being offered treatment that is suspected of being less effective. This issue can be addressed by offering full treatment to the patient at the end of the experimental trial.

Practice Effects and Number of Sessions

One apparent finding from reviewing the controlled studies done on clinical hypnotic analgesia is that researchers know little about the number of sessions needed to create clinical effects with patients. Various studies discuss treatment length ranging from 20 minutes to 1.5 hours. The number of sessions may vary from one or two sessions to multiple sessions occurring over weeks or months. Some investigators provide audiotapes for patients, others do not. Similarly, studies vary on whether patients are instructed to practice on their own.

It is fairly clear that acute pain can be treated with fewer and shorter sessions than chronic pain but that increased practice also benefits patients with acute pain. Chronic pain can rarely be addressed with limited sessions. Most investigators did not even consider the prospect of treating chronic pain without multiple sessions.

Determining how many sessions of hypnosis and how much practice is necessary to treat clinical pain remains a difficult empirical (not to mention clinical) challenge. One reason for this is individual differences in patients. Patients high in hypnotizability may require far fewer sessions and practice than patients who are low in such abilities. At this point, the hypnosis literature has only progressed to the point at which there are finally sufficient patient samples to detect meaningful differences in randomized controlled trials. Unfortunately, the very large sample size that could help determine the impact of variables such as the impact of the number of sessions remains elusive. There seems to be little question that patients benefit from both multiple sessions and the ability to practice audiotapes, but we know little beyond this.

Additive Effects of Hypnosis

A meta-analysis by Kirsch, Montgomery, and Saperstein (1995) indicated that hypnosis can substantially increase treatment effects beyond psychotherapy. Although Montgomery et al. (2000) reported the majority of patients benefit from hypnotic analgesia in their meta-analysis, we know little about how much hypnosis may have an additive effect as described by Kirsch and colleagues in the 1995 study. A compelling but unexplored notion is that hypnosis might be particularly effective when combined with other treatments of pain. In the area of acute pain, little is known about the potential synergistic effects of combining hypnosis and opioid analgesics for the treatment of procedures. More important, in the case of chronic pain, the potential impact of combining hypnosis with multidisciplinary pain treatment has yet to be determined. It may be that the greatest contribution of hypnosis is when it is provided in the context of multidisciplinary treatment; however, no studies have explored this possibility.

Melzack and Perry (1975) reported years ago in a small study that neither hypnosis nor biofeedback was effective in themselves for chronic pain, but the combination of treatments did demonstrate significant effects. The present review reveals that this notion remains almost completely unexplored in subsequent studies. While several trials have demonstrated that hypnosis is equal or superior to other pain treatments, a fruitful area for future studies will be to see whether it has additive or even synergistic effects with other pain treatments. Chapter 8 in this volume addresses the potential benefits of combining hypnosis with brief therapies such as motivational interviewing for pain control.

SUMMARY

In the 1980s, randomized controlled trials using hypnosis were virtually nonexistent, and reviews suggested that there was little evidence for the impact of hypnosis for clinical pain control. A review by Holroyd (1996) and a meta-analysis by Montgomery et al. (2000) demonstrated the emergence of a number of controlled trials that were more encouraging in their findings. A review of 17 acute pain and 12 chronic pain randomized treatment trials (Patterson & Jensen, 2003) reported that all but one or two of the studies reported that hypnosis was superior to control conditions and often was superior to alternative approaches. More recent reviews that my colleagues and I have done have been similarly encouraging (Elkins, Jensen, & Patterson, 2007; Stoelb, Molton, Jensen, & Patterson, 2009). The additional studies included in my review here continue to support this positive trend of results. Hypnosis continues to fare well in both controlled and randomized controlled trials. Further, it is proving useful with an expanded list of etiologies for chronic pain, including that from neuropathic etiologies (M. P. Jensen, Barber, Romano, Hanley, et al., 2009; M. P. Jensen et al., 2005; M. P. Jensen & Patterson, 2005). Moreover, the encouraging cost-offsetting data reported by Lang and Rosen (2002) have been replicated and extended to cancer pain. Hypnosis may have larger cost savings than were originally reported (Montgomery et al., 2007).

The empirical literature on clinical hypnotic analgesia still has substantial room for improvement. The largest studies that have been done use samples of 200 to 300 patients. Although perhaps barely adequate to determine outcome effects, such sample sizes fail to allow statistical modeling that can tell us more about what types of patients might benefit the most from hypnosis or such questions as the optimal number of sessions. Studies in this area seldom control adequately from the variety of nonspecific effects that might offer competing explanations for findings. Other potential areas that can be addressed include the impact of hypnosis when either combined with other treatments or examined above and beyond them.

Despite several areas in which the research can be improved, the evidence is overwhelming that hypnosis has a positive impact in the majority of patients when used to treat both acute and chronic pain. No longer can claims be made that hypnosis is nothing more than a placebo effect. As discussed in previous chapters, hypnosis has a rich body of laboratory studies, backed with carefully thought-out theory that supports its impact on analog pain. Further, the impact of hypnosis on pain has been demonstrated in psychophysiological studies, including those using sophisticated radiological techniques to monitor brain function. What is clear is that there are now in excess of 50 studies with patient samples that demonstrate the superiority of hypnosis over control conditions. Whereas once it was the anecdotal evidence that was overwhelming with respect to the number of pain etiologies that can be addressed by hypnosis, there now exists a body of controlled trials to support the impressive amount of laboratory and physiological studies on pain control.

4

ERICKSONIAN HYPNOSIS

Much of the discussion on hypnotic interventions for pain in this book is based on the work of Milton Erickson. Ericksonian approaches are sufficiently complex and enough of a departure from conventional hypnosis that a dedicated chapter detailing his work is warranted. Further, there is little in the literature that relates Ericksonian approaches specifically to pain control. In reading Erickson's work, one can find various brief chapters that mention pain or use pain control as an illustration of hypnotic technique (Erickson, 1948/1980a, 1983), but none of his many books were dedicated solely to this topic.

The main reason that an Erickson paradigm is used as a foundation for many of the hypnotic pain interventions discussed in this book is the number of options that it gives when "conventional" hypnosis fails. In the writings of many theorists and clinicians working with hypnosis, what will be observed is that the majority of them deal with the actual clinical problem addressed (e.g., anxiety, pain, depression); attention that is given to the actual induction is often minimal. If a patient does not respond to hypnosis, it is assumed that the patient is not hypnotizable, and the writer will recommend perhaps a nonhypnotic course. This indeed may be warranted with some patients. However, what is immensely appealing about Ericksonian techniques is that volumes have been written simply on the induction process in itself. With an Ericksonian approach, if one induction fails, the clinician has an endless array of alternatives. An additional benefit is that Ericksonian approaches are designed to enhance the rapport between clinicians and patients. In many cases both members of the therapeutic relationship will simply find the process to be more enjoyable. This chapter ends with an example of an Ericksonian hypnotic induction as used by Steven Gilligan in his workshops.

It would be presumptuous to assert that the essence of Ericksonian hypnosis will be captured in this chapter. On reading a series of chapters that describe Erickson's approach to hypnosis, one will discover that the accounts vary widely. Hammond (1988) captured this challenge well in an article titled, "Will the Real Milton Erickson Please Stand Up?" He pointed out the huge discrepancy that exists between speakers and writers who attempt to capture Erickson's approach. As is described in this chapter, Erickson did not entertain an overarching theory in the way he presented his work. Further, his writings changed over the course of his career. In the chapter that follows, much is made of Erickson's use of indirect suggestions. However, if one views tapes of his early inductions, it is apparent that he often used direct suggestions in his work. Descriptions of Erickson's work are largely shaped by the proclivities of the author attempting to describe it, and this chapter is no exception; it would most aptly be described as "a description of Erickson's work as seen through Patterson's personal history and approach to pain control."

The early part of this book places substantial emphasis on the science behind hypnotic pain control. Providing extensive attention to Ericksonian approaches may seem somewhat out of place in this respect. Ericksonian approaches have been criticized for lacking the empirical rigor that several other theoretical orientations have toward hypnosis. Admittedly, there are almost no laboratory studies that are based on this theoretical work; as discussed in Chapter 2 of this volume, most analog studies for hypnotic pain control come out of sociocognitive, neodissociative, or dissociated-control paradigms for understanding hypnosis. Further, few of the randomized controlled studies on pain control have been based on Ericksonian approaches. Milton Erickson has been described as atheoretical (Erickson & Rossi, 1979) and Ericksonian hypnosis as an approach without theory (C. R. Stern, 1985). As will be discussed, the manner in which Erickson recommended patients be approached, and hypnosis instituted, made it difficult to do the same intervention for two patients in the same way. This makes replication of results, one of the standards for clinical research, difficult. At best, a controlled study using an Ericksonian approach can only follow certain parameters; scripted, word-for-word inductions are in contradistinction to how he recommended hypnosis be approached (Erickson & Rossi, 1981; Erickson, Rossi, & Rossi, 1976).

Although much of my own career has been dedicated to conducting controlled clinical trials of hypnosis, an equal part of my professional time has been spent in clinical care and in training students. For clinical and training work, I have relied primarily on Ericksonian approaches. For one thing, the richness, depth, and creativity of Ericksonian approaches can be rivaled by few others in the hypnosis literature. In addition, such approaches are more promising for patients with less hypnotic talent or who are struggling in their ability to benefit from hypnosis. Many of the techniques that define Ericksonian hypnosis were defined for patients who appeared resistant to conventional hypnosis (Erickson & Rossi, 1979).

Further, although Ericksonian techniques have not been investigated nearly as thoroughly as more conventional hypnotic approaches, there is more scientific backing behind them that may be readily apparent. There is no theory associated with Ericksonian approaches that can be tested like sociocognitive or dissociated control theories (Bowers, 1992; Bowers & Davidson, 1991; Bradley, 1996; Chaves, 1989, 1993; Holzman, Turk, & Kerns, 1986; Kirsch & Lynn, 1995; Woody & Sadler, 2008). What Erickson wrote about was more along the lines of an overall approach that followed certain assumptions. This is very similar to motivational interviewing, which is discussed in Chapter 8 of this volume. Although Erickson's overall approach does not lead to a testable theory, there are a number of assertions behind the approach that are subject to scientific scrutiny. For example, much of Erickson's techniques are based on the assumption that the unconscious mind will continue to search for the solution to a problem after the conscious mind ceases to do so. He cited earlier cognitive studies to support this premise (Rossi, 1980), but there have been an number of more current studies to support that such cognitive problem solving continues over time (Sherman & Lynn, 1990; Zeig & Lankton, 1988).

Zeig and Lankton (1988) had long pointed out that many of the assumptions that lie behind Ericksonian approaches are rooted in the social psychology literature, which in turn is based on tightly controlled, theory-driven laboratory studies (see also Sherman & Lynn, 1990). As an example, Erickson frequently referred to establishing *yes sets* as a hypnotic induction technique (Erickson et al., 1976). Yes sets are a time-honored concept in social psychology (Sherman & Lynn, 1990; Zeig & Lankton, 1988). Social psychology has long taught us that if patients show a compliance with a series of requests, they will be more likely to reply with a request that follow. In much of Erickson's work, he used concepts that had been established in the social sciences to facilitate hypnosis. Another example is use of *seeding* in hypnotic inductions. Erickson wrote about the approach of *priming* in hypnosis, or using a word in an induction that would appear later, much in the way that foreshadowing occurs in literature. Seeding has an extensive empirical support in the social psychological literature.

Some of my work done at the University of Washington has provided empirical support for Ericksonian interventions for pain. In a series of studies, my colleagues and I have used the Rapid Induction Analgesia script designed and published by Joseph Barber (1977) as a means to standardize what is said to patients in the hypnotic induction. Examination of this script quickly reveals many components of Ericksonian hypnotic approaches. Seeding of suggestions is provided early in the induction; indirect suggestions for relaxation and pain control characterize the nature of the induction. What's more, this induction makes use of confusion and anchoring, both of which were interventions championed by Erickson (1948/1980a; Erickson et al., 1976). Using this script, my colleagues and I have published at least five controlled studies on reducing pain during burn debridement, one of the most painful type of procedures in the medical profession (Everett, Patterson, & Chen, 1990; Patterson, Everett, Burns, & Marvin, 1992; Patterson & Ptacek, 1997; Patterson, Questad, & Boltwood, 1987; Wiechman Askay, Patterson, Jensen, & Sharar, 2007). Our publications in the *Journal of Consulting and Clinical Psychology* that showed burn pain reduction in a randomized controlled trial using an attention-control group were ones that were based on rigorous science, and these were studies based on Ericksonian approaches (Patterson et al., 1992; Patterson & Ptacek, 1997). Again, although the overall theory may lack empirical support, many of the components have empirical backing, and a script that combines these various components is well tested in randomized controlled trials.

Erickson discouraged the use of scripts in hypnosis and encouraged clinicians instead to individualize each induction to a client's unique makeup and needs. As mentioned earlier, it is difficult to study inductions that vary with each patient. However, there is some evidence in the literature that tailoring each hypnotic induction to a patient's needs is more effective than generic approaches (Barabasz & Barabasz, 2006; Barabasz & Christensen, 2006).

ASSUMPTIONS BEHIND ERICKSONIAN HYPNOSIS

Given how esoteric an Ericksonian view toward hypnosis may appear to be, the assumptions behind it are surprisingly demystifying. First, Erickson did not see hypnosis as curative in itself. He saw nothing in hypnosis that transcended normal physiological abilities or offered miraculous curative powers (although he certainly acknowledged that an altered state occurs with hypnosis, as discussed later in this chapter). As Rossi put it, "the value of hypnosis from an Ericksonian perspective lies entirely in its use as a modality for facility healing processes by evoking psychological and physiological responses conducive to the well-being of the total person" (see Erickson, 1980b, p. xx). Consistent with what sociocognitive theorists have discussed, Erickson viewed hypnosis as a social ritual. What he regarded as being particularly important was the nature of suggestions, in particular, as they were tailored to the individual needs of a patient.

In contrast to sociocognitive theorists, however, Erickson and his students talked often about the existence of trance and its therapeutic value. Sociocognitive theorists generally fail to acknowledge the existence of trance and any special cognitive states arising through hypnosis. Certainly, if trance exists, they do not regard it as a special learning state. Erickson regarded trance as an everyday, normal experience. Steven Gilligan, whose interpretations and techniques based on Erickson's work are frequently discussed this book, views hypnosis as a "special learning state" (Erickson et al., 1976; Erickson & Rossi, 1980; Gilligan, 1985), a concept that was originally promoted by Erickson (1948/1980a). Erickson maintained that people go in and out of trance states often several times over the course of a day. Hypnosis was seen by Erickson as a social interaction designed to generate the naturalist phenomenon of trance. In other words, the clinician is often working to guide the patient into a natural state that happens quite naturally, independent of hypnosis. Kihlstrom's (2008) definition of hypnosis discussed in the introduction of this book does not use the term trance, nor does the empirical evidence discussed in the early chapters. However, it is difficult to discuss Ericksonian approaches and provide clinical examples without actually using the notion of trance, as well as the word itself.

Erickson taught us that conceptualizing trance as an everyday phenomenon can facilitate hypnotic work. Specifically, recognizing what a trance state is and how it occurs under natural circumstances can be useful to the clinician attempting to guide the patient into it through hypnosis. Trance states can occur through boredom or through absorption in an activity of great interest such as a book or movie. Anecdotally, Erickson was said to intentionally bore patients into trance states by telling stories about his grandchildren or watching TV with them. Trance states can also occur through the disruption of everyday patterns of thoughts and experience. One of the most salient examples of this is trauma. Trauma often leads to feelings or states of dissociation, and such states or derealization and/or depersonalization are similar to or can even be considered forms of trance. It follows that patients are highly suggestible after physical or emotional trauma. As is very much the case in a major trauma center (Patterson, Adcock, & Bombardier, 1997), patients are often anxious, focused, and highly suggestible. Even well-intended comments from health care professionals designed to help with pain control ("You will go to sleep and not feel a thing") may be taken literally by patients to suggest death and be terrifying to them. Conversely, positive suggestions can be received by the patients with a receptivity that is far greater than anticipated by the health care professional.

There are a number of other ways that understanding the nature of trance can be helpful to the patient in achieving hypnotic states. In Erickson's view, disrupting the patient's everyday thought process can facilitate a trance state, and this can help determine how hypnotic techniques are designed. One component of quick induction techniques is a gentle touch and push to the patient's forehead. Patients will often report that the unexpected nature of such touch helps lead to a different frame of mind. Along the same lines, surprising the patient and throwing him or her off guard can have similar effects. This was one of the premises behind Erickson's "handshake" technique in which he would pull his hand away from the patient in the middle of a handshake, leaving the slightly confused person's hand floating in the air (Erickson et al., 1976). Finally, confusion techniques, which is discussed in more detail below, are another means to disrupt the patient's everyday pattern of thinking, largely by overwhelming thought processes (Erickson et al., 1976).

Erickson's (1948/1980a) view of hypnosis was that it was a cooperative approach between the clinician and patient and that rapport was essential, although the term *cooperative approach* was introduced in Gilligan's (1987) writings. Many earlier approaches to hypnosis, dating back to Mesmer, have been known to embrace an authoritarian approach. Specifically, in early approaches to hypnosis, the hypnotist was seen as holding the power in the therapeutic relationship. Failure to respond to an induction was regarded as being caused by resistance from the patient (Stanton, 1985). Hypnotic suggestions were typically put very directly, for example, "When I count to five you will go into a deep, deep sleep." With E. H. Hilgard's theoretical work and scales designed to measure hypnotizability designed largely by Weitzenhoffer, the notion of trait theory began to come into play (Hilgard & Hilgard, 1975; Weitzenhoffer & Hilgard, 1959, 1962). In the trait theory view, hypnosis is seen as a function of abilities of a patient, and response to hypnosis, in turn, is largely a function of where patients fall on the continuum of measured hypnotizability (Hilgard & Hilgard, 1975; Spiegel & Spiegel, 1978). In this view, poor response to hypnosis is seen mainly as the patient having this type of disposition.

The cooperative approach views hypnosis as an interaction between the hypnotist and the subject. In this view, hypnosis lies neither exclusively within the clinician nor the client. Although direct suggestions and authoritarian approaches can induce hypnosis at times, such approaches are seen in the cooperative approach as resulting in less enduring behavior changes than those that are generated from the patients. Viewing the power of hypnosis as residing within the hypnotist is seen as inadequate. Nevertheless, the presence of a hypnotist is seen as necessary for the process of hypnosis to have a therapeutic effect in most instances. Although patients go in and out of trance states in their daily functioning, in this view, the guidance of the hypnotist and the impact of the social interaction are seen as typically critical to generating hypnotically generated change. Once again, the trance state in itself is not seen as special or curative; the therapeutic essence of hypnosis is the cooperation between the therapist and patient that allows the patient to generate solutions.

UTILIZATION

Central to Ericksonian hypnosis, and closely akin to the cooperative approach, is the concept of utilization. As mentioned, in the cooperative approach, effective hypnosis is a function of the relationship between the hypnotist and the subject. Trance is regarded as an everyday experience, and the role of the therapist is to facilitate the patient's ability not only to generate such trance states but also to use them in a manner that is therapeutic. In Erickson's view, every individual is unique, and hypnotic change is best facilitated by identifying and capitalizing on his or her proclivities. The most parsimonious tool available to individualize suggestions to the patient is utilization (Erickson, 1948/1980a).

Utilization involves taking what the patient offers in therapy and following that lead to engender therapeutic change. In the work of Erickson, as well as Gilligan, there are two major levels in this concept that can be applied to hypnosis and therapy. The first involves performing inductions. In this application, the therapist listens to and observes the patient, and then utilizes what the patient provides to facilitate and deepen trance. As a simple example, the hypnotist might make the suggestion that the patient's hand and arm are becoming lighter and will begin to float in the air. If, on examination, the patient's hand and arm appear to instead be heavy, then the therapist can use that information and make suggestions accordingly. The suggestion might reinforce the observation that the hand and arm feel heavy and relaxed (and perhaps will continue along this line).

The concept or utilization, as it is applied as a reinforcement of behavior during hypnosis, is often applied by most effective clinicians using hypnosis, regardless of theoretical approach. For example, if a patient's head slumps over in the middle of an induction, as long as he or she is comfortable, it is best to reinforce that behavior with statements along the lines of, "That's right, just noticing how your neck lets go as you become more relaxed." Patients may be wondering internally if it is acceptable to move while in hypnosis, and such reinforcements can reassure them that they are not "doing something wrong.". Erickson was far more intricate in his approach. In one of his writings, he discussed having a patient rest his hand on this stomach.

He would time statements such as, "Your hand is *rising* as you become more relaxed" with the patent's inhalations. Erickson, of course, knew that the patient's hand was going to rise as a function of inhalations.

The other, perhaps deeper, application of utilization goes beyond simple behavior during hypnosis to an overall conceptualization and expression of symptoms. In this view of utilization, symptoms are not regarded as something to be changed or eliminated but rather as a potential solution to the problem faced by the patient. For example, patients with a tremendous amount of sadness or other types of internal pain may use alcohol or drugs to suppress their internal pain. The concept of utilization might be used in the sense of the internal sadness as well as the alcohol and drugs used to suppress it. In therapy, the question becomes "What purpose are the drugs and alcohol serving?" In other words, the substance abuse is looked at as a form of utilization in which the patient is blocking unwanted pain. Along the same lines, the sense of internal pain is also utilized. Rather than the emotional pain being something that the clinician and patient attempt to eliminate, it becomes a guide for understanding the substance abuse. It is the process of fighting or suppressing the sadness that is leading the patient to destructive substance abuse problems. As such, through hypnosis, the patients learn to identify and, at a certain level, embrace their pain with an understanding that it will lead them to the solution of their substance abuse problem.

The reverse of this logic can also be true in that utilization can be applied to the addictive behaviors themselves. In this context, the avoidant behaviors become a clue to what the patient is suppressing. Much of the chapter on motivational interviewing discusses the negative consequences of attempting to force behavior change. Thus, the concept of utilization might lead the clinician not only to explore "what will awaken" in the patient if he or she does not pursue avoidant behavior but also to show greater acceptance of the pain (in this case, psychological pain) that the patient is attempting to suppress.

Utilization can thus refer to making use of practically everything the patient brings to the clinical situation. Inherent in this principle is that the clinician observes and listens to the patient very carefully. Also implicit in this approach is a nonjudgmental acceptance of the patient's symptoms and characteristics. There is certainly an element of unconditional positive regard seen in Rogerian and other humanistic psychotherapies. Further, the unconscious is regarded as a positive, problem-solving type of dynamic force in humans. However, Erickson takes this a step further (or certainly Gilligan does in his extension of this work) in that the therapist accepts the symptoms and the "dark side" with which the patient struggles and actually uses them in the course of hypnosis and therapy.

APPROACHES TO HYPNOSIS

There are a number of unique approaches to hypnosis that are borne out of the general concepts described above. These approaches have played a large role in defining the Ericksonian approach as being different from most other approaches to hypnosis. However, it should be noted that, particularly in his early work, Erickson did not necessarily use many of the unique induction techniques that defined his later work. Lankton (2008) provided a summary of some of the myths associated with Erickson's work. When a patient was responsive, Erickosn seemed content with using simple, direct statements. Many of his more creative and elaborate approaches seemed to be in response to patients who struggled to enter a hypnotic state. What follows are descriptions of some of Erickson's approaches that are more frequently discussed in the literature. This far from captures the almost endless, clinically rich approaches that he would use with patients. For example, one need not search extensively into his work to find elaborate examples of double binds (Erickson & Rossi, 1981; Erickson et al., 1976). Nevertheless, the examples below provide a useful illustration of his approach with more resistant patients as well as a foundation for many of the approaches that I discuss for pain reduction in the remainder of this book.

Indirect Suggestions

As described earlier, early approaches to hypnosis often used what is now referred to as the *authoritarian* approach. Hypnosis was typically administered using direct suggestions, or by "telling the patient what to do." Examples include statements such as "You are getting sleepy," "You are becoming relaxed," or "You are entering a deep trance." For a cooperative patient and one who is very receptive to hypnosis, such suggestions are usually effective in inducing hypnosis. Many of the examples of inductions for pain control discussed later in this book use direct suggestions, particularly for patients in hospital intensive care units who have limited cognitive abilities.

In their most simplistic form, indirect suggestions give patients the option of following a suggestion, as well as how he or she might follow it. Whereas a traditional direct suggestion might be, "Your right arm is becoming heavily," an indirect suggestion might state instead, "You may find that your right arm is becoming heavy in a moment, or maybe it will start feeling lighter. Either way, I would like you to notice if a very pleasant warm sensation spreads throughout that area of your body." Thus, rather than being told what they will experience, the patients are given the option of how to respond. Responding is put much more in terms of the patients' volition, and they are presented with a series of options about what that response might be.

It appears that Erickson developed indirect suggestions for a number of reasons (Erickson et al., 1976). The first reason, and the one that seems to be discussed most often in reference to Erickson's work, involves decreasing resistance. A direct command involves telling someone what to do. It is interesting that for very young children, direct commands are often preferred, at least in terms of generating compliance. A child who is given a choice and is still concrete in his or her thinking may refuse the command. As an example, if a 4-year-old is asked rather than told, "Would you come over here, Jimmy?," it is perfectly reasonable for him to respond with "No" or to ignore the request. After all, he has just been given that option; yet, adults seemed to be surprised when children refuse seemingly direct commands that are put in the form of questions. Although direct commands are often appropriate for children, for adults, they are often considered a form of rudeness. It is more socially appropriate to ask an adult, "Would you hand me the phone?" than to say, "Hand me the phone." Although many patients do not have a problem with direct commands when they are given in the context of hypnosis, it may be that for ones struggling with the process, the use of indirect commands may increase compliance simply by virtue of not forcing the patient and giving him or her freedom of choice in response. Further, at some level the patient may be thinking, "I am being told what to do and I don't like that." An indirect command avoids the potential that the patient may resist a suggestion for that reason.

A deeper, more theoretically complex reason to give patients indirect suggestions is that they serve to generate the hypnotic response (and solution) from the patients rather than giving it to them. According to this line of thinking, if a patient is told to experience a perceptual shift with a direct command (e.g., "You will feel your pain go away"), the patient may experience a short-lived reduction in pain. However, if the patient is led to generate a suggestion or solution him- or herself, the impact may be more long lasting. Indirect suggestions are theoretically unconscious directives that do allow patients to generate their own solutions. Erickson pointed out that cognitive research indicates that long after being posed with a problem, patients unconsciously continue to search for a solution (Erickson, 1948/1980a; Erickson & Rossi, 1979). More recent work on this "incubation" effect certainly suggests that problem solving continues in this manner (S. M. Smith & Blankenship, 1991; Yaniv & Meyer, 1987). Along these lines, Erickson (1967; Erickson et al., 1976) developed indirect suggestions because he believed that they served to generate unconscious searches and solutions in patients. Many of these indirect suggestions were put in the form of questions, for example, "And you have not quite yet realized how you will be able to reduce your pain for several hours, have you?" Erickson et al. (1976) maintained that putting a suggestion to the patient in the form of a question served more to generate unconscious searches for solutions and thus served more to generate solutions from the patient.

Multiple Choices

A particularly useful offshoot of indirect suggestions is the use of multiple choices. Erickson described this as covering all possibilities of a class of responses when giving suggestions. Gilligan (1987) expanded on this notion in this generative autonomy conceptualization. Providing multiple choices in hypnotic suggestions not only has the advantages of any indirect approach (not forcing a patient to accept a given suggestion) but also helps with the clinician's dilemma as to what suggestion to give to which patient at a particular time. No one really knows what suggestion is going to work with a given patient. The method of multiple choices is effective in this regard, not only because it provides several option for suggestions that the patient can choose, but also because it can include an implicit "forced choice" at the end of the statements. The essence of this forced choice is that patients receive the message that they are free to choose the path that will lead to improvement; however, what suggestion they follow must lead to positive change.

A multiple-choice suggestion format may be depicted as follows:

> You may experience "a."
> You may experience "b."
> Or you may experience "c."
> However, whatever you might experience, you will certainly experience "X."

Using this approach, patients are given several options for how they might respond but are then looped back to a suggestion for some type of benefit, regardless of which suggestion they follow. Using pain control as an example, patients might be told,

> You might notice that your pain alters from a dull throbbing to tingling sensation, you might notice that you look back and forget that you were experiencing discomfort all together, or you may find that you become so absorbed in your grandchildren that you cannot think about or feel anything else. What will be certain to amaze you is that you will feel surprisingly more comfortable.

As described by Gilligan (1987), if the clinician desires to maintain a type of continuous feedback loop with the patient, a step can be added to this format that allows for this by adding the italicized step below:

> You may experience "a."
> You may experience "b."
> Or you may experience "c."
> *And what are you experiencing now?*

Subsequent chapters in this volume elaborate how multiple choices can be applied to pain control. It is often useful to loop several sets of suggestions together. For example, the patient can go through three loops, each of which contains three suggestions. In addition, the suggestions can be layered so that each suggestion is hitting a potential level of the patient's pain problem. For example, one suggestion might focus on pain control itself, another on lifestyle changes, and a third on a core value of the patient that might lead to change. However, the clinician should also keep in mind that, at some point, the number of suggestions given can have diminishing returns. If a patient receives too many suggestions, ultimately he or she will likely become exasperated and will begin to lose those suggestions that might have proved helpful. Two to three loops, each containing three suggestions, should be adequate for this reason.

Truisms

Truisms are another Ericksonian technique of hypnosis that largely defined his idiosyncratic approach. Truisms are simply statements of "what is." If the therapist is facing a patient and the patient is sitting in a chair, a truism is that the patient "is sitting in a chair." In the hypnotic process, the statement would simply be, "You are sitting in the chair" (Erickson & Rossi, 1979).

Truisms offer a wonderfully simple means to facilitate a hypnotic state and to gain rapport with the patient. First, truisms present information to patients in a way that is no stretch to the patient's sense of reality, at least initially. The statement that the patient is "sitting in a chair" can hardly be disputed. However, even though that statement is patently obvious, the act of making it to the patient has a number of potential hypnotic effects. Although the patient knows he or she is sitting in a chair, that fact is very likely not this person's immediate awareness or focus of attention. When the patient hears that he or she is sitting in a chair, the patient's focus of attention is turned inward to a phenomenon that can be disputed. Few theorists in the area of hypnosis would dispute that a critical early step of hypnosis is to capture the patient's attention and to turn it inward. The use of truisms can often accomplish this in a very efficient manner.

A particularly effective use of truisms is to string a series of them together to create an induction. This is often referred to in the literature as *pacing* (Gilligan, 1987). As such, the patient might be told, "You are sitting in the chair, you are breathing in and out, and you are listening to my voice." What one hopes will occur is that patients receive three statements that serve to capture their attention and to turn it inward. However, the process of making repeated truisms allows the therapist to establish a rhythm, and sort of intuitive rapport, with the patient.

As will be discussed more in subsequent chapters, truisms are particularly effective when used in the following induction:

Pace (truism)
Pace (truism)
Pace (truism)
Lead (suggestion)

In other words, the patient is given three truisms and then a leading suggestion. Earlier in the induction, the leading suggestions are ideally less risky in terms of the clinician's interpretation of the patient's behavior. Using the present example, the therapist might say, "You are sitting in the chair, you are breathing in and out, and you are listening to my voice." The therapist then adds a suggestion such as, "And perhaps you are finding yourself becoming slightly more relaxed." Suggesting that the patient is becoming "slightly more relaxed" does not present much of a risk in terms of challenging the patient's internal sense of reality at that moment. For example, if the patient is told that he or she is becoming "deeply and profoundly relaxed" or experiencing a feeling "drifting" too early in the process, the patient's attention and sense of cooperation might be interrupted because the suggestion is discordant with his or her internal experience. As such, the leading statements made early in the induction are ideally more conservative and consistent with what the patient is likely experiencing internally.

As the induction process continues, the clinician continues to make three truisms and then a leading statement. As the induction continues and the patient ideally goes deeper into a hypnotic state, the clinician can then take more risk, and consequently guesses, as to what constitutes an effective leading statement. First, if the patient is profoundly relaxed and in good rapport with the clinician, as will often occur later in the induction, there is less of a chance that a leading statement will be disruptive. Second, at a later stage of the induction, the patient is likely simply more open to suggestions as a function of the process. Thus, as this pacing–leading induction continues, the clinician often is more adventurous in terms of the leading statements that are made. In addition, the process of providing repeated truisms can ideally create a sense of rhythm and rapport between the clinician and patient; hypothetically, the rapport that results under such circumstances can lead to suggestions that are intuitively generated by the clinician and phenomenologically accurate for the patient.

Erickson also used truisms in a more elaborate sense to provide suggestions to the patient. In this sense a truism is a simple statement of fact about behavior that the patient has experienced so often that it cannot be denied. Such statements can set in motion perceptual changes. Examples might include statements such as the following:

> "Most people can experience one hand as being lighter than another."
> "Everyone has the experience of nodding their head."
> "You already know how to experience pleasant sensations like the warmth of the sun on your skin" (Erickson & Rossi, 1979, p. 23).

Double Binds

Double binds are another type of relatively unique form of suggestion that has often been associated with Erickson's approach (Erickson et al., 1976; Erickson & Rossi, 1979). A premise of a double-bind suggestion is that it allows the patient's resistance to work against itself. As an example, years ago I was giving a lecture on hypnosis in a burn center. I finished the lecture and asked the audience if they would like a demonstration. They declined the offer of a demonstration with one of them as a volunteer subject but asked me to work with one of their patients with a burn injury instead. This patient was a very angry man in his 20s with a severe burn injury. His hostility was evident as I entered the room. I had sensed that this particular group of health care workers was skeptical about hypnosis and were quite certain that I was going to fail in attempting to use hypnosis with this particular patient. In fact, several staff members crowded inside the door and could barely suppress their smiles as they anticipated what was going to be an abject failure on my part (at least this was my perception). I approached the patient and asked him if he was willing to try hypnosis and he replied that he was. I then began the induction by asking if he would like to feel more comfortable in a moment. He quickly responded with a loud, "No!" At this point the staff were suppressing giggles rather than smiles. I saw a rare opportunity to use a double-bind suggestion with the patient. It was clear the patient was intent on defying me at this point, particularly with an audience consisting of a health care group whose care he had continually resisted. If I suggested to him that he would become more relaxed and pain free, he would have lost face in front of the burn team by complying with my suggestion. Consequently, the only option I had was to suggest the opposite of what I thought would be a desirable affective state for the patient, so I stated, "OK, as I talk with you I would like you to become more and more tense rather than more relaxed." If he allowed himself to tense up more, he would have been cooperating with my suggestion. The only way he could defy me at this point was to become more relaxed. Within about 30 seconds, the patient was deeply relaxed and snoring loudly, although still responding to suggestions about pain control.

Very clearly double binds have fallen out of favor because they can present difficulties with informed consent. For example, if a patient enters a therapeutic relationship and clearly expresses that he or she does not want to be hypnotized, it is not acceptable to use double-bind suggestions to facilitate hypnosis. Along the same lines, artful use of the patient's resistance against itself can reach levels of manipulation that can impair the clinical relationship. To put it another way, when a patient clearly says "no," that should be respected. That said, there is still a place for the use of double binds in current hypnosis. One example is to end inductions with a mild double-bind suggestion. Specifically, it can be useful to link to suggestions for eye-opening with acceptance of suggestions that were made earlier to the patient. So the therapist might state,

> And at the time your unconscious mind understands that you will know what to do to feel better, even though you conscious mind may not even realize this, your mind will give you a sign by allowing your eyes to open. And when your eyes open, you will find yourself awake, alert, refreshed, and awake.

The subtle double bind is that the subject is "not allowed" to open his or her eyes until the suggestion is accepted.

Erickson used double binds in a much more elaborate sense. For example, he described the conscious–unconscious double bind: "If your unconscious wants you to enter trance, your right hand will lift. Otherwise your left hand will lift." Or, "You don't have to listen to me because your unconscious is here and can respond to its needs in just the right way" (Erickson et al., 1976, p. 67). Along such more elaborate lines, he described double-dissociation double binds. "You can as a person awaken but you do not need to awaken as a body. You can awaken when your body awakes but without a recognition of your body" (Erickson et al., 1976, p. 67).

Metaphors

A final example of what characterized Erickson's approaches was the use of *metaphors*, also termed the *embedded* or *interspersal* approach (Erickson, 1948/1980a; Zeig, 1985). Erickson often provided suggestions embedded in the context of a story. In the context of utilization, metaphors are geared toward generating solutions from the unconscious. Erickson used a number of approaches to this end, including puns, paradoxes, and double entendres. However, under this rubric of techniques, he was certainly more recognized for his metaphors. More specific examples of Erickson's work in this area are presented in the next chapter.

Designing metaphors for pain control, particularly chronic pain, is challenging work. It is particularly helpful for the clinician to know the patient well and to be aware of the core values that drive the patient. There can be a number of potential advantages of using metaphors in terms of the overall Ericksonian approaches discussed in the chapter. First, the conscious mind and the logical thought that usually comes with the manner in which it processes information often resist sequentially presented hypnosis and/or direct suggestions. In other words, if suggestions are presented in a logical sequence, some patients (particularly adults) who are struggling with experiencing hypnosis may find that there is more to resist. In contrast, if patients are hearing a metaphor, very often put in the form of a story, it is far more difficult for them to struggle against the inherent suggestions.

For children, metaphors may be beneficial for other reasons. A child who is the subject of hypnosis often has not developed the capacity to process complex logical processing; this may explain why presenting inductions in the forms of metaphors is thought to be more effective with children (Barabasz & Watkins, 2005; Olness & Kohen, 1996; Scott, Lagges, & LaClave, 2008). As opposed to a formal induction, children will likely become more absorbed in, and cooperative with, hypnosis if they are asked to become a character in one of their favorite movies or TV shows.

SUMMARY

Prior to Erickson, approaches to hypnosis were largely dominated by inductions that tended to be straightforward, simple, and dominated by the agenda of the clinician performing the hypnosis. This largely remains the case today, and for many patients, particularly those who are more hypnotically talented, such approaches can be very useful. Although it is tempting to relegate Ericksonian techniques to some of the induction techniques he made famous (i.e., indirect suggestions, metaphors), using his approach successfully is much more a matter of taking a substantial shift in one's approach to the patient. It can be very difficult for a clinician to abandon a standard practice of providing a predesigned induction, which is what an Ericksonian approach requires. Not only does a stock approach to hypnosis not consider what may arise in the patient's unique history, but it also largely ignores what behaviors the patient shows and the experiences the patient has during the induction.

Ericksonian hypnosis is much more a matter of an intense effort on the part of the clinician to enter the patient's phenomenological world and to guide the patient to internally generated solutions. What may appear to be highly complex and elaborate (not to mention effective) hypnotic interventions out of this paradigm are often mainly borne out of carefully observing and following the patient. In turn, many of the unique types of induction techniques developed by Erickson, rather than being means to manipulate the patient, are actually means to enable the patient to guide hypnosis and generate solutions. Erickson recognized, as do modern-day therapists (e.g., W. R. Miller & Rollnick, 1991), that therapy solutions generated by patients are more likely to endure than those suggested to them externally. This chapter ends (see Appendix 4.1) with an example of an Ericksonian hypnotic induction as it is used by Steve Gilligan in his workshops.

APPENDIX 4.1: ERICKSONIAN INDUCTION EXAMPLE

The following example of an Ericksonian style is one that was developed by Steven Gilligan and one that he uses in his workshops. Gilligan notes that, during the induction, special attention should be paid to nonverbal patterning such as establishing and maintaining nonverbal rapport; developing eye fixation; using voice tonality that is resonant; using pauses, silence, and tempo shifts to absorb and reorganize conscious awareness; marking out key suggestions; keeping the underlying beat; and developing focused relaxation (i.e., absorption) in both hypnotist and subject. Also, each idiosyncratic aspect of experience—both positive and negative—should be welcomed and integrated within the induction.

Center, Set Intention, Open to Resources

I'd like to welcome you here today, and I'd like to suggest that we both take a minute or so to settle in and tune in and settle down to find that place inside that will support and allow some good, deep work to happen here today. If you'd like, you can close your eyes, and just take a few moments to breathe, to relax, to attune to yourself. Take these few moments to let go of anything that is not important and center into your own self. And as you do that, you can also take a few moments to set an intention for today's work. In the most simple terms possible, what is it that you would most like to accomplish here today?

The clinician, as participant/observer, attunes in a parallel, similar way.

You may find yourself expressing that intention in terms of a simple phrase or sentence, or maybe in terms of an image, or perhaps a feeling.

This can be elaborated.

And as you sense that simple but deep goal, you can also take a few moments to open to whatever resources in your life you'd like to call upon to support you and guide you during this process. It could be family members or close friends. It could be spiritual presences. It could be certain people who have been on this path before you, but it's nice to know that you can call upon different resources to support and help you on your journey today. And then when you're ready, you can open your eyes and come back into the room.

Get Feedback to Learn What/How to Support the Trance Work

Introduce Trance

This process of generative trance is one of learning and trusting your inner self to be the lead system in discovering how to achieve your deepest goals. There are so many different ways that you can learn to listen, to trust, to be guided by, to be helped by your own intelligence, much of which you don't yet know about. To learn what that means for you, I'd like to ask you to find a comfortable posture where you can be both relaxed and aware at the same time. A position that can open to relaxed absorption. Find a comfortable posture where you can feel your spine in alignment. Let your body relax, let your mind begin to be curious. Trance is a process of finding a balance point, a balance point where you can be totally relaxed and deeply attentive, a balance point where you can feel an inner connection and an openness to what's beyond, a balance point where you can breathe in and out, feeling both an experiential participation at a deep level and a gentle witnessing of the process. What Erickson used to call being "a part of and apart from," at the same time.

Join and Unfold Ongoing Responses: Suggestion Loop # 1

You can notice with curiosity whatever is happening for you at each moment. Take a few moments to further settle in and settle down; allow yourself to devote yourself to deep awareness to your inner self. Whatever you witness, whatever you become aware of, whatever you discover with that detached, absorbed curiosity, you can breathe that in. Allow it to relax and absorb you deeper into a beautiful, interesting inner trance.

You can notice your breathing moving in and out, in and out, in and out. That awareness of the rhythm of your breath, letting go a little more, letting go a little more, letting go a little more.

And as you experience that, you can notice other things. Different thoughts moving in and out, in and out, in and out. There's no doubt that some can be doubts, to be sure. Can't do it; will it work? Let go all of the way into trance? And as you notice those thoughts, your breath and the rhythm of the voice can allow you to go deeper and deeper, a little bit more down, a little bit more down, a little bit more comfortably in a trance.

You can sense different images, an image of yourself in the future, having achieved the goal, an image of yourself in a long forgotten pleasant childhood memory, an image of a favorite place you like to go to relax. And as you notice the images moving in and out, you can let yourself go a little bit deeper, a little bit deeper, a little bit deeper down into a comfortable trance.

Suggest "Parallel Autonomy" for Unconscious Mind

And as you go deeper, you can begin to witness your own creative unconscious mind. You can notice how it begins to lead you deeper and more comfortably into your own unique learning process. I can be talking out here, and you can notice that your unconscious can translate my voice into the voice of others. You can notice how your unconscious can translate my meanings into your own meanings. I may be talking about a bird in the sky, and you might find yourself experiencing something about a dolphin in the sea. I may be talking about eating a certain kind of food, and you may find your unconscious creating experiential images of lying in a hammock, because while we can remain connected in a trance, your unconscious has the capacity and the freedom to create its own meanings and your own path of healing and change. So just become so very curious about how as you relax deeper and deeper. That's it, deeper and deeper. That's it, deeper and deeper. That's it, allow your creative self to become more and more active, more and more active, more and more active. As you relax deeper into a trance, deeper into a trance, deeper into a trance.

Introduce Stories/Metaphors

So many times before you've had this experience. Now like other times, those times again now. For example, who has not sat in a classroom, listening to a lecture drone on and on. It is so hard to continue to concentrate on the external sounds, the mind begins to drift into internal associations. The mind naturally begins to drift into other worlds. You can be looking at a blackboard, watching something being written. Big A, little A; Big B, little B; Big C, little C, and elemental meanings begin to spell out new meanings.

A process of drifting into another dimension of reality, something in between the worlds, something beginning to develop within your worlds. When you dream at night now you recognize your unconscious dreams a dream and you're not really consciously noticing, but you are dreaming a dream of inner exploration. It happens again, and again. It isn't conscious thinking; it is becoming deeply immersed in unconscious thinking without really knowing it consciously until afterward.

Add more examples if needed.

Suggest Accessing of Goal/Future Self

Deep hypnotic awareness of room with a view, a space for experiences from four directions and more. Beginning with a goal, an intention, you can feel it beginning to return to this space, a door opening, the presence of the goal moving into awareness, a detached absorption of sensing. The door opens, and the future enters. Your future is within the deep hypnotic presence, a pearl within a shell, a jewel within a box, opening. You can feel it, you can sense it, a symbol, an image, a deep reality . . . enters . . . and the question of how, when, where that future will be created, achieved, lived, enjoyed, seen as a past achievement.

Suggest Resources for Realizing Future Self

A question of resources, which resources will come from which sources of creative intelligence? Dipping down into the well of wellness, the waters of creative knowing, swimming into deeper awareness, coming up to see the different resources, a beautiful source of resources. Over there . . .

Direct voice to left.

Over there . . .

Direct voice to right.

Sources of resources, different beings appear from the source of resources. Different people who know how to help, wise people, friendly beings, warm-hearted spirits, can be resources to open the source of inspiration for the future now being realized within a deep trance.

And resources of memories from the past, and memories of the future. Time turning on double helix axis, different memories from your lifetime, past-present-future time now to allow the creative self to dip into the source of resources.

This may be elaborated. [Note from Patterson: At this phase, suggestions for pain control can be provided/integrated.]

Integration of Resources

And as the axis turns, the past-present-future resources unfolding and unfurling in deep inner space, mixing, a meal of nourishment, a mosaic of wholeness, a dream of integration. The unconscious can begin to weave those resources, characters in a story, learnings in a sequence, songs on a CD, notes in a progression. Your unconscious can begin to weave these resources into an integration. That's it, a little deeper. Time changing, that's it. Time changing into a different dimension, all resources can move into integration, beginning two minutes of integration, soon, almost there, soon. Deep integration of resources all the way, beginning nowwwwwwwwwww.

Voice can move to "winds of change." During 2 minutes, hypnotist gives background support, for example:

letting   go . . . surrendering . . . opening . . . allowing . . . that's   it . . . time . . . future . . . now . . . present . . . integrating . . .

Future Orient

Deep breath.

And the integration integrating into breath, into future, into cellular awareness, into imagery. The integration integrating into now, future, present now is the future present in you, and it is something that you can continue to see now the future, a sense of opening beyond, opening to, opening through the held mind to the future held gently like a beloved, supported deeply by your presence. You can take a few moments to sense a commitment. You can make a vow. You can make a gentle promise, this future, this future, this future. You can make a gentle commitment to allow all your breath, your thoughts, your days, your dreams, to pave the way, to be the maze that can amaze in amazing mazes of ways, to align toward the spiral of unfolding, the future present now in the time.

Reorient

You can now take the time to begin the process of bringing a gentle close, a time to breathe into the body-mind a sense of "it's time." Amazing grace, the grace of completing the journey, the journey of now returning slowly, gently. Take a few moments, and then when you're ready, let yourself begin to orient back into the outer world.

5

ERICKSONIAN APPROACHES TO PAIN CONTROL

The richness inherent in Ericksonian approaches to hypnosis combined with a thorough knowledge of the field of pain control will prepare most clinicians to be highly effective in reducing pain and suffering. The key highlight of the Ericksonian approach is that it is cooperative and individualized to the patient. Hypnosis is seen as an interactive approach between the therapist and patient, and certainly not something that is "done" to the patient. In terms of individualization, the therapist is often following the patient and capitalizing on the strengths that he or she may have. In this view, resistance is seen as a problem of the therapist rather than the patient. Specific to pain control, the Ericksonian approach emphasizes what every good clinician knows: that how a patient responds to pain has to do not only with the present but also with the patient's historical responses to pain, as well as anticipatory responses likely to occur in the future. Ericksonian concepts may seem frustratingly complex to the clinician who wants to intervene quickly with a patient in pain. However, the process of truly listening to patients and reflecting back to them what they need is also often simple. One way of looking at this approach is that the patient is giving the clinician the answer to the test before the clinician even takes it.

One chapter cannot do justice to the breadth of hypnotic suggestions for pain relief, be they from Erickson or from any other source. A central theme of this book is that drastically different interventional approaches are warranted by different types of pain. Whereas acute clinical pain can respond well to simple direct hypnotic interventions without many potential complications, chronic pain typically requires far more intricate assessment and intervention; the thoughtless application of hypnosis to chronic pain may exacerbate the problem more than help it. Whereas some types of chronic pain are held in place by the environment, lifestyle, and personality factors, other types of chronic pain may be more a matter of some type of disease process or ongoing nociception feeding into the patient's suffering.

Much of this book has to do with understanding how pain and related psychological factors cause the patient to suffer. Some chapters discuss how to address pain and suffering that primarily requires a change in lifestyle. Most clinicians working in pain control are anxious to have a series of suggestions that have a direct impact on reducing the pain itself, and providing this information is a primary purpose of this section. However, it is critical that clinicians understand that adequately treating pain usually goes far beyond suggestions for pain control. Again, understanding a biopsychosocial approach to pain control and how hypnosis fits into it is far beyond the scope of this chapter and is discussed in greater detail later in the book.

The most comprehensive and creative list of hypnotic suggestions for pain control in the literature has arguably evolved from Erickson's writing, and these are the focus of this chapter. In discussing such approaches, it is useful to understand how Erickson himself viewed hypnotic approaches to pain. It is interesting to note that, as powerful an impact that Erickson had on the field, his expectations for the effect that hypnosis might have on pain were usually quite modest. Erickson viewed eliminating all pain though hypnosis as an untenable, unrealistic goal in most circumstances. At one point, he gave the example that an increase in scholastic test scores from 70% to 85% might be a joyous accomplishment but that clinicians do not seem to be satisfied with a 15% reduction in pain in their patients.

Erickson frequently wrote about a fractionalization approach to pain reduction in which pain was gradually reduced (e.g., Erickson, 1983). Much of Erickson's work in hypnotic pain reduction reflected the time-honored behavioral concept of *successive approximations*. Seldom did he try to remove all pain at once. Instead, he saw pain control as being on a continuum, and he tried to move the patient to the range of more comfort. Perhaps one of the classic examples of this is a patient who had excruciating abdominal pain from malignant cancer. Erickson was able to treat this by suggesting to the patient that he would experience an irritating mosquito bite where the pain was located. So rather than eliminating all sensation, or even all unpleasant sensation, he was able to substitute a more acceptable sensation for one that the patient could not tolerate. Erickson also cited this example with a patient who has severe breast cancer pain who was provided with the suggestion for an annoying, minor itching-burning sensation in the sole of her foot (Erickson & Rossi, 1979).

TYPES OF SUGGESTIONS FOR PAIN CONTROL

What follows is a series of hypnotic procedures for reducing pain that were described by Erickson. His original description of these techniques can be found in his book *Innovative Hypnotherapy* (Erickson, 1980b) as well as his chapter in Rossi's edited volume of Erickson's collected papers (Erickson, 1948/1980a, Volume 4, Chapter 24).

Direct Abolition of Pain

As described previously, Erickson generally discouraged direct abolition of pain as a type of hypnotic approach. Sweeping suggestions for the elimination of pain go against the successive approximations of pain reduction, which is a far more realistic way to approach this clinical issue. Also, he felt that direct suggestions for pain control could interfere with the self-generated solutions that arise out of indirect suggestions.

Suggestions for complete removal of pain is an approach that clinicians should avoid, except in rare circumstances. The expectations that clinicians put on themselves and communicate to their patients have a great deal to do with their clinical effectiveness (Kirsch & Lynn, 1995; Turner & Chapman, 1982); certainly, going into a patient relationship with an expectation that one can reduce pain will potentially increase clinical effects. However, communicating to the patient that all pain will be removed raises hopes and expectations beyond what is reasonable and will be of little benefit to the therapeutic relationship. Clinicians should communicate realistic expectations to the patient; any clinician who asserts that hypnosis will remove all pain—in even a small number of patients—is likely being disingenuous. Even Erickson seldom reached this benchmark in his work.

Erickson stated that direct suggestions for pain abolition could be useful in some rare circumstances; an example of this is with major surgery. Hilgard and Hilgard (1975) reported more than 20 different types of major surgery that have been done with hypnosis as the sole anesthetic. The majority of these cases likely used direct suggestions for the elimination of all pain. It is also likely that the majority of these patients were highly hypnotizable.

A clinical scenario in which direct suggestions for pain relief, not necessarily total pain elimination, come into play is the intensive care unit (ICU). In the ICU typically there is a narrow window of time to work with patients before confusion or drug effects dominate their conscious presentation. With a reduced sensorium, patients are often incapable of grasping the subtleties of indirect suggestions; they are quite literal in their thinking. Thus, short inductions with direct suggestions are often preferable. In the ICU scenario, the suggestions actually can be targeted to pain elimination, but it is important that the patient is left with some sensation to replace pain. Stating to patients who fear for their survival that they will "feel nothing" or "feel no pain" might elicit death anxiety, so stating that they will "feel nothing but comfort" is preferable. As such, in the ICU situation, it is far preferable to make suggestions along the lines of "you will feeling nothing but comfort and complete relaxation."

Permissive Indirect Hypnotic Abolition of Pain

Erickson was more comfortable making suggestions for complete abolition of pain when they were done in a permissive rather than direct fashion. His writings did not describe exactly how he would recommend doing this for pain, but, of course, he wrote volumes on permissive, indirect approaches. This would often involve the use of questions, which Erickson believed would stimulate patients' searching into their unconscious resources. An example of this might be, "And you don't know exactly how the pain will be suddenly eliminated, do you?" Beyond this example, it is difficult to describe permissive, indirect suggestions, because they are much more a matter of the entire interaction with the patient rather than a matter of a few statements. As described earlier, when the cooperative approach is used, the entire process is designed to elicit problem solving from the patient. This involves not only the use of questions but also utilization and other techniques to draw upon the patient's resources.

Amnesia

An increasingly popular drug that is used during brief threatening medical procedures is midazolam (Versed), which has no impact on pain itself but can be administered before a medical procedure as an amnestic. Patients are conversant and cooperative while the medical team is at work, but they come out of the procedure with no recall and no pain, providing that no tissue damage has occurred. If a patient goes through a surgery on Versed alone, he or she will wake up in pain from the residual trauma to the body. At its best, hypnotic suggestion can work in a similar manner. Erickson pointed out that more threatening or emotionally salient events can cause patients to forget their pain. Certainly, this can pertain to a soldier in a combat situation, which has gained recognition as a concept through Beecher's (1959; see also Melzack & Wall, 1965, 1973) work. As mentioned in an earlier chapter, Hoffman and colleagues have reported that patients sufficiently captivated by an immersive virtual reality environment seem to forget about their pain (Hoffman, Doctor, Patterson, Carrougher, & Furness, 2000; Hoffman, Patterson, & Carrougher, 2000; Hoffman, Patterson, Carrougher, & Sharar, 2001).

Erickson advised that such amnesias can be partial, selective, or complete. There is a wide range of wording that can be used to accomplish amnesic suggestions, such as, "And wouldn't it be interesting if you found yourself so absorbed in your comfort that you seemed to forget about everything else?" Or, "I am wondering how it would feel if several hours passed and all you seemed to remember is how pleasant you seemed to feel during that period?"

Analgesia

Analgesia has to do with reducing pain, and it captures most drugs used to treat pain, such as aspirin, nonsteroidals, and opioid analgesics. Like this class of drugs, hypnotic analgesic suggestions reduce pain rather than eliminate it. Like amnesia, suggestions can be partial, complete, or selective. Analgesic suggestions are often accomplished by introducing sensory modifications to the patient: "Perhaps you will be pleased to notice feelings of growing warmth and heaviness in your back." Or, "You may find that the only thing you are able to notice is a deep, profound relaxation, and everything else seems to go away."

Anesthesia

Anesthesia is the elimination of pain. Erickson was seldom in favor of using such suggestions, just as he did not usually recommend the total abolition of pain. Common anesthetics such as lidocaine work by numbing an area, with the hope of eliminating any sensation of pain.

Glove anesthesia is a common hypnotic suggestion and can be used in this context. The patient might be told,

> And as I continue talking with you, notice if you begin to feel a sensation in your right hand here where I am lightly touching it. It is as if your skin is becoming covered with an electrician's thick leather glove, an increasing feeling of numbness. You might remember the sensation of your hand falling asleep and that is what seems to be happening now.

Once a glove anesthesia is accomplished, this sensation can be moved to different parts of the body. The line between anesthesia and analgesia can become difficult to distinguish at this point, but ultimately, the distinction is not important.

Hypnotic Replacement and Displacement of Pain

As discussed earlier, Erickson was fond of replacing or changing a sensation rather than trying to eliminate pain altogether, so this category of suggestions is one that typified his work. Erickson offered a nice example of how he provided suggestions for replacement or substitution of pain to a patient with cancer:

> For example, one cancer patient suffering intolerable, intractable cancer pain responded most remarkably to the suggestion of an intolerable, incredibly annoying itch on the sole of her foot. Her body weakness occasioned by the carinomatosis and hence inability to scratch the itch rendered this psychogenic pruritus all absorbing of her attention. Then hypnotically, there were systematically induced feelings of warmth, of coolness, of heaviness and of numbness for various parts of her body where she suffered pain. And the final measure was the suggestion of an endurable but highly unpleasant and annoying minor burning-itching sensation at the site of her mastectomy. This procedure of replacement substitution sufficed for the last six months of the patient's life. The itch of the sole of her foot gradually disappeared, but the annoying burning-itching at the site of her mastectomy persisted. (Erickson & Rossi, 1979, p. 134)

Hypnotic Displacement of Pain

Erickson liked to use the displacement technique to transfer pain from an area of the body that was perceived as threatening by the patient to one that was less so. One example he gives is of treating a man with intractable abdominal pain from cancer. Given that the patient perceived that the pain in the abdomen could destroy him, experiencing pain in his left hand was far more acceptable to him. For the 3 remaining months of his life, the patient experienced pain in his hand rather than his abdomen, and Erickson (1980b) reported that this promoted his functioning and relationship with his family.

It is well understood in the cognitive–behavioral literature that changing the nature or location of pain facilitates the patient's perception of control of pain overall. Any time a patient is able to change qualities of the pain experience, this will likely lead to improved pain control because to change pain sensations is to exert at least some control over them. Thus, when patients are successful in changing their pain through hypnotic suggestions, it has the benefit of enhancing the patients' sense of control; such control, in turn, can lead to the ability to create other sensory modifications.

Hypnotic Time and Body Disorientation

Patients who have experienced chronic pain for extended periods of times may have difficulty remembering periods when they were pain free; this is also the case in people with long-term depression. Patients experiencing very severe, untreatable pain lose all perception of what it is like to be pain free. In such cases, Erickson recommended orienting patients to periods in their life when they were either pain free or when the pain was certainly less of an issue. Patients do have such memories and resources within them, and accessing them can be a powerful form of pain control. Having patients return to such an earlier time to access such resources and then having them bring them to the present can be a very powerful technique. Similarly, patients can also be trained to imagine a future in which their pain is absent or more manageable. A later chapter presents a technique in which resources from the past are tied to images of comfortable functioning in the future.

Body disorientation was another type of suggestion discussed by Erickson, and it is likely that such suggestions will often be limited to highly talented hypnotic patients or to those who are in so much pain that dissociative tendencies begin to come easily as a way to escape.[1]

> Thus one woman with the onset of unendurable pain, in response to posthypnotic suggestions, would develop a trance state and experience herself as being in another room while her suffering body remained in her sickbed. This patient explained to the author when he made a bedside call, "Just before you arrived, I developed another horrible attack of pain. So I went into a trance, got into my wheelchair, came out into the living room to watch a television program, and left my suffering body in the bedroom." And she pleasantly and happily told about the fantasized television program she was watching. Another such patient remarked to her surgeon, "You know very well, Doctor, that I always faint when you start changing my dressings because I can't endure the pain, so if you don't mind, I will go into a hypnotic trance and take my head and feet and go into the solarium and leave my body here for you to work on." The patient further explained, "I took a position in the solarium where I could see him (the surgeon) bending over my body, but I could not see what he was doing. Then I looked out the window, and when I looked back he was gone, so I took my head and feet and went back and joined my body

[1]Excerpt reprinted from *The Collected Papers of Milton Erickson on Hypnosis: Vol. IV. Innovative Hypnotherapy* (pp. 242–243), by M. H. Erickson (E. L. Rossi, Ed.), 1980, New York, NY: Irvington. Copyright 1980 by the Erickson Foundation. Reprinted with permission.

and felt very comfortable." This particular patient had been trained in hypnosis by the author many years previously, had subsequently learned autohypnosis, and thereafter induced her own autohypnotic trance by the phrase, "You know very well, Doctor." This was a phrase that she could employ verbally or mentally at any time and immediately go into a trance for the psychological–emotional experience of being elsewhere, away from her painful body, there to enjoy herself and remain until it was safe to return to her body. In this trance state, which she protected very well from the awareness of others, she would visit with her relatives, but experience them as with her in this new setting while not betraying that personal orientation. (Erickson, 1980b, pp. 242–243)

Hypnotic Reinterpretation of a Pain Experience

Reinterpretation of a pain experience has become a hallmark of cognitive–behavioral treatment of pain. In fact, in sociocognitive conceptualizations of hypnotic pain control, there seems to be little difference between altering such cognitions and hypnosis (T. X. Barber, Spanos, & Chaves, 1974; Chaves, 1989; Chaves & Barber, 1976; Spanos & Chaves, 1989a, 1989b, 1989c). Inducing hypnosis is not even regarded as necessary for such suggestions to be useful (Chaves, 1993). In the cognitive–behavior literature, catastrophizing has become a central concept in pain control. *Catastrophizing* refers to excessively negative thoughts about the meaning of pain. If a patient experiences a pain sensation and is convinced that it will lead to his or her death, or can never be changed, those thoughts will have a great deal to do with how he or she is able to cope with that pain. Modifying such cognitions can reduce pain, and such modifications can certainly be done in the context of a hypnotic induction.

Burn pain, one of the most intense and difficult-to-treat forms of nociception, provides a good example of how reinterpretation of sensations becomes particularly salient with burn injuries. It is well known that full-thickness burns are not necessarily painful because the depth of the tissue damage is severe enough to destroy the function of nerve endings. As full or partial thickness (i.e., second-degree) begin to heal, it is common for skin buds to appear on the epidermis. Such buds are extremely sensitive to touch and pain. This leads to some important reinterpretive messages to patients, both in and out of hypnosis. Patients can be told that the presence of skin buds is a sign of healing and the return of viable, nonscarring skin. It might very well suggest that the patient will heal without the need for a skin graft. This is excellent news for the patient, and while it may not make the pain go away, it certainly casts a more positive light on it.

This leads to a concept that is critical in the chronic pain literature: the difference between *hurt* and *harm*. If patients experience pain and believe that it is harming them, their reaction will often be to guard themselves and restrict movements. Decreased movement typically leads to biomechanical problems and disuse syndromes that will only worsen chronic pain, but ultimately may be the only factors that keep it in place. If patients can be convinced that the pain they are experiencing, while hurting them, is not causing harm, this has profound implications for their participation in rehabilitation. Certainly, this is where a thorough medical workup is essential, because pain is often indeed a warning signal, and suggesting movement when protection is necessary can worsen the problem.

One of the better examples of reinterpretation of pain sensations came from a nurse working with patients with amputation pain. She explained to them that phantom limb pain or sensations can be overwhelming at first. However, she likened these experiences to going camping along a noisy creek. Initially, all one hears is the sound of the water, but eventually the sounds tend to move into the background of perception. Inherent in this suggestion is that phantom sensation is part of the hurting that goes with amputation and is no longer serving any type of warning or functional purpose.

Hypnotic Time Distortion

Erickson cited Cooper (Cooper & Erickson, 1959) as being one of the first to report time distortion techniques for pain control and discussed one compelling case as an example. A patient presented with "intractable attacks of lacerating pain" that occurred day and night for periods of 5 to 10 minutes, every 20 to 30 minutes. Between each episode, the patient lived in dread of the next attack. The patient was taught amnesia for the periods of the attacks. He was then taught to experience all of the pain in a 10- to 20-second trance state and then to forget that this might have happened. Thus the patient would be talking to his family, would go into a trance state, would scream in pain, and then would resume his conversation as if nothing had happened. It is interesting to note that, as discussed earlier, there was no attempt to eliminate all of this patient's pain.

Time distortion can be an effective suggestion for chronic pain, particularly when combined with confusion and amnesia. A patient may be told,

> Some time in the future—it might be a few hours from now, or perhaps a few days—you will look back and be surprised at the amount of time that you have been in a comfortable state, maybe initially that will be only for a few minutes, or maybe it will actually be a few hours. You might also find that the times during which you are in pain simply seem to shrink rapidly. What once seemed to be an hour will seem like 10 minutes or even 10 seconds. We have all had the experience of being so wrapped up in a wonderful activity that time seems to fly by,

and that is how it will seem, only the periods in which you are comfortable will just seem to slow down. Ultimately, you will look back and be amazed that you have difficulty remembering the last time you actually experienced pain.

Hypnotic Suggestions Affecting a Diminution of Pain

For patients who are not fully responsive, Erickson recommended suggestions for diminution of pain—specifically, that the pain would diminish imperceptibly, hour after hour, without the patient's awareness. He argued that suggesting that the pain diminished imperceptibly made it harder for the patient to refuse what occurred in hypnosis. He stated that the diminution of the pain (or parts of the pain) would not be noticeable, that a 1% reduction would not be noticeable, nor would a 2%, 3%, 4%, or even 5% reduction. Over sessions, the amount of pain reduction is increased, but in gradual increments that are designed to be imperceptible to the patient.

Patients often respond well to the concept of a "dial" or "rheostat" that they can use to turn down their pain in an imaginative sense. They can be given the suggestion that there is a dial on their abdomen, back, or other part of their body, and that by turning down the dial they are able to reduce their pain, much like they are able to with a dimming light switch.

Metaphors/Interspersal Technique

Erickson's use of metaphors to deliver suggestions, an approach that he often called the *interspersal technique*, was discussed in the previous chapter. In brief, suggestions for pain control are embedded in the context of a story or narrative. Erickson's most famous pain metaphor was reported with his treatment of a florist with terminal cancer pain and is reprinted below.[2]

> The author began: "Joe, I would like to talk to you. I know you are a florist, that you grow flowers, and I grew up on a farm in Wisconsin and I liked growing flowers. I still do. So I would like to have you take a seat in that easy chair as I talk to you. I'm going to say a lot of things to you but it won't be about flowers because you know more than I do about flowers. *That isn't what you want.* (The reader will note that italics will be used to denote interspersed hypnotic suggestions, which may be syllables, words, phrases, or sentences uttered with a slightly different intonation.) Now as I talk and I can do so *comfortably,* I wish that you will *listen to me comfortably* as I talk about a tomato plant. That is an odd thing to talk

[2]Excerpt reprinted from *The Collected Papers of Milton Erickson on Hypnosis: Vol. IV. Innovative Hypnotherapy* (pp. 269–271), by M. H. Erickson (E. L. Rossi, Ed.), 1980, New York, NY: Irvington. Copyright 1980 by the Erickson Foundation. Reprinted with permission.

about. It makes one *curious*. *Why talk about a tomato plant?* One puts a tomato seed in the ground. One can *feel hope* that it will grow into a tomato plant that *will bring satisfaction* by the fruit it has. The seed soaks up water, *not very much difficulty* in doing that because of the rains that *bring peace and comfort* and the joy of growing to flowers and tomatoes. That little seed, Joe, slowly swells, sends out a little rootlet with cilia on it. Now you may not know what cilia are, but cilia are *things that work* to help the tomato seed grow, to push up above the ground as a sprouting plant, and *you can listen to me Joe* so I will keep on talking and *you can keep on listening, wondering, just wondering what you can really learn,* and here is your pencil and your pad but speaking of the tomato plant, it grows so slowly. *You cannot see* it grow, *you cannot hear* it grow, but grow it does—the first little leaflike things on the stalk, the fine little hairs on the stem, those hairs are on the leaves too like the cilia on the roots, they must make the tomato plant *feel very good, very comfortable* if you can think of a plant as feeling and then, *you can't see* it growing, *you can't feel* it growing but another leaf appears on that little tomato stalk and then another. Maybe, and this is talking like a child, maybe the tomato plant does *feel comfortably and peaceful* as it grows. Each day it grows and grows and grows, *it's so comfortable Joe* to watch a plant grow and *not see* its growth *not feel* it but just know that *all is getting better* for that little tomato plant that is adding yet another leaf and still another and a branch and it is *growing comfortably* in all directions. (Much of the above by this time has been repeated many times, sometimes just phrases, sometimes sentences. Care was taken to vary the wording and also to repeat the hypnotic suggestions. Quite some time after the author had begun, Joe's wife came tiptoeing into the room carrying a sheet of paper on which was written the question, "When are you going to start the hypnosis?" The author failed to cooperate with her by looking at the paper and it was necessary for her to thrust the sheet of paper in front of the author and therefore in front of Joe. The author was continuing his description of the tomato plant uninterruptedly and Joe's wife, as she looked at Joe, saw that he was not seeing her, did not know that she was there, that he was in a somnambulistic trance. She withdrew at once.) And soon the tomato plant will have a bud form somewhere, on one branch or another, but it makes no difference because all the branches, the whole tomato plant will soon have those nice little buds—I wonder if the tomato plant can, *Joe, really feel a kind of comfort.* You know, Joe, a plant is a wonderful thing, and *it is so nice, so pleasing* just to be able to think about a plant as if it were a man. Would such a plant *have nice feelings, a sense of comfort* as the tiny little tomatoes begin to form, so tiny, yet so *full of promise to give you the desire to eat* a luscious tomato, sun-ripened, it's so *nice to have food in one's stomach,* that wonderful feeling a child, a thirsty child, has and can *want a drink, Joe* is that the way the tomato plant feels when the rain falls and washes everything so that *all feels well.* (pause) *You know, Joe,* a tomato plant just flourishes each day *just a day at a time.* I like to think the tomato plant can *know the fullness of comfort each day. You know, Joe, just one day at a time* for the tomato plant. That's the way for all tomato plants. (Joe suddenly came out of the trance, appeared disoriented, hopped upon the bed, waved his arms and his behavior was highly suggestive of the sudden surges of toxicity one sees in patients who have reacted unfavorably to barbiturates. Joe did not seem to hear or see the author until he hopped off the bed and had walked toward the author. A firm grip was taken on Joe's arm and then immediately loosened. The nurse was summoned. She mopped perspiration from his forehead, changed his surgical dressings, and gave him, by tube, some ice water. Joe then let the author lead him back to his chair. After a pretense by the author of being curious about Joe's forearm, Joe seized his pencil and paper and wrote, "Talk, talk.") "Oh yes, Joe, I grew up on a farm, I think a tomato seed is a wonderful thing, *think, Joe, think* in that little seed there does *sleep so restfully, so comfortably* a beautiful plant yet to be grown that will bear such interesting leaves and branches. The leaves, the branches look so beautiful, that beautiful rich color, *you can really feel happy* looking at a tomato seed, thinking about the wonderful plant it contains *asleep, resting, comfortable, Joe*. I'm soon going to leave for lunch and I'll be back and I will talk some more. (Erickson, 1980b, pp. 269–271).

SUMMARY

A premise of this book is that directly focusing on pain reduction during hypnosis may not always be the best way to facilitate the patient's comfort and well-being. Using hypnosis to change the patients' lifestyle, encourage him or her to move therapeutically, or simply improve his or her sleep may ultimately have the strongest impact on the well-being of a patient reporting chronic pain. However, there are many instances in which focusing on pain can be of tremendous benefit, particularly if the pain is driven by some type of lesion or ongoing nociceptive signals. Even if the goal is to get at lifestyle changes of the patient or underlying dynamics that are driving the pain, using hypnosis to increase comfort can increase rapport and invest the patient in the more comprehensive treatment process that is often necessary to control pain.

It is interesting to note that the creative list of hypnotic analgesic suggestions developed by Erickson seldom had the purpose of eliminating pain. Rather, the goal of his suggestions was usually to change the perception of pain and gradually reduce rather than eliminate it. What we still do not know is what type of suggestion is going to work with a given patient at a particular time. The several types of creative suggestions offered by Erickson can be put in a multiple-choice format as is consistent with indirect suggestions.

6

ACUTE PAIN, CRISIS, AND THE HOSPITAL SETTING

This book generally divides pain into acute and chronic categories, each of which requires markedly different approaches with respect to medical and psychological treatments, including hypnotic analgesia. Acute pain, in turn, can be further subdivided into different categories that are useful when considering specific hypnotic approaches. The acute pain settings addressed in this chapter include settings in which patients are already experiencing acute pain (typically in as hospitalized inpatients) at the time clinicians choose to use hypnotic techniques. Such inpatient treatment settings can also include the intensive care unit (ICU). Not only is the ICU an environment in which patients experience frequent acute pain and anxiety, but it also presents unique environmental and cognitive challenges (and opportunities) for the use of hypnosis. The chapter also discusses procedural pain—acute pain that occurs in response to medical procedures. Such procedures are a common source of acute pain and anxiety and are particularly amenable to hypnosis because of their predictable timing. The approaches in this chapter have been discussed in a number of earlier publications (M. P. Jensen & Patterson, 2008; Patterson, 1996, 2009; Wiechman Askay & Patterson, 2007), although none of them has addressed this topic in the detail put forth here.

THE NATURE OF ACUTE PAIN

Acute pain occurs in the presence of tissue damage. At the site of tissue damage, receptors for pain called *nociceptors* are activated by heat, pressure, and other forms of injury. Such nociceptors transmit afferent pain signals through sensory neurons of two general types: A-delta fibers and C fibers. A-delta fibers are small and myelinated, and therefore transmit information rapidly (sometimes called *fast pain* fibers). This is why, for example, when one stubs a toe, a quick, initial, and transient pain signal is received in the brain suggesting that "this is really going to hurt." In contrast, C fibers are thinner and unmyelinated; hence, sensory signals are transmitted more slowly through them (hence they are sometimes called *slow pain* fibers). Thus, when one stubs a toe, the initial burst of pain is followed shortly thereafter by a dull, throbbing, and more long-lasting pain due to C fiber transmission. One important message here is the strong association between actual tissue damage and the pain signals that are transmitted to the brain in settings of acute pain. In contrast, such association is not always present in chronic pain. It should also be noted that acute pain serves as a useful warning sign. If one is using a table saw and feels a painful sensation in the hand, this suggests that it is a very good idea to pull the hand away before the entire limb is severed. In this way, acute pain serves a very adaptive purpose.

Not only does acute pain often warn a person that something might be terribly wrong, it also initiates a series of evolutionally adaptive physiological and emotional responses. Often, the flight-or-flight response will be evoked, mediated by the release of excitatory neurotransmitters (e.g., epinephrine) from the adrenal glands. In behavioral terms, a patient in acute pain may become physically agitated and combative, may attempt to flee the situation, or may experience a type of "freezing and withdrawal." Such responses are all adaptive in evolutionary terms. Particularly when a person is being attacked, such fight-or-flight responses increase the chance of survival. Importantly, psychological treatment for acute pain often involves teaching the patient that such responses are no longer necessary or useful. However, convincing patients of such concepts is often not easy because the clinician is working against a cascade of instinctually driven physiological responses.

Another important feature of acute pain is that it activates arousal and vigilance. If our ancestors felt the pain of an arrow piercing their arm, it would immediately suggest the presence of a significant threat in their environment and that actions to detect the source of the threat and escape it (if not fight it) would be advisable. Such responses serve an obvious adaptive purpose. However, as discussed earlier, in the absence of a clear threat, such responses to acute pain are often counterproductive in psychological terms. Specifically, heightened vigilance and arousal are often precursors to anxiety, which both accompany and exacerbate acute pain. Similarly, acute pain elicits anxiety. Thus, acute pain and anxiety can cyclically interact so that they both are exacerbated. The sympathetic neuroendocrine response that accompanies anxiety can serve to heighten the sensitivity to painful stimuli and to amplify the pain experience. In our own research, my colleagues and I have found that providing anxiolytic drugs such as lorazepam (Ativan) in conjunction with opioid analgesics reduced pain during burn wound care (a form of acute procedural pain) better than did opioid analgesics alone (Patterson, Ptacek, Carrougher, & Sharar, 1997). Such findings demonstrate that anxiety can accompany acute pain, and that by treating it appropriately, one can more effectively reduce the pain experience.

Although an initial burst of acute pain can serve as a useful warning sign, ongoing acute pain can have a number of dire consequences. Patients receiving care for painful conditions (e.g., burn injuries, cancer, fractured bones, nonhealing wounds) may be subjected to acute pain repeatedly and/or over an extended period of time, due to associated therapeutic procedures or the condition itself. Such pain has been associated with a number of negative physiological effects.

As is the case with any type of trauma, both functional and emotional recovery can be hindered by the presence of acute pain. Burn pain provides a good example of the physiological side effects of acute pain that can contribute to an adverse stress response. These include (a) sympathetic neuroendocrine system activation resulting in the release of catecholamines, (b) sympathetic system influences on immune function, (c) adrenergic stimulation of bacterial growth, (d) norepinephrine regulation of myelopoiesis; and (e) release of glucocorticoids (Bonica, 1990; G. Smith & Covino, 1985). Remarkably, the severity of acute burn pain has been shown to influence posthospitalization emotional recovery to a greater extent than the size of the burn, the length of hospitalization, or even the patient's preinjury mental health. Ptacek and colleagues (Ptacek, Patterson, Montgomery, Ordonez, & Heimbach, 1995), for example, reported that early, postinjury pain scores were associated more strongly than any other predictor variable with distress and quality-of-life scores 1 month following hospital discharge. Another study suggested that this relationship held at 1-year posthospitalization (Martin-Herz, Patterson, Ptacek, Finch, & Heimbach, 1998). Future studies will likely substantiate the practical utility and importance of adequate burn pain treatment.

Whereas untreated pain can have negative physiological effects, successfully treated pain can likely improve health outcome. There is evidence that good pain treatment can improve immune and cardiovascular function (Chapman, 1985; Chapman & Bonica, 1983; Mackersie & Karagianes, 1990). Further, there is some preliminary evidence that when children with burn injuries receive more opioid analgesics (e.g., morphine), they not only experience less acute pain but also later demonstrate fewer symptoms of post-traumatic stress disorder (Saxe et al., 2001). Thus, there is substantial evidence to indicate the benefits of treating acute pain not only for immediate humane reasons but also because of long-term benefits to the patient's eventual health and well-being (J. T. Smith, Barabasz, & Barabasz, 1996). It should be noted that patients being treated for acute pain in the hospital potentially enter the setting with drug and alcohol problems (Wiechman Askay, Bombardier, & Patterson, 2009); often this can be a reason to provide more medication to patients early on, given their increased drug tolerance and anxiety, but also to manage medications carefully, particularly at discharge.

THE HOSPITAL ENVIRONMENT

Little has been written on the psychological impact of hospitalization. This is unfortunate because the hospital environment can have a great impact on a patient's emotional state and potential response to hypnosis, and hypnotic treatment for the acute pain will often occur in the hospital setting. It is difficult to provide any universal description of a hospital environment because such environments differ widely. Trauma hospitals, for example, are often dominated by surgical services and may focus on ortho-pedics, neurosurgery, and general surgery. General hospitals tend to focus more on illness, with internal medicine as the dominant form of medicine. Other hospitals have almost an exclusive focus on cancer treatment, with oncology as the dominant form of medicine. The type of diagnosis and the specialty of medicine have much to do with what the nature of the hospital environment will be and what challenges it might present to the patient emotionally. Hospitals also vary substantially in terms of size, socioeconomic status, and demographics (e.g., urban vs. rural setting). The experience of a patient in a large-county urban trauma hospital will vary markedly from one in a small rural general hospital.

There are also basic commonalities among hospital environments. First, if a patient is in a hospital, there is almost always some sort of threat to health. Such threat may range from a life-threatening disease to the outcome of a minor surgery; in either case, some degree of uncertainly accompanies being in that environment. Even if the reason for a particular admission does not involve a threat, the patient may still respond negatively to hospitalization. The hospital environment, much like the courtroom, can become a conditioned stimulus for anxiety for many patients. Environmental characteristics of hospitals include sterility, blandness, and the smell of antiseptic and other chemicals. Almost certainly, patients in the hospital are removed from the established comforts of home, including their clothes, bed, food, and recreation.

An interesting feature of hospitalization is that patients usually face a series of requests or demands that they will seldom experience at any other time in their lives. Over the course of a hospitalization, patients may be asked to change into gowns, take new medication, go through multiple tests, defecate into bedpans, change fluid intake, eat a restricted diet, and undergo any number of potentially painful procedures or surgeries. To cope with hospitalization, patients must go through what might be regarded as an adaptive dependency. In other words, they will respond willingly to a number of requests or subtle demands without questioning them, ones that they would typically not dream of acquiescing to in everyday circumstances.

Ironically, such adaptive dependency is a process that will facilitate hypnosis rather than work against it. If a patient has agreed to take off his or her clothes in a strange setting, tolerate a needle being stuck in the arm, or provide a stool sample, it is difficult for the patient to regard hypnosis as being an equal challenge, in terms of unpleasantness. Being asked to relax and follow beneficial hypnotic suggestions seldom rivals the typical level of challenges that patients face in the hospital environment.

However, other characteristics of the hospital environment might potentially impede hypnosis. Sedating medication can interfere with the attention necessary for patients to respond to an induction. Poor sleep, nausea, illness, and pain are all factors that may make hypnosis more difficult to perform. Hospitals are notoriously noisy and disruptive settings, and clinicians should anticipate potential interruptions to inductions.

INTENSIVE CARE

The intensive care unit (ICU) takes many of the above features of the hospital environment to an extreme. While hospitalization may elicit some sort of vague general sense of anxiety in patients, ICU care often can be interpreted as a threat to their lives. High-technology equipment in the ICU is often noisy and disruptive to sleep. Because of illness, medication, disturbed metabolic factors, and poor sleep, patients are often fatigued and overwhelmed. ICU psychosis (delirium) is common, not only because of the aforementioned factors but also because some patients mentally "check out" as an adaptive response (Patterson, Ehde, & Ptacek, 1994).

Because of these variables, there are a number of ways that hypnosis should be conducted in the ICU to make it more successful. First, patients in the ICU seldom have the attention or vigilance for a long induction. A 20-minute induction with deep relaxation will be more likely to put the patient to sleep as much as anything. Second, ICU patients are often straightforward and simple with respect to their cognitive functioning. Inductions that contain elaborate or confusing language will often be lost on this patient population. Often, family members, and even some staff, do not realize that the patient's ability to process and retain information during intensive care is extremely limited. It is common for patients to have minimal recall of even extended stays in the ICU.

Not only is it easy to overestimate a patient's cognitive capacity in the ICU, but it is also a challenge to appreciate how basic psychological needs are. Certainly, when patients are overwhelmed, their focus may be much more on moment-to-moment survival or reducing pain rather than long-term adjustment concerns. It stands to follow that it might be tempting to assume that a patient with a traumatic amputation is attempting to cope with their limb loss, when their true concern is if they will live to see another day. Accordingly, the goals of hypnosis will likely have much more to do with simple comfort and reassurance than to address long-term issues.

The hypnotic induction and related commentary in Appendix 6.1 are designed for the patient on the ICU. The appendix addresses several of the environmental and patient issues described in the section above.

ACUTE NONPROCEDURAL PAIN (EMERGENCY ROOM CARE)

Most acute pain comes from trauma (e.g., blunt force injuries, cuts), flare-ups from disease processes (e.g., sickle cell anemia), or health care procedures. Pain from trauma or disease processes usually occurs without warning and presents a significant sense of suffering and anxiety for the patient. If the pain is from trauma, the patient's mental state will show many of the characteristics discussed previously. He or she may withdraw, show self-protective behavior, and be limited in cognitive resources. Although such injuries will typically have no enduring effect on cognition, patients typically will be in survival mode; they will be focused only on escaping the pain or addressing the threat that is creating it. They may show dissociative functioning if the threat is of enough significance. Although it is not possible to predict patients' cognitive state, the main point here is that their capacity to manage complex information will be hindered. Their behavior will be directed toward the goal of eliminating their pain or the threat that is causing it.

It follows that hypnosis with this population should usually be quick and simple. The patient will have neither the capacity nor the desire to follow any sort of long, complex induction. However, unlike the typical ICU patient described above, these patients will likely have less medication in their system and will show more capacity for cognitive functioning. As such, hypnotic intervention for a patient in acute pain or crisis differs from the ICU model described above.

The somewhat dated transactional analysis model of psychotherapy (describing parent, child, and adult ego states) or more recent writings on ego state therapy (Barabasz & Watkins, 2005; H. H. Watkins & Watkins, 1997; J. G. Watkins & Barabasz, 2008) provide a useful framework for intervening in crisis (Berne, 1975). What is useful from this model for crisis intervention is that the patient is often in a "child" ego state when in acute pain. The nature of the trauma or pain often leads the patient to be emotionally regressed and dependent on those around them. Effective clinical intervention often requires the clinician to take on a "parent" role. Specifically, the clinician often must be directive rather than permissive. Patients in this situation do not want choices; they need to be focused on activity and often must be told what to do. Elisabeth Kübler-Ross, author of *On Death and Dying* (1969), related the story of a mother who was at home when her husband and children were killed in a car crash. A friend went over to comfort her. The mother was clearly distraught and in crisis. The friend's response was to instruct the mother to organize her shoe collection. She had quite a large collection and was able to remain calm when simply given the task of organizing them; this allowed her at least to get through the immediate emotional crisis.

The point here is that when one is working hypnotically with a patient who is in crisis, it is important to model calmness and to give the patient something to do. Thus, in talking with a distraught patient, the clinician calmly repeats a message over and over. If the patient is emotionally out of control, it may be necessary to match his or her affect first, with a directive comment, and then begin to model calm affect. For example, if a patient is screaming "I am hurting!" and the clinician cannot get his or her attention, the clinician may reflect the statement, "You are hurting! And you are also able to hear my voice and do exactly what I say." Appendix 6.2 provides an example of hypnotic induction for acute pain and crisis.

PROCEDURAL PAIN

Another type of acute pain is that from medical procedures such as dentistry, surgery, burn wound care, or cancer treatment. Although labor and delivery pain is not caused by a health care professional, it shares most characteristics of such procedural pain. Unlike most other forms of acute pain, pain caused by procedures is usually predictable at its onset. Procedural pain typically creates a significant amount of discomfort that is fortunately limited in duration.

The fact that procedural pain is usually a predictable event is both a hindrance and an advantage in terms of treatment. Because patients are usually aware that they will be undergoing a painful procedure, they have the opportunity to build up a great deal of anticipatory anxiety. This is particularly the case with children. As discussed in Chapter 2, children have been known to develop conditioned phobic responses to hospital scrubs (typically green in color). They become anxious when the person wearing green enters the room. Often, and particularly with children, the anxiety associated with a painful event becomes a more significant management problem than the pain itself. Moreover, as noted early on in this chapter, anxiety and acute pain have a cyclical relationship, and anxiety can exacerbate the pain. As mentioned, in our own research, we have discovered that giving patients with burn injuries benzodiazepine-class drugs (i.e., tranquilizers) can reduce the amount of pain they report during procedures.

The predictability of a procedure also presents an advantage to treatment. Specifically, knowing when patients are to undergo painful procedures provides a window of opportunity to prepare them for both pharmacological and psychological interventions. For example, if we know that patients are going to have their burn injuries cleaned at a particular time of the day, they can be medicated 30 minutes before with a tranquilizer that will offset anticipatory anxiety. For the procedure itself, a highly potent, short-acting opioid agonist pain medication, such as synthetic morphine (Patterson & Sharar, 2001), can be used.

The predictable nature of procedural pain has similar advantages with the application of hypnosis. In fact, hypnosis with procedural pain and anxiety is one of the more effective applications of hypnosis for any type of health care issue (see Elvira Lang's seminal work in this area; e.g., Lang, in press; Lang et al., 2000). If we know a patient has an impending procedure, we can do a hypnotic induction—even several inductions—well before the procedure is scheduled to occur. Working with a patient before the procedure often has the advantage of the patient largely being free from the effects of large doses of pain medication or anxiety.

A useful paradigm for using hypnosis for reducing pain from medical procedures is to transform the stimuli that would normally elicit anxiety into cues for comfort and relaxation. This is done effectively in the Rapid Induction Analgesia technique described by J. Barber (1977). For any medical procedure, there are going to be some absolutes for the patient in terms of the environment. For example, in the case of patients undergoing surgery, it is a given that they will enter a health care facility, interact with health care professionals, and have an intravenous (IV) line placed. Normally, as the time for a medical procedure nears, each one of these events will be a cue for increased anxiety. When patients walk into a hospital the day of an invasive procedure, their heart rate and blood pressure likely increase, and when a nurse walks into the room with an IV line, their anxiety will likely increase more. If these very cues can be ones that elicit deep relaxation rather than anxiety, then there can be a potential benefit to the patient. Not only will he or she have a cue to experience comfort and analgesia at an important moment before the procedure, but the trend of escalating anxiety often occurring before a threatening procedure can be mitigated or interrupted.

An important advantage to this paradigm, and generally the use of posthypnotic suggestions, is that the hypnotist does not have to be physically present at the procedures. Unless the hypnotist is the surgeon, anesthesiologist, or some other clinician who is present for the procedure on a regular basis, it will seldom be practical or possible to be present at the actual procedure. Using the approach described in the next section, the clinician can train the patient before the procedure and build in cues for posthypnotic suggesting that the patient cannot miss.

HYPNOSIS FOR MEDICAL PROCEDURES

The characteristics of procedural pain described in the previous section allow for a simple but effective paradigm for using hypnosis. The steps are discussed in this section.

Identifying the Impending Threatening Event and the Affective State That the Patient Desires to Have During It

The first step is to identify the procedure that the patient finds threatening (this will usually, of course, be the referral issue). Typical issues might include surgery, cancer treatment procedures, dental procedures, or childbirth. However, this approach can be used to address many sorts of anxiety-producing future events, for example, courtroom appearances, public speaking, and exams. Once the event is identified, the clinician can determine how patients predict how they will affectively experience the event. Presumably, they will want to feel deeply relaxed and comfortable, but it is a good idea to have the patients report how they would like to experience the procedure.

Eliciting Comfortable Imagery From the Patient

Generating positive imagery is often very useful in hypnosis, but clinicians should not assume that one patient's relaxing imagery is good for another. For example, one might assume that the beach is a desirable location, but some patients find that imagery to be threatening. Therefore, it is a good idea to ask patients where they like to go to relax. A surprising number have told me that they like to relax "at a chair in their home" and prefer this over some sort of exotic nature imagery. In any case, it is also useful to find some descriptors associated with the patient's favorite place to relax. If a patient says she likes to go to the mountains, the clinician should have her describe what the mountains are like, whether there are trees and water, and so on.

Identifying Cues Associated With the Medical Procedure

An important step before the induction begins is to identify cues associated with the medical procedure. However, it is not sufficient to say to a surgical patient, "When you go into surgery, you will feel completely relaxed." The cues have to be carefully selected on the basis of what the patient will consciously experience and also in a way that accounts for potential last-minute changes. To tell the patient that she will be relaxed when she is rolled into the surgical room may not be useful as she may be amnesic from sedation by that point. Further, suggesting that "seeing Dr. Jones" will be the reminder for comfort may not account for last-minute changes unless it is assured that surgery will take place only with this particular doctor.

Consequently, posthypnotic cues should be based on absolutes. If a patient is having a chemotherapy treatment, it is almost certain that it will be in a given facility. The patient will have to go through doors to enter the facility. At some point, the patient will experience an IV line being inserted into a vein. In the case of surgery, it is almost certain that the patient will enter a hospital or treatment facility. He or she will have to change into a hospital gown. The nature of the cues is going to differ given what the procedure will be and who the patient is. The important step at this point is to gather several environmental cues that will reflect the reality that the patient experiences.

Using Hypnotic Induction With an Emphasis on Deep Relaxation

The type of induction used is largely a matter of what the clinician and patient find useful. However, for the purpose of procedural pain control, it will almost always be beneficial if the induction involves deep relaxation. Ultimately, the patient will be given hypnotic suggestions to return to a state of deep relaxation during the procedures, so if such experiences can be generated during the induction, the intervention will likely be more useful. Typically such inductions will include counting for deepening and progressive relaxation of body areas. For a greatly abbreviated example, you might say, "I am going to count from 1 to 10. As I count each number, you will find yourself becoming deeper and deeper relaxed." Then, as the patient is counted down, he or she is brought through a type of rapid progressive relaxation: "One, you can feel relaxation on the top of your head and it starts to spread down through your forehead like warm pancake batter. Two, down through your face, your mouth and jaw, down into your neck. Three, deep comfortable warmth spreading down into your shoulders." This obviously can be done with more indirect hypnotic suggestions or different imagery. The point is that the induction will likely be most useful if deep relaxation is part of the suggestions.

Linking Posthypnotic Cues to the Cues Associated With the Procedures

When the patient has reached an adequate level of depth of relaxation, his or her imagery can be introduced, "And now that you are deeply and comfortably relaxed, you find yourself at your favorite spot in the forest (or at the beach, at home, etc.). Notice what the trees look like around you (enter in imagery based on the patient's report)." At this point, the link with the medical procedure can be introduced. This is where posthypnotic suggestions are linked with the environmental cues surrounding the procedure. Labor pain and delivery are used in the following example.

> And now that you are in your comfortable place, profoundly relaxed, without a care in the world, you begin to realize some amazing things. Wouldn't it be interesting if you found yourself returning to this very comfortable state whenever it might be the most important to? I wonder what it might take to remind you to suddenly be again in the comfortable place you are right now? Perhaps you will find that when you are in the hospital and your contractions become strong and regular, that will be the signal for this to happen. Perhaps being told to push will have a very interesting effect on you, that you find yourself breathing slowly and regularly, like you are now, and it will all seem so easy. Wouldn't it be interesting if the realization that you are delivering a baby becomes the signal? That understanding, that you are actually delivering, suddenly reminds you to return to all the comfort that you have right now. Maybe you will become profoundly relaxed when you enter the hospital, maybe it will be when your contractions grow, or maybe it will be the actual process of delivery. I don't really know, I only ask you if it would indeed be of benefit if all the comfort you are experiencing now came rushing back with really no effort at all.

The link between environmental cues and posthypnotic suggestions can be put in a number of ways. For a highly hypnotizable patient or one who is fairly concrete in thinking, the suggestions can be more direct. "When you enter the surgery area on the day of surgery, all the comfort you are experiencing now will come back instantly. This will be your cue for deep relaxation." The example in the previous paragraph reflects more indirect styles of giving hypnotic suggestions.

Alerting

After providing the posthypnotic suggestion, the clinician can return patients to their relaxing place. Before bringing them out of the hypnotic state, it is a good idea to provide the patients with the opportunity for completion. If patients are having a pleasant experience with hypnosis, they often are reluctant to leave this state. In addition, the hypnotic suggestions may have not hit the area of core importance for the patient. For this reason, it is often useful to allow patients to provide any self-suggestions they would like.

> In a moment you will find yourself slowing returning to an awake state. Before we start, however, I would like to give you the opportunity to experience anything you would like or to even give yourself some suggestions. What I will do is to give you 30 seconds of silence to experience anything you would like, 30 seconds of silence, starting now.

The clinician can then bring the patient out of the hypnotic state using counting or whatever means fits into the initial induction.

SUMMARY

Acute pain differs from chronic pain because it is short-lived but often practically unbearable and intertwined with anxiety. Because it tends to occur at predictable times, using hypnosis to reduce acute pain is one of the most practical, as well as empirically supported, applications of this treatment. Clinicians can become hardened to the fact that hospitalization is an extremely unpleasant, anxiety-provoking experience for patients. Not only are patients removed from practically everything that is rewarding in their lives, but they are also often dealing with a major threat to their health.

Hypnosis is very much underused as a means to reduce pain, anxiety, and suffering in this context. It can and should be used much more frequently, although the clinician should be aware of the challenges faced by hospitalized patients (i.e., medications, health issues, sleep deprivation, etc.). The other prominent application of hypnosis to acute pain is for patients undergoing medical procedures. Dentistry, surgery, child delivery, burn care, and other invasive procedures are all capable of causing pain and anxiety. Hypnosis can be used efficiently for procedural pain by working with the patient before the procedure begins and working to build in posthypnotic suggestions for comfort, relaxation, and analgesia during the procedure. The use of hypnosis for acute pain is often straightforward, and even clinicians who are novices in its use should consider attempting this modality.

APPENDIX 6.1: HYPNOTIC INDUCTION FOR THE INTENSIVE CARE UNIT

The following is an example of a hypnotic induction designed for the patient on the intensive care unit that is based on an induction reported by Patterson (1996).

> You have been through quite a trauma and I'm part of the team that focuses on getting you out of the hospital and back to work as soon as possible. I am also interested in making you as comfortable as possible as you go through the remainder of your care.

Comment: The implicit message is that with regard to survival, the patient is over the worst. The possibility of the patient's not surviving is not raised.

> As a way to make our patients more comfortable, we often offer hypnotic treatment in addition to their pain medication. I wanted to see if you would be interested in this type of approach. Would you like to begin right now?

Comment: The statement that many patients go through hypnotic treatment normalizes this approach. Patients often fear that we will reduce their pain medication but may be afraid to admit this; therefore, hypnotic treatment is offered as an addition to analgesic drugs. It is rare for patients to refuse hypnotic treatment on the ICU, as long as they are aware that their pain medication will not be reduced. Often this offer is met with statements such as, "I'll try anything to get rid of this pain."

> Now, will it be OK if, as a result of our talk, you find yourself going into a comfortable sleeplike state from which you can awake at any time?

Comment: Some patients will need to be hypervigilant about their care or may not respond to a dissociative hypnotic suggestion, for whatever reason. This question is designed to assess such concerns in layperson's terms. Note that the patient's choice regarding waking up is offered to counteract the patient's perceiving sleep as a metaphor for death.

> Good, now where do you like to go to relax?

Comment: A description of the patient's favorite place to relax is elicited, including descriptors that will later be used to stimulate imagery from a variety of sensory modalities.

> Fine. Now close your eyes, take a deep breath, and let it out very slowly.

> (As the patient lets his or her breath out, I put my hand on the patient's forehead and gently turn the head to one side.)

> That's fine.

Comment: The instructions are brief, straightforward, and simple. Moving the patient's head is designed to surprise the patient, capture the patient's attention, communicate the therapist's willingness to actively intervene, and facilitate the induction.

> Now I am going to count from 1 to 10. With each number I count, allow yourself to become deeper and deeper relaxed. When I reach 10, you will find yourself in a very deep, very comfortable state of relaxation. Are you ready to begin? One, two, three . . . that's right, find yourself becoming more and more relaxed as the numbers grow larger. Notice how slow your breathing is. Four, five, six . . . Good, just letting yourself sink deeper into the bed. Just listening to the sounds of my voice, becoming more and more relaxed, really slowing down your breathing now. Seven . . . your head and neck are so deeply relaxed now. Your arms and legs, your whole body just heavy and relaxed. Eight . . . the only thing you can hear is my voice . . . the only thing you can notice is how comfortable you are. We are almost there. Nine . . . really noticing that deep feeling of relaxation, heaviness, and comfort, really feeling your breathing slowing down. Deeper and deeper, and now ten.

(At the count of 10, the therapist puts a palm on the patient's forehead and move it gently to one side again.)

Comment: The counting begins at a relatively quick pace. As the induction progresses, it slows and the pauses between statements lengthen.

> That's right, deeply, deeply relaxed. It's as if you are asleep but you can still hear my voice. And as I continue talking, you find that you are at your relaxing place.

(The patient's identified relaxation scenario is specifically identified.)

> Notice what you see there . . . what does it smell like? You are absolutely comfortable when you go to your place.
>
> Now, as you remain in your comfortable place, I would like you to notice how comfortable it feels to be this way, and how you can become more and more relaxed and you continue breathing slowly . . . now. I would like you to go to a level where you are absolutely comfortable, a state of mind where your body will know just what you need to do to get yourself better.
>
> As you continue to move closer and closer to the special state of mind, I would like you to know that when you get there, a special part of your mind will give us a signal. Specifically, when you are at a place where your mind will really help you feel comfortable, safe and knowing what you need to know to heal your wounds quickly, it will signal us by allowing this finger to rise seemingly on its own power.

Comment: The notion of a "special part of the mind" can be substituted for the "unconscious," or whatever metaphor is comfortable to the clinician and patient.

(Upon seeing the finger rise)

> Good. Now as you remain at this very special place, notice how good it feels to know that deep inside you know what it will take to move through your care comfortably and safely.

Comment: This finger signaling allows the patient to be the judge of what constitutes his or her optimal level of comfort and to quicken the pace of the overall induction. The patient almost always provides this signal. However, if no finger signal occurs, the therapist can work around this by assuring the patients that they can benefit no matter what their current experience is or that they may actually reach their optimal level some time in the future.

> . . . that you will heal quickly and that you will move through care with only those sensations that you need to have. In fact, it will be perfectly okay if the only thing that you feel during your care is a sense of well-being and relaxation.

Comment: Some patients may need to have some experience of pain, so it is desirable to give them control over the amount of analgesia they will experience.

> You are doing very well. Now just continue to stay in the state of mind where you find out that there are things you can do to recover in a rapid and comfortable fashion. You may stay in this comfortable state for as long as you would like.

Comment: At this point, any other hypnotic suggestions that the patient may need can be implemented, such as suggestions for increased performance in therapy or improved appetite.

> In fact, at the time you are ready to return to a wakeful state, we will allow your finger to signal us once again by slowing rising up again.

Comment: The patient is left to decide when to return from the induction via this signaling. Patients often need these instructions repeated, particularly if they are in a deep state of relaxation.

> That's very good. In a moment I will begin counting back so you can return to a temporary state of alertness. Before I do, however, I want you to remember a couple of things. First, whenever I touch you on the forehead like this, whenever the nurse touches you on the forehead like this, or whenever your [spouse] touches you on the forehead like this, you will become relaxed as you are right now. Even more comfortable that you feel right now.

This sequence can be repeated for emphasis.

I also want to remind you that you can return to your comfortable place whenever you want. As a matter of fact, you will find yourself counting from 1 to 10 and going to your place before all of your future dressing changes. Now, I am going to count from 10 back to 1. When I reach the number 1, you will find yourself alert, awake, and comfortable. However, you will also know that you can return to a deeply relaxed state from now on, whenever it will benefit you.

The patient is counted back up with hypnotic suggestions for wakefulness.

Comment: The presence of the signal is reinforced by the response, "That's very good." This is a very important reassurance and encouragement to the patient. On the ICU, it is often desirable to have close family members observe the induction and participate in the posthypnotic suggestion.

With hypnotic treatment on the ICU, states of wakefulness are regarded as being as transient as hypnotic states. The patient is given the message that he or she will be alert until the next painful procedure. Occasionally, patients are left in the hypnotic state with the instructions that they will return to an awake state when they are fully rested and ready to continue their care in a comfortable matter.

APPENDIX 6.2: INDUCTION FOR ACUTE PAIN AND CRISIS (AND THE EMERGENCY ROOM)

This induction combines all of the major elements of quick inductions, including Ericksonian technique and ideomotor signaling. Designed for situations in which the clinician does not have much time to work with the patient, examples may include patients in the hospital emergency room or intensive care unit, or those who are in acute pain or anxiety when the clinician reaches them. Frischholz (personal communication, June 25, 2009) correctly pointed out the many similarities between the early part of this induction and Spiegel and Spiegel's (1978) induction that is part of the Hypnotic Induction Profile. When hypnosis is done rapidly, there is the risk of bringing the patient out too quickly, which may in turn cause unpleasant confusion or headaches. What is effective about this induction is that it relies on patient feedback at every stage, which allows the clinician to work quickly but with the assurance that the patient has reached the various states that are desired. The induction should begin with the patient sitting comfortably in a chair, or upright in a bed, with his or her hands resting on each thigh (or on either side, if in bed). It is good clinical practice to alert patients that they will be touched, particularly as their wrist may sit in their lap at the beginning of the induction. Having the patient begin to have the arm get lighter sets the stage for hypnotic suggestions to come.

> I am going to help you quickly reach a hypnotic state that will allow you to control your pain (anxiety, itching, nausea, etc.) more effectively. Are you willing to follow all of my instructions? Good. At some point, if it is OK with you, I will be touching your wrist here. I would like you to begin by just getting the sense that this hand (wrist, arm) is becoming lighter, like it is hollow and filled with warm air.
>
> Very good. I now want you to roll your eyes up and look at my finger (the finger rests on the forehead, in between the eyes, about an inch above them). Now, as you keep your eyeballs up, I want you to take a deep breath. Hold your breath, and keep you eyes looking up. As you keep your eyeballs looking up, I now want you to close your eyes and let your breath out. Very good.

At this moment, put the flat of your hand on the patient's forehead and gently push, perhaps tilting the patient's head back slightly. The eye roll and the touch on the forehead are quick induction techniques. The touch on the forehead surprises patients and breaks their habituation patterns.

> Now, as you continue to become more and more relaxed, I would like you to notice if your arm here is becoming lighter and lighter. So light that I am going to take your wrist now and wouldn't it be interesting if that hand and arm float up in the air all by itself?

At this point, the clinician takes the patient's wrist and gently lifts up the arm so that it is about eye level. A slight jiggle is given to the wrist so that there is an implicit hypnotic suggestion for the arm to remain in the air.

Comment: Having the arm float in the air is another quick induction technique. If the patient's arm remains in the air, then they are very likely following hypnotic suggestions and doing well with the induction. If the arm feels heavy and doesn't seem to want to lift in the air, then it is best to follow that lead with a statement such as, "Or perhaps you are finding that your arm has become heavier and wants to sit at your side."

> Very good. You notice how that hand is floating comfortably in the air. And, all the time you are becoming more and more comfortable and focusing more and more on the sound of my voice. Now, after your hand stays in the air for a certain amount of time, isn't it natural for it to become heavier and slowly move down? You may notice that happen now, the hand is moving down ever so slightly. And as it moves down, that can be a signal— a signal from your mind to you. That the farther the arm moves down the more comfortable you will feel. So that eventually, when your arm rests on your leg (or bedside), that will be your mind's way of letting you know that you are just as comfortable as is going to be useful to you right now.

Comment: This is a particularly good technique for a patient who is struggling with resistance. Once in the air, the hand may move down, move up, or stay in the same place. Using the principle of utilization, the clinician follows the patient's lead ("Or perhaps as you become more relaxed, your hand seems to float upward"). In most cases the hand moves downward and becomes a contingent hypnotic suggestion. When it rests on the lap, that becomes a signal for relaxation.

As the hand moves downward, the clinician makes hypnotic suggestions for increased relaxation and comfort. At the time it rests at the patient's side, the clinician reinforces this.

> Good! Deeply, deeply relaxed, deeper with every breath you take. Now, as you continue to breathe slowly and comfortably, I would like to talk to the part of your mind that is a friend to you. It is the part of your mind that allows you to keep breathing and keep your heart beating, even when you are not aware of it. It is the part of your mind that can be a tremendous resource when you need it to be. It may be that you find the rest of your mind going off to a nice comfortable beach, or just sitting in the chair here, or even listening to my voice, but it is the special part of your mind that I will talk to now.

Comment: The "special part" of the mind can be a metaphor for the unconscious and can reflect whatever theoretical comfort the clinician and patient have for this material. In any case, much of the language here is geared to create dissociation. There are also elements of mild confusion to help work with patients who are trying to track cognitively the induction too aggressively.

> What I would like to ask that part of your mind to do now is give you a signal. That at the time you have become just as relaxed as you need to be right now, your mind will let you know by allowing this finger to move up in the air (indicate finger with a touch). It will be as if a string is tied to that finger, pulling it up in the air; the rest of you mind may not even be aware that it is happening.

Comment: Note that the finger signal is suggested in a manner that elicits dissociation and automaticity in behavior. I do *not* say "raise your finger when you are comfortable." When the patient raises his or her finger, be sure to reinforce it, "That's right! Absolutely relaxed." A small percentage of patients do not show a finger signal. In such cases it is fine to go ahead with the induction and not focus on it. Do not let the lack of a finger signal throw you off, as I have had a great deal of success in most of the inductions where I do not get it. Whether or not you do get the finger signal, you can move to the next step.

> I now want to ask that special part of your mind to help you again. Specifically, I want your mind to give you a signal when it knows at a very deep level that it knows what to do to control your pain. It may be that it allows you to forget that you were ever in pain in the first place. It may be that you find that the area where you once felt pain is becoming cool and numb. Perhaps you will become so absorbed in whatever is happening around you that you won't have time to think about what you were experiencing. I don't know. I only know that you will feel surprisingly more comfortable. And when your mind knows this, it will signal you by allowing this finger to raise up in the air once again, as if the finger had a mind of its own.

Comment: The second finger signal is to verify that the patient "gets" the hypnotic suggestion at a deep level. In this example, I provide three potential ways that the patient might manage pain with a "forced choice" that the patient will feel more comfortable. It is not essential to provide these hypnotic suggestions with the model I am using here.

> Good! I am now going to ask your mind one more request. At the time where your mind feels that we have done the work that we need to do today, it will give you one more signal. So, you may have any experiences you would like to have deep in the privacy of your own mind right how. And at the time when your mind feels that you are ready to start coming back into awake state, it will signal you by allowing this finger to pull up into the air one final time.

Comment: With the quick induction technique, it is important to get the signal from the patient that he or she is ready to return. If a couple of minutes pass with no signal, then it might be useful to query the patient at this point.

I notice that we are not getting a signal right now. Just remain in a comfortable state, and notice that you are able to talk at the same time. Let me know what you are experiencing now.

Upon getting the last signal, the clinician states,

You are doing very well. We are now going to begin returning to a conscious state. Just notice yourself becoming more alert and awake. At some point, but not yet, not until you are ready, you will find your eyes open. And your eyes opening will be a signal from your mind. This will be a signal that you are ready to come back feeling awake, alert, refreshed, and safe. You will come back knowing at a very deep level about how to make yourself more comfortable. Take all the time you need, but realize that your eyes will open only when your mind says they are ready to open.

Comment: The pace of the patient's return is left to the patient. The process of opening the eyes becomes a contingent hypnotic suggestion—that the patient is only allowed to open his or her eyes when the patient has completed the process and internalized useful suggestions.

7

CHRONIC PAIN

Hypnosis is perhaps best known for its efficacy for treating pain; certainly, the largest number of research studies have been performed in this area. Yet pain is often treated in the hypnosis literature as a single entity rather than a collection of many different processes and problems. When one discusses the use of hypnosis for pain management, it is important to be clear about which of many types of pain problems one is considering (e.g., pain from dental or medical procedures, childbirth, arthritis, fibromyalgia, headache). Each type of pain or pain problem warrants different medical and psychological treatments approaches.

ACUTE VERSUS CHRONIC PAIN

As previous chapters have emphasized, one crucial distinction is whether the pain problem being addressed is acute or chronic. The differences between these types of pain problems, especially with respect to treatment, are so dramatic that they should actually be considered two different treatment entities. In many cases, the treatment approaches that are most effective and useful for acute pain can cause greater pain and disability in individuals with chronic pain.

Acute pain control was discussed in Chapter 6. In brief, *acute pain* can be defined as pain that is generated by tissue damage or active nociception, and that is expected to resolve once healing from that damage is complete (often within hours or days, sometimes within weeks or months). Acute pain usually serves the critical survival purpose as a warning of damage or potential damage. For example, the pain from a broken arm is a signal that immediate immobility is in the best interest of survival. Once the warning associated with acute pain is understood and appropriate action is taken (it would not be of benefit to ignore the pain from a ruptured appendix or a broken leg), then treatment can be focused on removing as much of the pain as is possible. It serves no purpose, for example, for patients to experience the pain from a root canal or a burn wound debridement. Reducing or eliminating painful sensations that result from acute pain, often through the use of analgesics and immobility, is often appropriate and effective. It should be mentioned here that this is one of the few areas that hypnosis can potentially be harmful. If acute pain is serving as a warning signal, and a patient masks it with hypnosis, the results can be deleterious. As Piccione, Hilgard, and Zimbardo (1989) reported, a highly hypnotizable student came close to death when he used hypnosis to mask symptoms of a burst appendix.

Chronic pain, in contrast, is often not associated with an identifiable lesion. By definition, it is the pain that remains or continues after healing (from an injury) has taken place, usually by 3 months, but certainly by 6 months after an injury (L. Jacobson & Mariano, 2001). Chronic pain can also result from ongoing damage or developing lesions (i.e., ongoing acute pain) or from disease processes such as cancer, arthritis, or multiple sclerosis. Chronic pain is notoriously refractory to traditional biomedical interventions. For example, outcome data show that the response to surgical interventions for chronic low back pain is not uniformly positive, despite increased efforts over the years to select patients who are deemed most likely to benefit. One review paper, for example, found that only 65% to 75% of patients receive satisfactory clinical outcomes following spinal fusion, with poorer outcomes associated with increased number of fused levels and the use of instrumentation (Turner et al., 1992). With some types of chronic pain, a focus on pain reduction on elimination in itself often is not only futile but may also serve to worsen the patient's condition. Continued focus on ineffective biomedical treatments may distract patients from seeking and obtaining training in the psychosocial approaches that they truly need, that is, learning skills that would help them more easily engage in valued life activities despite pain.

In short, the most effective treatments for chronic pain are often the opposite of those for acute pain. A classic example of this is the fact that immobility and rest are usually important for acute pain treatment. In contrast, for chronic pain, inactivity can lead to increased pain and dysfunction (via muscle and tendon atrophy), whereas activity and exercise can contribute to less pain and improved function over time.

Chronic pain is a major public health issue and far more complex to treat than acute pain. It is among the most common physical conditions in the United States, with an estimated 70 million people suffering from one or more pain syndromes, and with many of these individuals permanently disabled (L. Jacobson & Mariano, 2001). Not only does chronic pain adversely affect patients' physical and psychological well-being, but it also costs society an estimated $125 billion in health care, disability compensation, lost productivity, and tax revenue. Unlike acute pain, chronic pain responds poorly to biomedical interventions and is typically maintained by factors that have little to do with the original tissue damage. These factors include emotional distress, excessive focus on physical complaints, a conviction for a physical cure, secondary gain, and atrophied muscles resulting from reduced activity.

NEUROPATHIC AND NOCICEPTIVE PAIN

Chronic pain can have a number of primary underlying causes, although one (or both) of two types is usually present in patients presenting with chronic pain: (a) *neuropathic* pain, or pain resulting primarily from damage or disruption in peripheral or central nerves; and (b) *nociceptive* pain, or pain resulting primarily from ongoing signals from nerves that detect and communicate pain from the periphery.

Neuropathic Pain

Damage or disruption to the central nervous system and periphery can result in nerves that continue to transmit pain signals, even though the surrounding tissue (e.g., muscle, bone) has either healed or remained intact in the first place. One example of neuropathic pain is the pain that can result from a shoulder avulsion (when a shoulder is traumatically pulled from the socket), which often causes nerve damage that then results in ongoing neuropathic pain. Spinal cord injury can also result in chronic, below-injury-level neuropathic conditions such as dysathesias. Individuals with multiple sclerosis have ongoing nerve lesions as a part of their illness, some of which result in chronic neuropathic pain.

The standard biomedical treatment for neuropathic pain is medication. Currently, neuroleptic agents (gabapentin, pregabolin) and sometimes antidepressants (given for their effects on nerve function) are considered first-line treatments for neuropathic pain (Dworkin et al., 2007). Opioid analgesics are also sometimes used, but there remains significant controversy over their limited efficacy for neuropathic pain, as well as their potential for long-term negative health effects (Dworkin et al., 2007). Exercise and activity are not usually specifically recommended for such conditions because the problem is nerve related and exercise/activity has its greatest benefit on muscles and tendons. However, to the extent that the patient with neuropathic pain is becoming, or has become, deactivated (i.e., has stopped moving), then that patient may be at risk of developing a nociceptive pain problem as a result. In this case, exercise and reactivation is an important treatment component to consider.

Nociceptive Pain

Chronic nociceptive pain is the result of ongoing nociceptive input in nerves that are otherwise intact and acting normally; these nerves detect and signal damage or potential damage. The most common examples of nociceptive pain are osteo- and rheumatoid arthritis. Pain due to repetitive stress or injury (e.g., shoulder pain in people with spinal cord injury who use a manual wheelchair for years) and pain from chronic muscle spasms or trigger points (often seen in people with low back pain and fibromyalgia) are other types of nociceptive pain.

Usually, the most effective treatment for nociceptive pain is physical therapy that focuses on strengthening and stretching muscles and tendons, especially those that surround the area perceived as painful by the patient; often such areas of the body have been immobilized for some period of time. While this treatment approach can be a challenge for some patients, especially those who are fearful of any painful sensations associated with reactivation, a large body of research supports the efficacy of reactivation treatments for chronic nociceptive pain (Chou & Huffman, 2007; Henchoz & Kai-Lik So, 2008). Supportive cognitive–behavioral therapy may be provided along with reactivation treatments to address fears of reactivation (Chou & Huffman, 2007).

EVALUATING THE PATIENT WITH CHRONIC PAIN

Chronic pain almost always presents challenging evaluative issues, especially when compared with acute pain. With acute pain, the specific cause of the pain can often be readily identified, and an effective treatment approach, even if it is simply to take advantage of the healing that occurs with time, is almost always available. With chronic pain, however, the specific source (or sources) of the pain is rarely easily apparent, and the most effective treatment approaches for that pain problem (or problems) are not always obvious.

Consequently, a critical first step when considering treating any patient with chronic pain is to provide a thorough evaluation of the patient and the pain problem, ideally using a biopsychosocial perspective.

The primary goal in the initial evaluation is to identify the factors that may be contributing to this particular patient's pain and suffering. From the perspective of a biopsychosocial model, and given the way health care is currently organized, the "bio" piece of the evaluation should be performed by a physician or health care provider with medical training. The "psychosocial" piece of the evaluation is usually performed by a psychologist. The structure for the evaluation procedures suggested here is derived in large part from the work of Mark Jensen (e.g., M. P. Jensen & Patterson, 2008).

Biological Factors

Biological factors refer to the physiological or anatomical characteristics of the patient that might be contributing to the patient's chronic pain. A critical issue for the biological evaluation concerns the extent to which the pain has neuropathic and/or nociceptive components, and whether there may be plastic changes that may have occurred in the nervous system that are also contributing to pain and suffering. The term *plastic changes* refers to neuroplasticity, or the process through which chronic pain seems to become imprinted in a patient's neurological processing even after tissue damage or other causative factors have gone away. As indicated earlier, such factors are usually best assessed by a physician or health care provider with medical training, ideally with training that includes how to evaluate and treat chronic pain (training in this area is sadly lacking in medical schools currently). It is well beyond the scope of this chapter to describe the specific components that should be included in a thorough medical valuation of chronic pain. Loeser (2001a), however, provides a good resource for this.

Clearly, a thorough medical evaluation is a prerequisite to the use of hypnosis or any other treatment for pain; problems that need immediate medical attention such as undiagnosed cancer or other illnesses, tumors, or lesions that might respond well to surgery must be ruled out. Although undiagnosed medical problems for which treatment provides a dramatic relief of pain may be infrequent, medical evaluations are important to identify those biomedical factors that may potentially respond to treatment. In addition, they will help by providing an opinion about the types of pain involved (i.e., nociceptive, neuropathic, plastic, or some combination of these), as well as those medical treatments that are indicated. It is important to keep in mind, however, that the presence of a treatable medical condition that is the source of the pain does not preclude the use of hypnotic approaches; often, hypnosis and teaching individuals self-hypnosis can make patients who are in active treatment more comfortable.

The most effective chronic pain treatment often consists of an interdisciplinary approach that combines medical and psychological interventions (including physical therapy and rehabilitation counseling). In addition, even if medical issues are deemed to not play a large role in the patient's pain, if such issues are not evaluated and ruled out with a thorough evaluation, patients may be less likely to entertain more psychological/social models for understanding and ultimately addressing their suffering. Some patients with chronic pain have a biomedical focus, an intense fixation on the belief that there is something medically wrong with them that requires a medical fix. If this is not ruled out, and it may require a thorough medical evaluation to do so, patients may reject suggestions for psychosocial approaches for pain management, such as hypnosis.

Psychological Factors

With the provision that the medical causes of a patient's chronic pain have been thoroughly assessed, the clinician's task is to then assess the potential psychological and social contributions to pain and suffering. Such information ultimately becomes the target for treatment. The remainder of this section addresses how to perform such an assessment in a way hypnosis can be targeted toward those specific factors that may be contributing to the patient's pain and any suffering associated with pain. The core of this evaluation would include basic historic information about the pain problem, including the pain onset, treatments attempts and the patient's perceived efficacy about treatment, education, marital/relationship status, history of drug or alcohol use/abuse and treatment, previous psychological treatment, and cognitive status. These factors would be assessed in any evaluation prior to consideration of a psychological intervention for any medical issue. Following the collection of such historical information, some of which may yield important information about factors that could be influencing pain or pain behavior (e.g., a patient who complains of pain as a socially sanctioned way to express suffering associated with depression or a history of above), the assessment can be geared toward assessing the other psychosocial factors that may be contributing to the pain and pain behavior (and that can be treated through hypnosis).

Assessing the Pain Experience

At some point, the pain experience of the patient should be assessed. Often, the clinician may elect to assess this early in the evaluation as an indirect way of communicating that the clinician views the patient's experience as both important and real. As listed in Table 7.1, the global intensity and unpleasantness/bothersomeness of pain should be assessed (I have found that 0–10 numerical scales are most useful for this, but categorical scales [e.g.,

TABLE 7.1
Pain Assessment and Hypnotic Suggestions

Problem/issue	Treatment options	Hypnotic suggestions for . . .
High pain intensity	Appropriate medication management, appropriate exercise, hypnosis	See Chapter 6
Pain bothersomeness	Cognitive restructuring, acceptance therapy, hypnosis	Decreased bothersomeness of pain, ability to ignore pain
Illness conviction/ biomedical focus	Education, hypnosis, appropriate exercise, cognitive restructuring	A broader understanding of the biopsychosocial nature of pain
Use of maladaptive coping strategies/ lack of use of adaptive coping strategies	Education, motivational interviewing modeling, operant therapy, hypnosis	Imagining effective use of adaptive coping strategies, age progression to higher functioning
Catastrophizing	Cognitive restructuring, hypnosis	Imagining adaptive cognitions in response to pain flare-ups through age regression
Sleep disturbance	Elimination of inappropriate long-term sleep agents (e.g., benzodiazepines), consider medications that might help with sleep (e.g., some antidepressants), sleep hygiene education, exercise, hypnosis	Sleep onset, duration, acceptance of sleep interruption, good sleep hygiene
Lack of social support	Couples therapy, communication training, in-counseling/analysis if related to personality disorder	Hypnosis not indicated
Presence of reinforcement of pain behavior, or discouragement of well behavior	Education, couples therapy or education, operant therapy	Hypnosis not indicated

Note. From *Hypnosis and the Relief of Pain and Pain Disorders* (p. 518), by M. P. Jensen and D. Patterson, 2008, New York: Oxford University Press. Adapted with permission.

none, mild, moderate, severe] may be preferred by some patients and are often as useful as 0–10 scales for tracking pain over time), as well as its location(s). It is important to be aware of time characteristics, including duration and frequency of pain flare-ups and time course of pain in a typical day, when developing treatment strategies. Knowledge of pain variability (i.e., worst and least pain intensity) is important because the level of least pain provides a clear indication of how low pain intensity can get without any additional medical treatment; maximizing the time spent at this low level can be an initial first goal of treatment (if a reduction of perceived pain intensity ends up being a treatment goal in this particular case).

The clinician should assess state (current) and trait (usual) anxiety levels, depression, and sleep problems, all of which can influence pain and suffering, as well as the psychological resources that might or might not be available for learning new self-management strategies. Patients who are highly anxious or depressed, or who are not getting adequate sleep, have fewer resources for learning new skills. When depression, anxiety, or sleep problems are issues, they need to be directly addressed (using both hypnotic and non-hypnotic interventions, as appropriate) with treatment to facilitate overall improvement.

It is also important to assess the patient's own understanding of the causes of his or her pain, what treatments the patient has tried that have worked (or have not worked), and how the patient copes with or manages pain. Further, the content of thoughts the patient has in response to pain (looking, in particular, for catastrophizing or alarming cognitions as opposed to realistic and reassuring cognitions [see below], as well as a global attitude of pain "acceptance"), the effects of the pain problem on significant relationships, and the responses of others (in particular, close family members or partners with whom the patient lives) to patient pain behavior all can play a role in treatment.

Assessing Patients' Thoughts About the Cause(s) of the Pain Experience

Knowing the patient's ideas about the cause of his or her pain experience is extremely important. If the patient believes that the pain is solely the result of ongoing tissue damage, or if he or she believes that the only way to reduce pain is through surgery, then the patient may not be open to hypnotic or other psychological approaches for pain management. The patient's model for his or her pain can be ascertained by simply asking the question, "What do you think is causing your pain?" Or, alternatively, "What have you been told is causing your pain?" followed up with the question, "Do you agree with this?"

The clinician can incorporate important information concerning the patient's model of his or her own pain problem into the hypnosis treatment (see below). In addition, the clinician can evaluate the patient's current acceptance of a purely biomedical model versus a more complex biopsychosocial model of pain. This is important to understand early in treatment, because if the clinician presents an explanatory model of pain that varies widely from that which the patient holds, the patient may hesitate in working with the clinician or may not even return for the next session.

If the patient's explanation for the cause of pain is consistent with the medical evaluation, then it is unlikely that illness conviction is contributing to the problem. *Illness conviction* is a steadfast belief held by the patient that a serious health problem is causing the pain that can only be fixed with a biomedical intervention, such as surgery. If the patient with painful diabetic neuropathy states that the pain is caused mostly by the result of diabetes, then illness conviction is not likely to be a serious concern. Similarly, a patient with a complex low back pain problem that has no clear explanation who says, "None of the doctors have been able to tell me what is causing this pain, and I do not really care. I just want to get better. If that means exercising more, I will exercise more. If that means learning to use hypnosis, I will do that," that patient is not demonstrating an illness conviction. On the other hand, if the patient expresses vague, nonspecific concerns that physical damage or a lack of healing is causing the pain (despite a clear record that the medical tests for physical damage are negative), then illness conviction may be a significant issue and probably needs to be addressed before treatment based on a biopsychosocial model can proceed.

Another useful question for assessing possible illness conviction and biomedical focus is "What treatments have you tried for your pain?" This can be followed up with "Which of these were effective and which would you like to try again?" Some patients will present a long history of biomedical treatments and will be interested only in attempting such approaches in the future. This suggests that the patient has a biomedical focus and may not be receptive to hypnosis or other types of psychological approaches for pain management. Patients with a biomedical focus may require a great deal of patience from health care professionals; in this case, the best course of action may be to give the patient some time to come to terms with the fact that pain relief does not necessarily lie in a biomedical treatment, or at least be willing to learn some effective strategies for pain management to use *until* an effective biomedical intervention is identified. To help facilitate a patient's openness to nonbiomedical treatments, motivational interviewing can provide a nonconfrontational approach that can help assure that the patient considers options in addition to only biomedical ones (see Chapter 8, this volume).

Assessing Pain Coping Strategies

Asking patients about the coping strategies they have used for pain management provides a wealth of clinical information that can guide treatment decisions. All patients do something to cope with pain, even if this involves nothing more than being passive and inactive. For example, watching television and sleeping, to the extent that patients do these as a means of distracting themselves from pain, can be considered pain coping responses. These particular passive responses are generally maladaptive; that is, they can lead to increases in pain and disability over time.

The distinction between adaptive and maladaptive coping (Boothby, Thorn, Stroud, & Jensen, 1999) is a useful one. Although every patient is unique, and what is adaptive or maladaptive for one may not necessarily be adaptive or maladaptive for another, adaptive (usually active) coping responses are usually associated with better long-term adjustment. Examples of adaptive coping for chronic pain might include participating in a regular exercise program, pacing one's activities (i.e., avoiding very high or very low levels of activity), practicing relaxation or self-hypnosis strategies on a regular basis, and learning to maintain activity despite pain—an overall "acceptance" of pain and willingness to engage in valued life activities regardless of pain.

Maladaptive (usually passive) coping responses tend to be focused on immediate pain reduction (e.g., rest; avoidance of activities that increase pain, even when those activities are otherwise reinforcing; pain-contingent analgesic use) but typically do not benefit the patient in the long term and can, in fact, lead to poorer function over time. Rest, guarding (limping or holding a body part still), and inactivity, in particular, can put the patient at risk of long-term deactivation and contribute to muscle atrophy, disability, and increased pain (Bortz, 1984). Inactivity after pain unfortunately often arises from patient reactions to acute pain and even medical advice. While potentially adaptive at first, patients can develop a fear of movement that borders on phobic dimensions (Patterson, 2005). Other forms of dysfunctional coping for chronic pain include guarding body parts (e.g., keeping one's neck stiff or limping), cessation of vocational activities, and use of strong analgesic medications on a pain-contingent basis, despite increasing tolerance for their effects.

Coping strategies can be assessed simply by asking the patient what he or she does to deal with pain; however, some patients may struggle with the concept that what they are doing or not doing can actually be considered as coping strategies, and so they may need help in identifying different coping responses. One can also assess coping by asking patients how significant people in their life know they are experiencing pain. The patient's response to this question ("I go to my room to rest," "I have a few beers," "They don't know because I don't tell them and just keep going") can provide important information about coping responses.

Adaptive coping responses that are rarely used, or maladaptive ones that are frequently used, can be a target for intervention, with or without hypnosis. The primary intervention for maladaptive coping techniques is education and social reinforcement for incompatible coping responses (e.g., reinforcement of exercise and daily walking for someone who rests in response to pain), although motivational interviewing can be used with patients who are particularly struggling with such changes (M. P. Jensen, 2002).

If a patient is aware of deficits in coping and is motivated to learn new approaches, it might be easy to teach and encourage adaptive coping. For example, one of the most powerful approaches to dealing with problems associated with pacing (a maladaptive response to pain involving overuse) is to teach the patient to use an operant-based quota system (i.e., exercise or activity is conducted within the range of endurance rather than to a point that causes pain and fatigue). In the multiple-choice technique of giving hypnotic suggestions described at several points in the book, effective and adaptive pain coping strategies can be woven into hypnotic suggestions for pain relief.

A particularly vexing maladaptive response to pain is catastrophizing. *Catastrophizing* refers to exaggerated and extremely negative automatic cognitions that can occur in patients with chronic pain (Sullivan & D'Eon, 1990; Sullivan et al., 2001). Such thoughts, even when patients are unaware of them, demonstrate consistent negative associations with pain and functioning. Examples of catastrophizing thoughts include "This pain is horrible," "It will never go away," or even "This pain means I am going to die." Treatments that decrease catastrophizing cognitions are associated with decreases in pain and improvements in functioning. In chronic pain treatment, the goal is to help patients learn to replace or alter these thoughts into more reassuring ones: "I would prefer not to experience pain, but I can deal with this," "My experience of pain comes and goes, and I am learning to have an effect on that experience," and "This pain does not really mean anything. It is just there now, and it will lessen in the future."

Albert Ellis (1961, 1980, 1995) was one of the pioneer cognitive–behaviorists who helped to identify some of the key words that indicate a patient is operating with dysfunctional cognitions. Words such as *should, must,* and *can't* were ones that he argued can lead to neurotic behavior and distress. For example, "I must pass the test. I can't stand making Cs." Ellis jokingly referred to such thoughts as "musturbatory" thinking. By listening carefully to a patient with chronic pain, clinicians can identify similar language triggers. Words such as *never* and *always* or excessively negative views of the impact of pain can help alert the clinician that the patient is operating with catastrophizing cognitions. Simply asking the patient what thoughts go through his or her head during a flare-up or onset of pain can go a long way to determining the flow and content of cognitions.

The presence of significant catastrophizing can suggest the possibility of depression or depressive symptoms. Depression is a common issue with chronic pain and has been estimated to occur in 33% or more of patients with this diagnosis, compared with significantly lower rates in an otherwise healthy population (Romano & Turner, 1985). When depression is present, it is important to address it for a number of reasons. First, complaints of chronic pain can be at least a partial expression of depression, and treating the affective disorder may have a large impact on the suffering associated with the pain. Second, adaptive pain management almost always requires motivation and activity. With the anhedonia that accompanies depression, the clinician will likely be facing a struggle when trying to activate a patient with depression and chronic pain. With older adults, who may have been raised in a time when depression was viewed as a personal weakness, it may be easier to communicate suffering through physical pain.

Patients with chronic pain often suffer from sleep disturbances, and these in turn interfere with a large variety of functional activities. Sleep disruption (both too much or too little sleep) has also been associated with increased pain (Tang, Wright, & Salkovskis, 2007; Wilson, Eriksson, D'Eon, Mikail, & Emery, 2002). Moreover, restorative sleep has been shown to predict subsequent resolution of chronic widespread pain (Davies et al., 2008). Thus, sleep disorders should be addressed as a part of any pain management program. It is unfortunate that sedative medications are being increasingly used to help patients sleep, given their negative effects on sleep architecture.

The most appropriate first-line treatment for sleep management is sleep hygiene training. Sleep hygiene interventions are centered largely on stimulus–response approaches. For example, the bed should be a stimulus for sleep and not a stimulus for staying awake. It follows that patients should not go to bed until they are sleepy, should not have televisions or other distracting stimuli turned on in the bedroom at bedtime, and should leave the bed after 15 or 20 minutes if they are unable to get to sleep. Further, they should be advised to wake up at the same time each morning, even after a night of poor sleep. Other components of good sleep hygiene include avoiding naps or avoiding caffeine-containing products (including many popular carbonated beverages and chocolate), keeping to regularly scheduled daytime activities (e.g., eating at the same time), and developing a relaxing and consistent going-to-bed ritual (e.g., brushing one's teeth, checking to make sure all doors are locked, reading for a specified period of time). The basic idea is to train the brain and body to expect to go to sleep at about the same time every night by developing a consistent pattern. As discussed in Jaffe and Patterson (2004), it is only after these and other such approaches have failed that medications should be used.

When medications must be used, the mixed agonist receptor benzodiazepines are recommended because they demonstrate quick onset, clear from the system relatively quickly, and are known to be associated with good sleep architecture (Jaffe & Patterson, 2004). If patients still have great difficulty staying asleep or have accompanying depression, trazadone is often a good option (Jaffe & Patterson, 2004). Hypnosis is also a good option, not only to reduce pain that interferes with sleep but also to address the insomnia itself. Elkins, Marcus, Palamara, and Stearns (2004) described how hypnosis can be used with an effective sleep hygiene program.

Social Factors

It is interesting that social influence can have both positive and negative effects on a patient's ability to adapt to chronic pain. As far as facilitating the ability to cope with pain, general positive social support has long been known to be one of the most important buffers to the negative effects of chronic illness as well as pain (Kerns, Rosenberg, & Otis, 2002; Lopez-Martinez, Esteve-Zarazaga, & Ramirez-Maestre, 2008). The specific mechanisms by which social support improves adjustment are not known. Certainly there are benefits to having a supportive listener when one is suffering (as long as that listening is not provided on a pain-contingent basis), particularly when such a person might be able to use this as a way to facilitate problem solving.

However, social support has also been suggested to benefit people with illness or pain in more practical ways. Having an individual to remind patients or to drive or accompany them to medical appointments is an example of this. M. P. Jensen et al. (2002) linked social support with more positive mood in patients with chronic pain as well as with a lack of pain interference with activities. As mentioned earlier, depression is a common issue with chronic pain, and social support may also reduce the negative impact of depressive disorders. For this reason, it is useful to gain an understanding of what types of social support networks patients have in their lives and facilitate the development of caring and (nonpain-contingent) supportive relationships.

In the assessment of social issues with respect to pain, it is useful to determine who the primary person in the patient's life is and ask that person to participate in the initial evaluation. Some patients will have a limited social network, and improving this area of their life can be an important part of treatment, even if the focus of care is on pain control. Interventions to enhance social relationships can extend from social skills training to goal setting or analytical therapy for patients with deeper rooted areas (Baker & Nash, 2008).

Although adaptive social support can provide an important buffer to alleviating the impact of chronic pain, maladaptive social interactions can also contribute to ongoing pain and dysfunction. Of particular concern are solicitous responses from significant others, especially when they are provided on a pain-contingent basis. Fordyce (1976) has long taught that pain behavior is strengthened when the consequences that follow it are positive, or if its increase can avoid an unpleasant consequence. So, if a wife responds to her husband's pain complaints by giving him a massage or other sympathetic response, including the taking over of some unpleasant activity or chore (e.g., washing the dishes), the reinforcing nature of such attention may serve to increase the husband's pain behavior through operant conditioning. Indeed, this phenomenon is so powerful that Flor and colleagues have even demonstrated that the presence of a spouse is capable of causing the areas of the brain that process and reflect pain experience to show more activity in people with chronic pain (Flor, 2003; Flor, Kerns, & Turk, 1987; Flor, Knost, & Birbaumer, 2002; Flor, Turk, & Rudy, 1989). This effect can also be seen if significant others somehow discourage a patient's efforts to show well behavior. As an example, a spouse may show worry or criticism when a patient begins to exercise, a dynamic that can undermine improvement (Schwartz, Jensen, & Romano, 2005).

A number of specific questions may be used to help determine how interpersonal factors may influence pain behaviors (M. P. Jensen & Patterson, 2008). Specifically, the patient can be asked the following during the evaluation: (a) "How does your spouse/family member/roommate know that you are hurting?" (the response to this question can provide information about the specific pain behaviors shown by the patient); (b) "What does your spouse/family member/roommate do when you appear to be in pain?" (this assesses possible positive reinforcement for pain behavior); and (c) "What does he/she do when you try to exercise or do chores even when you are in pain?" (this assesses possible discouragement of well behaviors).

Other questions that assess possible pain behavior reinforcers include "What do you no longer do because of your pain?" and "What do you do less of . . . ?" Responses to these questions may provide information about adverse activities that a patient is able to avoid because of pain. For example, if that patient dislikes mowing the lawn or doing the dishes and pain allows the patient a socially sanctioned way of avoiding these activities, this negative reinforcement (avoidance of an aversive activity can be reinforcing) may be contributing to the maintenance of pain behavior. It follows that the clinician should consider not only what increases after (and possibly rewards) pain behavior but also what decreases as a function of pain (the avoidance of which may serve as reward).

Finally, a thorough pain evaluation should consider other types of mental health diagnoses. As mentioned previously, a large percentage of patients with chronic pain suffer from major depression and treating such affective disorders can also help address the pain, or at least the suffering that often accompanies pain. Patients with chronic pain also have a host of other psychological disorders, particularly along the lines of anxiety and stress, as well as somatoform disorders. Not only will treating such issues often diminish pain and suffering, but failure to address them will often thwart any treatment plans that are developed.

Not only are these *Diagnostic and Statistical Manual of Mental Disorders* (4th ed., text rev. [*DSM–IV–R*]; American Psychiatric Association, 2000) Axis I disorders important, but the Axis II (character) disorders must also be considered. Even though *DSM–IV–R* Axis II disorders are challenging to treat, knowledge concerning the presence and severity of these disorders helps one to understand and predict patient response and helps guide how treatment should progress. Patients who have histrionic tendencies, for example, may have a tendency to dramatize pain complaints. A clinician using hypnosis may be disappointed in a seeming failure to reduce reports of pain and suffering in patients showing such Axis II tendencies, when the presentation is much more a factor of the patient's personality style. Similarly, unanticipated improvements and lauding of the clinician may also be a function of a dramatic presentation, and the clinician must be careful not to be seduced by unrealistic improvement and flattering compliments.

MATCHING HYPNOTIC TREATMENT TO CHRONIC PAIN ISSUES

Clinicians should keep a number of issues in mind when developing a treatment plan for chronic pain management, including treatment plans that involve hypnotic interventions. First, every treatment plan, whether or not it contains hypnotic components, should be targeted to all of the (modifiable) factors that have been identified (in the evaluation) to be contributing to pain and dysfunction, not just the experience of pain. Mirroring, perhaps, many health care practitioners who focus attention and treatment on biomedical factors only, there is a tendency in the field of hypnotic treatment for chronic pain problems to focus treatment on the experience of pain itself. However, pain and pain-related suffering can be the end result of a number of factors (maladaptive coping, inactivity, sleep dysfunction, depression, anxiety, social interactions), and pain can then have an impact on each of these factors in turn. Focusing on pain alone is an inefficient way to address all of these negative effects. M. P. Jensen et al. (2006) reported that hypnosis focused on pain control often has beneficial side effects on these types of issues.

The most common factors associated with chronic pain include (a) high pain intensity, (b) significant pain bothersomeness, (c) illness conviction/ biomedical focus, (d) use of maladaptive coping techniques, (e) underuse of adaptive coping strategies, (f) presence and particularly excess of catastrophizing, (g) sleep disturbance, and (h) operant factors that keep pain behaviors in place. As described in the previous section, a large part of the initial evaluation and case formulation is deciding how much each of these eight factors might be contributing to patient dysfunction. When treating chronic pain with hypnosis, the clinician who understands this clinical issue will seldom focus only on pain reduction and might not even include suggestions for sensory pain reduction (suggestions for an ability to engage in valued life activities are much more common). The following sections describe how hypnosis can be used to address each of the factors that might emerge as important during the evaluation, listing specific hypnotic suggestions that might be important. This approach was designed by Mark Jensen, with some collaboration (M. P. Jensen & Patterson, 2008).

Severe Pain Intensity and Pain Bothersomeness

Reducing the global magnitude of pain and its bothersomeness often comes first to mind for patients and clinicians who are considering using hypnosis for chronic pain management. This is not completely unreasonable, although, as discussed above, it might be a disservice to the patient to consider this the only or even always the primary goal of treatment. Chapter 6 of this volume lists a number of approaches that Erickson suggested for reducing pain, and pain reduction is the most common application of hypnosis that is discussed in the literature. Erickson's hypnotic suggestions for pain reduction and management included suggestions for amnesia, analgesia, anesthesia, replacement or substitution of sensations, sensation displacement, time or body disorientation, reinterpretation, and the use of metaphors for diminution of pain.

When considering hypnotic inductions, it may be useful to remember that the perception of muscle tension often accompanies chronic pain. Therefore, hypnotic suggestions for deep relaxation and comfort are beneficial for many patients, even those who have minimal hypnotic abilities. For this reason, it is often useful to begin hypnotic inductions with suggestions for deep relaxation when working with patients with chronic pain.

However, there are some important provisions to this. First, not all patients respond well or enjoy hypnotic suggestions for deep relaxation; it is important not only to accommodate patients' preferences and individual responses but also to tailor inductions to suit these as the clinician gains more experience with each patient. Second, although many patients benefit from relaxation-based inductions, for some patients it may be important to alter the inductions over time to help keep them engaged in the hypnotic process. To a significant degree, effective hypnosis requires that clinicians are able to capture and hold a patient's attention and interest. Moreover, with chronic pain treatment in general, and hypnotic interventions in particular, it is a good idea to disrupt patterns of everyday (especially maladaptive) thinking with surprise and novelty. Thus, although some patients may improve their hypnotic responsiveness by practicing the same inductions over time, others may require that clinicians capture their attention with altered (and sometimes surprising) approaches at each session.

It is also not always easy to predict ahead of time which hypnotic suggestions are going to work best with any one given patient; it is far better for the patient to teach the clinician what works with him or her rather than for the clinician to try to dictate ahead of time what will work. It is common in clinical practice, when given a range of hypnotic suggestions, that patients will report that one of the suggestions that may have been given as an afterthought by the clinician, and not as a primary suggestion, was the one that patients later reported as most useful. Sometimes patients report that a particular suggestion, which may not even have been directly given, "really worked well." This may be due to the fact that clinicians often provide indirect suggestions that the patient's "mind will provide just the right suggestion for your comfort and well-being" (see below). Thus, in many cases, it is the patient's own interpretation of the hypnotic suggestions given, rather than the suggestions themselves, that has proved beneficial. Often the patient takes a kernel of a hypnotic suggestion given and then, through fantasy and imagination, creates what is useful for pain control.

That said, when clinicians use hypnosis for chronic pain management, it is usually beneficial to begin with an induction that is relaxation based. Following this, when a goal of the session is to help the patient learn how to create pain relief or comfort, M. P. Jensen and Patterson (2008) recommended providing a series of hypnotic suggestions for pain reduction, enhanced relaxation, and perceived control over pain. Over the first few sessions, patients are given a number of different hypnotic suggestions (see, e.g., Table 7.1) and then asked to provide feedback concerning their effectiveness, often during the hypnotic session (J. E. Barber, 1996). Specifically, while in hypnosis, the patients are told,

> And now, while allowing the muscles of your voice to become activated while still remaining relaxed, and deeply focused, please tell me on a 0-to-10 scale, with 0 being "no pain sensation" and 10 being "pain sensation as intense as I could imagine," how would you rate the current intensity of any uncomfortable sensations you are felling now?

One of the more difficult concepts for novice hypnotists to grasp is that it is acceptable to talk with a patient while he or she is having a hypnotic experience (J. E. Barber, 1996). Although the depth of the hypnotic state could potentially lighten when the patient is queried, it is always possible to return the patient to a deeper state. In any case, identifying the most useful types of hypnotic pain suggestions early in a course of treatment is an extremely effective approach. Obviously, what the patient finds most useful can be repeated later in treatment and audio-recorded for home practice.

For the treatment of chronic pain, posthypnotic suggestions are particularly important. In the case of acute pain, hypnotic suggestions are typically targeted for a particular time or event (see Chapter 6). Chronic pain, being an ongoing perceptual experience, is a much more difficult challenge. First, one should make hypnotic suggestions that any pain relief obtained during the session will endure for a time period after the session (in making this suggestion, clinicians give patients a selection of options, e.g., "for seconds, minutes, hours, days, or even weeks and months . . . and can become something your mind does automatically, all the time . . . without having to think, like breathing or walking . . . ," both to enhance a sense of control and to make it easier for them to comply with the suggestions). The natural course of chronic pain is that it comes and goes and becomes of greater of lesser intensity over time. Clinicians should capitalize on this phenomenon when providing hypnotic suggestions. For example, it is not that useful to tell patients that their relief will last for 24 hours; rather, it is more useful to say, "You may be pleased to notice that your comfort lingers on far beyond the session today. Perhaps this will be for a matter of minutes, hours, day, weeks, or even years." Another way to state this and to make use of amnesia is to say, "At some point you may look back, hours or even days from now, and notice that you are pleasantly surprised at how long you have gone on experiencing a sense of comfort after the session was over."

Second, the patient can be given some type of trigger to induce posthypnotic suggestions for comfort after the session (i.e., teach the patient self-hypnosis): "You may find that whenever you close your eyes and count to 10 that these feelings of deep comfort come rushing back" or "You can notice that profound comfort returns just when you slowly release your breath." Third, posthypnotic suggestions can be built into further inductions and practice sessions. Patients can be told that each time they go into a hypnotic state the degree level of analgesia will be more profound and last longer; the same can be suggested for the use of practice tapes.

Far more than with acute pain, chronic pain management is a skill that is practiced and maintained. Although a few patients can attain significant relief with minimal practice, many patients will require ongoing practice to obtain long-lasting pain relief. This is also the case for the number of sessions with the clinician. Enduring reductions of pain will typically require multiple hypnotic sessions and then ongoing practice by the patient, usually with audiotapes or CDs. One approach is to meet with the patient for an initial four sessions of hypnosis and self-hypnosis training. This is often enough for patients to achieve significant reductions in perceived pain and to have learned what they need to continue practicing self-hypnosis on their own. Those patients who obtain no relief at all after four sessions may decide to discontinue treatment. Others might experience significant benefit, but both the patient and clinician believe that more could be gained with additional sessions. Consequently, treatment might extend to 10 sessions total, or even more if many issues related to the pain surface and require ongoing intervention. In short, there is really no standard protocol for pain management in the clinical setting. Each patient is unique and requires individualized therapy.

Following each session, the clinician should obtain feedback from the patient regarding the efficacy of the hypnotic induction used and suggestions given. The clinician should ask the patient about his or her responses to the induction in a nondefensive manner (it is important that the patient is not trying to please the clinician with his or her impressions). Such information is used to modify future inductions and hypnotic suggestions. It is useful to identify at least one, and often more than one, nonpain goal for the patient to show improvements that may help, indirectly, contribute to pain relief and improved functioning (e.g., improved sleep, confidence, or well-being). As discussed several times throughout this book, identifying a core value of the patient is often central to pain control, as well as any other sort of behavior change. If what drives a sense of joy in the patient is being a good mother, showing pride in one's work, being a good athlete, or being a valued grandparent, this is useful for the clinician to know. At times, working on a nonpain goal may be the greatest factor in creating long-term pain reduction and reductions in suffering.

The hypnotic suggestions that the patient finds to be the most effective in the first few sessions can form the basis of the suggestions used in later sessions, but at any point during treatment the clinician might decide to try a new suggestion, especially if additional issues come to light. Soon after treatment begins, if not from the very first session, the sessions should be audio-recorded. The patient is then given a copy of the recording (usually on a CD) and encouraged to listen at least daily, but more often if the patient is able and finds the CDs helpful. It is ideal if the patient can listen to the CDs without interruption. As the patient is given more CDs, he or she can develop a personalized library of these from which to select as needed. Often, one or more are found to be particularly helpful for the patient, and the clinician should encourage the patient to listen to these the most often. However, patients should also listen to the other recordings ever so often, because they might contain hypnotic suggestions that the patient could find helpful in the future. Finally, patients should be encouraged to practice self-hypnosis on their own without the use of the recording, and they should be told that their ability to successfully achieve comfort with self-hypnosis will improve over time and with practice.

Using a protocol similar to that described above, M. P. Jensen et al. (2005) found that the great majority of patients report significant pain relief that lasts beyond the treatment sessions. They have also found that the benefits of hypnosis exceed those of either progressive muscle relaxation or electromyogram-assisted relaxation training, even though these other interventions engendered the same degree of positive outcome expectancies; in other words, even though outcome can be influenced by "nonspecific" components such as expectancy and motivation, hypnosis has specific effects beyond these nonspecific effects (M. P. Jensen, Barber, Romano, Hanley, et al., 2009; M. P. Jensen, Barber, Romano, Molton, et al., 2009). Jensen and colleagues have noted that the protocol used in these studies was more rigid and standardized that that used in the clinic, given that it was developed as part of a study. Moreover, they found that even if patients report that their pain intensity does not decrease, many report that the pain bothers them less, and they feel more in control over the pain and its effects (M. P. Jensen et al., 2006).

However, as should be clear, many patients with chronic pain are not going to obtain the most relief using hypnotic techniques that focus only on pain reduction. As discussed, a number of factors contribute to the ongoing maintenance of pain and suffering. If patients continue to remain sedentary, for example, or have social or financial disincentives for improvement, progress may be short-lived. Under certain circumstances, focusing on the pain reduction may even be counterproductive. For patients presenting with significant illness conviction or who have a biomedical focus, hypnosis might be viewed as a "magic wand," one more treatment that is done to them (such as surgery) as opposed to a skill that they learn to use themselves to manage pain. However, hypnotic suggestions for analgesia will likely present a problem with such patients only if the clinician ignores the overall picture. If patients are willing to entertain a biopsychosocial model for their pain and the lifestyle changes that come with it, hypnotic suggestions for analgesia do not carry the same risks (e.g., diverting the patient from what is important in treatment, creating false expectations). The following suggestions discuss how some of these associated issues can be treated with or without hypnosis.

Illness Conviction and Biomedical Focus

When patients are convinced that their pain means something is medically wrong with them and requires a biomedical "fix," this suggests the presence of significant illness conviction and a biomedical focus. When patients are too fixated in this direction, any attempts to address a number of factors that keep suffering in place can be impeded. A first line of approach for patients who present with illness conviction is education (to teach the biopsychosocial model) as well as approaches that shift the patients' model of illness.

Explaining the biopsychosocial model in terms comprehensible to laypeople is a challenge but a necessary prerequisite. It is important that this be done in a manner that does not threaten patients with the perception that their pain is solely psychologically determined. In fact, it is advisable to begin by pointing out that injury and tissue damage have certainly played a role in their pain experience, particularly early on in the process. Other educational information might involve the difference between "hurt and harm," this is, that movement might hurt initially but is not actually doing damage to them (provided this is medically substantiated).

One of the most effective ways to enable patients to shift their position about health care is through the use of motivational interviewing. Motivational interviewing is a process through which the clinician will start by carefully understanding and acknowledging the patient's position on pain. Through the process of (selective) reflective listening, the clinician enables the patient to weigh the pros and cons of his or her approach to pain, gently encouraging discussion and acceptance of a more complex (but more accurate) biopsychosocial understanding. The following are some examples of motivational responses to patient concerns, providing they reflect accurately what the patient has said: "So far, seeking medical interventions for your pain hasn't seemed to make a difference in the amount of comfort you are experiencing" or "Increasing your exercise seems like a good idea for you but you never seem to be able to get started." Chapter 8 of this volume discusses how hypnosis can be helpful in the context of a motivational interviewing approach.

As one example, motivational interviewing uses a "menu of options" for how patients might consider change; for example, they can continue to pursue biomedical consults, increase or change their medication another time, or consider a shift in their entire approach to pain control. Hypnosis might be used to suggest to the patient that a dramatic change in perspective might be of use at this time. The following is an example of hypnotic suggestions along these lines:

> I wonder what your dog would do in this situation? I bet you that if there was a fenced-in area and your dog was trying to run through it, he would not keep running into a blind alley over and over again. We humans are funny, will run down a blind alley over and over again. We will kick or shake the candy machine when it does not give us what we want. Most dogs, on the other hand, would just find another way to the bone.

Another way this is applicable is to put the menu of options in the terms of an Ericksonian range of choices during hypnosis:

> It may be that you continue visiting new doctors, or you may try something different with your medication, or maybe you will try something brand new that doesn't involve any of these things. The point is that you never seem to give up, and this should be a deep source of pride for you.

Another potential area of intervention under the rubric of biomedical focus is fear of movement from chronic pain. People with ongoing chronic pain often reduce their level of activity, often for fear of reinjuring themselves or making their experience of pain worse. Over time, activity can become more and more constricted, leaving the patient at greater risk of injury, muscle spasms, and subsequent pain flare-ups. Although the original injury to tissue may have healed, plastic changes in the nervous system may be making the patient exquisitely sensitive to input (such that the brain interprets that input as pain), or there may remain significant muscle weakness or spasm/trigger points that continue to send nociceptive signals, even though any threat of actual physical damage is long gone. Thus, some patients may develop a fear of pain that reaches phobic levels (Vlaeyen & Linton, 2000; Vlaeyen et al., 1999). Standard treatment for these fears involves a very graduated increase in exercise/activity using an operant (reinforcing activity with rest) program. A similar approach, called *in vivo reactivation*, has recently been developed that focuses specifically on increasing activity in just those muscles or for those activities that produce the greatest fear (De Jong et al., 2008; Leeuw et al., 2008; Linton et al., 2008). Hypnosis has long been known to be effective with anxiety and phobias. Provided, of course, that the exercise or reactivation program has been cleared by the appropriate medical personnel, patients can be given hypnotic suggestions for confidence, safety, and motivations for such activity.

Use of Maladaptive Coping or Lack of Adapting Coping

As discussed in detail previously, many patients experiencing chronic pain use less adaptive coping techniques; perhaps the most nefarious is responding to pain with rest or inactivity. Guarding or protecting an area of the body is another example of maladaptive coping, as is using alcohol or tranquilizers as a primary means of analgesia. In contrast, exercising regularly and developing the ability to identify and correct negative cognitions are adaptive coping techniques that should ideally be built into the patient's repertoire. Fordyce's (1976) quota system, discussed earlier, is one of the more productive means of building adaptive movement.

In the use of the multiple-choice, layered format that is discussed throughout this book, a suggestion for adaptive coping is often included in the three suggestions that are provided. Thus, the clinician can provide two alternatives for pain relief and then one for adaptive coping. It might be suggested that the patient will develop a strong desire to see his or her physical therapist and cooperate successfully with the therapy, or that the patient will find exercise to be effortless and enjoyable. As clinicians, we need to understand not only what hypnotic suggestions will reduce our patients' pain but also what coping responses will cause long-lasting changes in their ability to control it.

Age regression and progression can be hypnotic approaches that provide the patient with more resources for coping. Patients may have been in pain for so long that they have difficulty even imagining what it feels like not to be in pain. Age regression can be used to have a patient picture him- or herself at a time before the pain began to occur. Similarly, with age progression, patients can picture themselves in the future, in good health and with pain so low as to be essentially inconsequential. With respect to coping, in both regression and progression, patients can imagine themselves in a number of activities when they are experiencing less pain. Those activities often constitute what will be effective coping for the patient.

Catastrophizing

One of the most consistent findings in the chronic pain treatment literature is how catastrophizing is negatively associated with good outcome (Sullivan & D'Eon, 1990; Sullivan, Sullivan, Stanish, Waite, Sullivan, & Tripp, 1998; Sullivan et al., 2001). Cognitive restructuring is a desirable first step in addressing this issue with patients. Most patients will have no awareness of the negative thoughts they have and what their impact is on their pain experience. With cognitive restructuring, patients are first taught to identify their catastrophizing or other maladaptive thoughts, and then to replace them with, or alter them into, more adaptive and reassuring ones. Although patients need to understand the concept of catastrophizing through normal conversation (it is easy to overlook how many patients may not grasp this concept), the principles that we are trying to get across can be strengthened through hypnotic suggestion:

> And I want to remind you that your thoughts can be a wonderful thing for you. I mean you went to school to develop your thoughts. At least at first you need your thoughts to follow directions home. However, we both know that some of the thoughts that you have about pain are not so useful, like the automatic thoughts that just make you unhappy. At first, you can't stop having those thoughts; you feel a twinge of pain and the thought comes. Maybe the thought is that the pain is awful, maybe that the pain will not go away, or maybe that the pain means you are going to die. None of the thoughts are true, but your mind does whatever it wants. Wouldn't it be interesting if, when the automatic thoughts appeared, a big flashing light appeared in your brain that said, "That is not true!" I don't know how your mind will react to the automatic thoughts, maybe it will just find them funny, even ridiculous. I do know that more and more, you will begin to recognize when your thoughts try to play silly tricks on you and how untrue they really are.

Another way to address catastrophizing thoughts is to use the concept of applying acceptance therapy and chronic pain. In essence, the transitory nature of thoughts is discussed in an induction with the purpose of allowing the patient to detach from the emotional impact of the thought. This part of this induction might sound like this:

> And I wonder what you are thinking right now. Think about what you are thinking right now. I would argue that you can't grasp what you are thinking about right now because as soon as you try to think about it, the moment is passed, and you are actually thinking about a memory, not a thought that is happening in the present. And what follows from all of this is that you actually cannot hold on to single thoughts. Your thoughts enter and leave your mind. One thought appears, only to be replaced by another,

and then another. As we discussed, you may have thoughts about your pain when your pain occurs. Thoughts that it won't go away, thoughts that you can't do anything about it, thoughts that it will always be there. I don't know. But I do know that these thoughts are no less transitory than any other thought that comes into your mind. So the thoughts you have about your pain are only thoughts and ones that are going to go away. No thought that you have is going to stay with you for too long. If you watch the sky long enough, you will realize that it will never stay the same; it may be cloudy one moment and then it will become sunny. It will never stay the same for any length of time.

Sleep Disturbance

Disturbed sleep is a common issue with chronic pain. The issues can be cyclical, as pain can impair sleep, and, in turn, the patient who is sleep deprived is less able to cope with chronic health issues. As mentioned, the best approach to sleep issues, certainly before considering medication, is sleep hygiene education. Putting patients on a more regular sleep–wake cycle (in particular, having them wake up at a consistent time), encouraging the use of the bed as a stimulus for sleep (e.g., removing television and games from the bedroom), encouraging exercise at favorable times, and avoiding caffeine in the afternoon are examples of sleep hygiene approaches.

Once a sleep hygiene program has been established, hypnotic interventions can follow the model described for acute pain in Chapter 6. Specifically, the patient is hypnotized with an induction that ideally emphasizes deep relaxation. Posthypnotic suggestions are geared toward whether the problem is sleep onset (which is assessed beforehand) or sleep maintenance. When relaxed, the patient is given posthypnotic suggestions that are tied to the proper stimuli associated with sleep. If problems with sleep onset are an issue, the patient might get the following suggestion.

> What you will find is that you will not go to bed until you are sleepy. When you lie down in bed and your head rests on the pillow, you will find a feeling rush over you, a feeling of profound comfort and relaxation. Indeed, you may find yourself so deeply relaxed that nothing else matters.

If the issue is remaining asleep, then the patient might get a hypnotic suggestion of this nature:

> You may not know this, but over the course of a night of normal sleep, we go through periods of very deep sleep and very light sleep. When we undergo the light stages of light sleep we are close to a state of drowsy wakefulness. People with normal sleep might go through a brief awakening, but they will ignore it and go sleep. What you used to do is have the same brief wakefulness, only instead of going to sleep, you say to yourself, "Oh my

gosh, I am awake and will never get back to sleep." I wonder what it would be like if, from now, when you have the normal stages of light sleep and brief awakening that your mind reacts by telling you that you are almost still asleep, you are just going through a phase of lighter sleep. Soon you will fall back into a deep sleep. When you do experience such brief awakenings you will be filled a sense of deep comfort and the knowledge that you will drift back to sleep. And even if you don't drift back to sleep this time, you will the next time.

Axis I (Depression and Anxiety) and Axis II Diagnoses

It is beyond the scope of a discussion on pain control to describe how depression and other issues might be addressed with or without hypnosis, if they become manifest during a chronic pain assessment. As we have emphasized in the assessment section, addressing Axis I disorders are often critical to pain control. Not only will such treatment often reduce some of the pain, it will also remove barriers that the patients have to following a pain treatment program. That said, Michael Yapko (1992) and Assen Alladin (2008) have published extensively on the use of hypnosis for depression management, and the clinician working in this area is strongly encouraged to reference their work.

Social Support

As discussed earlier, the issue of social support plays a role in treating chronic pain in two different ways. First, a helpful social support network, including at least one individual who knows the patient well and provides steady and nonpain contingent support, provides an important role in how well a patient copes with pain. Helping a patient develop a greater social support network is an ongoing psychotherapeutic/social skills training issue. A clinician highly skilled in hypnosis can apply hypnosis to such issues, but, in general, this falls more in the realm of psychotherapy or social skills training.

It is interesting that work with family members of a patient with chronic pain shows that family members have often reached some type of understanding about operant influences on pain on their own. They are often relieved to hear that minimizing discussions of and attention to the patient's pain can have therapeutic effects. The concept of extinguishing pain behavior might seem inhumane, but it is important to understand that the concept is ignoring pain behavior, not ignoring the patient. Social interactions that center largely on pain can burn out the most patient family members; in contrast, making other topics the focus of the relationship can improve the quality of relationships. Further, focusing less conversation and less attention to pain often does indeed result in less suffering for the patient.

For these reasons, involving family members in treatment can be an important component of chronic pain care. There is a role for hypnosis in this respect. However, it is important to note that family members can often sabotage treatment, often unintentionally, for a variety of reasons. Patients need a certain amount of time and privacy to practice self-hypnosis. Further, although hypnosis is becoming more mainstream, hypnosis may still cause a certain amount of ridicule from a family member who is not familiar with it. For this reason, it may be helpful to explain to family members the role of hypnosis in pain control. Also, it might be particularly useful to show family members pictures of brain scans of patients receiving hypnosis for pain. Such images are capable of swaying the opinions of a skeptical scientist and should certainly help convince a wary layperson.

Mindfulness, Acceptance Therapy, and Hypnosis

It is important to discuss the integration of hypnosis with acceptance therapy and mindfulness as an approach to chronic pain, given the clear similarities between mindfulness and hypnotic approaches. Chapter 1 of this volume already discussed some of the research done in the area of mindfulness and acceptance therapy, particularly that of McCracken and colleagues (McCracken & Eccleston, 2003, 2005; McCracken, Vowles, & Eccleston, 2004). The point was also made that many of the principles of acceptance therapy are inherent in Fordyce's (1976) work.

A large part of the mindfulness literature focuses on the practice of meditation. There is a large variety of meditation approaches, and many of these have been associated with improved management of chronic pain (Kabat-Zinn, 1982; Shapiro & Carlson, 2009; Shapiro, Oman, Thoresen, Plante, & Flinders, 2008). There are also studies to suggest that meditation can change the manner in which the brain responds to a number of types of negative affect and suffering (R. J. Davidson et al., 2003). One key appears to be the benefits of practice and meditation over a long period of time (Kabat-Zinn et al., 1992; Ludwig & Kabat-Zinn, 2008; Shapiro et al., 2008). Similarly, Jensen and colleagues have emphasized the benefit of practicing self-hypnosis outside of the therapy session for chronic pain (M. P. Jensen, Barber, Romano, Hanley, et al., 2009; M. P. Jensen, Barber, Romano, Molton, et al., 2009; M. P. Jensen, Nielson, & Kerns, 2003; M. P. Jensen & Patterson, 2006). Although self-hypnosis and meditation are not the same thing, there are a number of similarities (e.g., their common goals of using focused attention to achieve a specific psychological state), and an effective therapist can facilitate integration between these two approaches. The integration between hypnosis and meditation is a wide-open field at present, in terms of both clinical application and research.

There are at least two major ways that mindfulness and acceptance therapy can be integrated into hypnotic treatment of pain. One, which has been a general theme of this book, has to do with acknowledging that chronic pain is part of a patient's perceptual experience and can be difficult to change directly, and should therefore not be considered a focus of treatment; rather, pain relief and relief from suffering are best thought of as side effects of adaptive pain management. This focus has been noted in outcome research with multidisciplinary pain treatment centers, where outcomes are often manifested in increased quality of life, return to work, and more enjoyable activity, rather than actual pain reduction (Turk & Okifuji, 1998a, 1998b). As discussed in this chapter, patients with chronic pain may be best served by hypnotic suggestions focusing on sleep, on increasing activity, or on goals that do not focus on pain reduction per se. One such nonanalgesic suggestion that can be made to patients is to develop practices such as meditation or yoga.

Hypnotic inductions for pain relief and mindfulness/acceptance therapy can also be integrated in a more direct manner. The acceptance model holds a number of underlying assumptions such as the impermanence of thoughts, perceptions, and experiences, as well as the notion that resisting chronic pain can lead to increased suffering. Rather than fighting chronic pain, patients can be given suggestions that pain and suffering are both natural outcomes of living (as are comfort and joy), and that all experience and sensations are things to accept rather than things to struggle against. Often, this acceptance may be a useful precursor to additional steps through which the patient can move sensations to the background of their experience. Similar to dissociative hypnotic suggestions, acceptance therapy treatments encourage patients to deidentify with the contents of consciousness (Shapiro & Carlson, 2009). In simple terms, the patient is taught, "If I can see or feel it, then I must be more than it." Along these lines, the patient can be taught, not to fight pain, but to acknowledge it in a nonjudgmental manner when it is present, and then understand that there is more to existence and consciousness than the pain. The actual hypnotic suggestion could be:

> I wonder if while you are in this state, and perhaps long after, you can reflect on what is part of you without trying to change it. For example, while you are listening to me, you might be having thoughts. You cannot *not* have thoughts, they just seem to come and go. This is the case with pain as well. No matter how badly you have felt pain before, it has never remained the same. And even if you are experiencing pain now or in the future, you have to wonder who is experiencing the pain. There is a bigger part of you that is observing the pain. So as you begin to realize and understand that you may not always be able to make the pain go away, there is part of you that is much bigger; you are not your sensations—you can watch them come and go from a distance.

Mindfulness (meditation) and acceptance therapy is a complex approach regarding discipline on the part of the patient and therapist. Although not yet considered by many from either field, there is a great deal of potential for hypnotic procedures to be integrated into acceptance-based approaches and vice versa.

SUMMARY

The empirical evidence supporting the application of hypnosis to treat chronic pain has blossomed over the past decade. Hypnosis is unquestionably a useful approach for chronic pain, but clinicians have to consider the complexity of this clinical issue. First, every patient must be evaluated independently with the intent of teasing apart the multiple factors that might be contributing to the patient's pain. What clinical interventions, both hypnotic and nonhypnotic, that are used with the patient often go far beyond reducing the pain itself. It might be that what ends up making the greatest difference with patients is increasing their activity, improving their sleep, or reducing depression. If clinicians apply hypnosis within the context of a biopsychosocial model for understanding pain, the probability of having a long-term impact on pain reduction and increased function will be greatly enhanced. Appendix 7.1 provides an induction example in its entirety for using hypnotic suggestions for integrating lifestyle changes for patients with chronic pain.

APPENDIX 7.1: INTEGRATING SUGGESTIONS FOR LIFESTYLE
CHANGES INTO HYPNOTIC SUGGESTIONS FOR PATIENTS
WITH CHRONIC PAIN: A SAMPLE INDUCTION

One of the strongest messages of this book is that focusing hypnotic suggestions for chronic pain analgesia may not be the most effective way to go and may also be counterproductive to good clinical care. With many types of chronic pain, what that patient experiences as pain sensation is not under the control of nociception or tissue damage. In other words, there is not some sort of tissue damage or illness process contributing to the patient's sensation of pain. Instead, the perception of pain in such patients may be better explained by a variety of alternative factors, such as deconditioning and lack of movement, poor biomechanics, misinterpretation of symptoms and catastrophizing thoughts about pain, or neuroplasticity (essentially, rewiring of neuropathic signals so that the patient responds as if in pain without the presence of tissue damage).

In such cases, the goal of treatment is often to enable the patient to adopt a biopsychosocial model for understanding the conceptualization and treatment of pain. One outcome that arises from such models is that pain reductions may not be the best goal of treatment; increasing activity and more participation in life activities, such as work and recreation, may prove to be superior goals for the patient.

When it comes to hypnotic inductions then, reducing patient suffering may be a matter of providing a series of hypnotic suggestions that do things such as increase their activity or motivation for treatment. When taking the tack of increasing motivation, it is important to integrate the core values of the patient. Specifically, and in keeping with the discussion of motivational interviewing (see Chapter 8, this volume), what are the core values that might come into play in motivating behavior change? A patient with chronic back pain may find that her pain is limiting the time that she is able to spend with her grandchildren, and her desire to change this is a good example of a core value that can be integrated into hypnosis.

The example of an induction below is for a patient with back pain that appears to be moderated by musculoskeletal processes and lifestyle issues, such as deconditioning, inactivity, and failure to follow through with medical and physical therapy advice. This tends to be the hardest type of pain to address with hypnosis. Examples of hypnotic induction scripts that are used with specific pain syndromes are included in the appendix at the end of this book. Further, M. P. Jensen and Patterson (2008) provided a nice summary of suggestions for chronic pain beyond those found in this volume. The induction presented below that leads into the hypnotic suggestions applies the "pace, pace, pace, lead" approach, or one that uses three truisms and a suggestion.

When adequate levels of relaxation, rapport, and a sense of rhythm are achieved, then hypnotic suggestions for pain control driven by the above considerations are provided. Essentially, the example alternates between suggestions for well-being, lifestyle changes, and eliciting motivation from the patient's core values.

For the induction phase, it is far better that the hypnotist uses what he or she senses in the moment rather than following this particular script. Truisms are statements of what is, such as the fact that the patient is sitting in the chair (see Chapter 4, this volume). Stating that the patient is "becoming more relaxed" is a hypnotic suggestion. Suggestions during the initial stage are best based on changes that can be observed in the patient (e.g., slowing of breathing, eye blinking). The following is useful only as an example for how the clinician might interact with the patient; it is not meant as a script to be used clinically.

> OK, Ms. Lee, let's begin by having you sit here comfortably, keeping your eyes open for now. You may find it interesting that it doesn't seem like there is a thing you have to do. I am going to be talking about what seems to be happening right now, and then I might make some suggestions about your relationship with what is happening to your back.
>
> You are sitting in the chair
> You are breathing in and out
> Your feet are on the floor
> And perhaps you are listening to my voice
> I don't know exactly what you are experiencing but
> I do know that you are
> Sitting in the chair
> You are breathing in and out
> Your feet are on the floor
> And maybe you find that you are listening to my voice even more clearly
> I am not sure exactly what you are experiencing but I do know that you
> Have your feet on the floor
> You are sitting in the chair
> You are breathing in and out
> And perhaps your breathing is slowing down ever so slightly
> I can't tell exactly but I am aware that
> Your eyes are beginning to blink [*stated only if this is occurring*]
> You are sitting in the chair
> Your feet are on the floor
> And maybe you are finding your eyes becoming tired and wanting
>   to close.

This induction can continue for another 5, 10, or 15 additional minutes. The nature of the exact truism used is not important, but it is essential that whatever truism that occurs is actually happening. For example, once the patient closes her eyes, then "Your eyes have closed" can become a truism. This induction will be more effective if the hypnotist picks up on behavior changes demonstrated by the patient and reinforces them (e.g., "Your neck is letting go, perhaps as you are beginning to relax"). As this progresses over several minutes, the hypnotist can take more guesses with suggestions; often, this might be a function of what we sense the patient is going through (e.g., "Perhaps you are finding yourself developing a sense of drifting, or maybe you are finding that the evaluative voice in your head seems to have largely gone away").

Once a nice rhythm has been established and the patient is showing indications of deep relaxation and other signs of a hypnotic state, the next step is to introduce the concept of an internal resource. This could be viewed as the unconscious, an inner voice, a "friend inside," or whatever concept is comfortable to both hypnotist and patient. An important purpose for including this concept is to facilitate dissociation and/or automaticity in response. The notion of a third party can create that type of dissociative gap between the patient and her actions. Rather than her having to do something, it becomes a matter her unconscious resource doing something. In this case, we will use a friendly part of the mind as a resource.

> You are breathing slowly and deeply
> You are completely supported by the chair
> You are responding to suggestions that are useful to you
> And as this continues, perhaps you begin to become aware of a profound resource in your mind. Part of our mind allows us to breathe, even if we are not thinking about it. Part of our mind allows our heart to beat. This part of your mind can be a tremendous resource when you need it to be.
> Perhaps you find that this part of your mind is allowing you to breathe slowly and comfortably.
> This part of your mind allows you to feel completely supported by the chair.
> This part of your mind allows you to respond to suggestions that are useful to you.
> And wouldn't it be wonderful if this part of your mind enabled you to begin to do things that make you far more comfortable in life?
> I don't know exactly how your mind might allow you to do this, I only know that it is quite powerful and can serve you in a variety of different ways.
> Your mind may serve you now by allowing you to notice how comfortable your body has become and perhaps allowing that to go on longer than you might have ever imagined.
> Perhaps your mind will serve you by allowing you to suddenly realize that you already know what you need to do to make yourself more active.

Or maybe you have a sudden picture of what it is like to be with your grandchildren and totally enjoying their company.

I don't know exactly how your resources will serve you.

It may be that you begin to notice a type of cool numbness in your back, or some other interesting and pleasant sensation that never seemed to be there before. Along with this, is there now a sudden urgency to see your physical therapist and take care of yourself, a sense of knowing that the work you do with her is such an important link to spending time with your grandchildren, that you might find yourself excited about attending the sessions. You are indeed excited about seeing your grandchildren.

Maybe this is how your mind will serve you or perhaps it will make you feel more comfortable in other ways.

Perhaps you will experience the sensation of a dial in your back, one with which you can turn up or down the sensations of your back. Just as you turn a dial on the wall to make the lights become dimmer, you find that the sensations in your back dim in a similar manner. What your mind might do instead is remind you of the wonderful pleasure that can come with taking short walks. How good it feels to be outdoors, smelling the flowers and feeling the sun shine down on you, and never knowing who you might bump into while on a walk, what pleasant surprises might await you.

It may be that you put your pain in a box. What type of box? Perhaps looking in front of you, you see a shiny box, about the size of a shoebox, only it is square in shape. You put your pain in there. I don't know how, it just happens. Now you are going to take that box and put it in a slightly bigger box; nothing can get out of that box. Now take the bigger box and put that into an even bigger box, and that in turn goes into a bigger box. Finally, the box gets so big that you are looking at it in the back of a train, and now the train is slowly chugging away, farther and farther into the distance. Just watch the train disappear into the distance.

Yes, your mind can serve you in so many different ways.

It may be that several hours after we have talked, or maybe it will be a couple of days, I am not sure how long it will be, you look back and are amazed at how comfortable you have been. It will seem as if you can't remember the times that you were not comfortable or that somehow they have gone by very quickly in your mind. It may be that this comes out in your suddenly wanting to do so much. And enjoying what you do, as long as it is safe for you. What begins to become the focus is what you can do and the special people you can do things with.

So many resources inside of you that you seldom are aware of. Just as you breathe in and out, just as your heart beat, your mind continues to be a friend to you in ways you might not have imagined.

And now you might find that if given some silence for 30 seconds, you are able to give yourself whatever type of suggestions that will serve you;

30 seconds of silence to gain a sense of completion, starting now (allow 30 seconds).

Yes, isn't it interesting how your mind can serve you.

For just as you are sitting in the chair

You are listening to my voice

And are breathing in and out

Your mind is perhaps remembering the things that might be useful to you and forgetting those that aren't. No matter what you remember, you are surprisingly more comfortable, more relaxed, and more capable.

And as you sit in the chair

And listen to my voice

And you are breathing in and out

Perhaps you gain the sense of becoming more alert

Yes, sitting in the chair

Listening to my voice

Breathing in and out

And becoming more and more awake

Moving around in your chair now

Becoming more awake

Just knowing what you will bring back with you

More and more alert now

Feeling more refreshed

More and more aware of the gifts you have

And perhaps feeling your eyes beginning to open.

Obviously, the rate at which the patient is brought out must be matched to the behavior/experience of the patient, as is the case with this entire example.

8

MOTIVATIONAL INTERVIEWING

There are a number of reasons why a chapter that focuses on the integration of Ericksonian approaches and motivational interviewing (MI) is a fitting culmination for a book on hypnotic approaches to pain control. The first reason arises from the shared focus of both chronic pain treatment and MI treatment: lifestyle behavior change. The management of chronic pain is a challenging task from any clinical perspective. Often, the most parsimonious route in improving the quality of life in such patients is to help them decrease their use of pain medications, reverse a sedentary lifestyle, and engage in challenging physical therapy exercises. A number of hypnotic suggestions enable patients to alter their perception of pain; yet effective treatment also requires that patients follow through with disciplined adherence to behavioral programs that focus on changes in lifestyle. MI is an evidence-based approach that enhances patients' intrinsic motivation to entertain alternative models and pursue behavioral treatment strategies.

Previous chapters have argued that Ericksonian hypnosis holds promise as an evidence-based treatment for pain control because many of its underlying principles have been substantiated by social–psychological research. Both MI and Ericksonian hypnosis share empirically supported components of brief therapies, such as exchanging information with patients to change perceptions, offering a menu of options rather than a single suggestion to reduce resistance, and emphasizing that the patient is free to choose whether to change. Accordingly, a second reason to consider blending MI and Ericksonian hypnosis is that a large body of scientific evidence supports the feasibility and effectiveness of using MI in combination with treatment as usual for behavior change. At least two systematic reviews of MI outcome research have shown that MI's effects are stronger (Dunn, Deroo, & Rivara, 2001) and longer lasting (Hettema, Steele, & Miller, 2005) when used additively to enhance another treatment.

Perhaps the most compelling reason to blend MI and Ericksonian hypnosis is the untapped but potentially powerful synergy from combining two clinical approaches that are complementary in task and similar in their styles of being with patients. Both styles are regarded as being easy on the patient and the clinician. Both approaches remove the struggle between the therapist and the patient by tailoring clinician statements to patients' needs and viewpoints. Not only does the interpersonal style of MI mirror that of Ericksonian hypnosis, but each therapy seems to pick up where the other leaves off. Hypnosis, for example, by evoking perceptual changes, confusion, or disequilibrium, aims to help patients release rigid viewpoints ("all of my suffering comes from my pinched nerve") and embrace alternative views or insights ("there's a lot I can do to reduce my own suffering"). Once new perspectives render patients more accepting of lifestyle change, MI can significantly enhance their motivation to initiate and sustain behavior change. Successful lifestyle behavior change is characterized by chronic relapses to both old behaviors and old viewpoints, hence the need to alternately deploy these two complementary treatments with such compatible interpersonal styles. The potential additive effects of combining MI and Ericksonian hypnosis are ones that should be explored thoroughly on a theoretical and clinical basis. This chapter offers a tentative agenda for such an endeavor.

BACKGROUND OF MOTIVATIONAL INTERVIEWING

MI is a brief therapy approach that had its genesis largely in the treatment of people with alcohol and substance abuse issues. In noting how people often struggled with giving up destructive habits, W. R. Miller (1983) became interested in studying the phenomenon of change itself. Investigators (e.g., Curry, Wagner, & Grothaus, 1990; DiClemente, 1999; Miller & Rollnick, 1991) have noted that often, even despite multiple external forces that might encourage change, such as families, the legal system, and psychotherapy, people typically make intentional behavior change only after making a decision to do so; thus, although external factors are indeed important in initiating and sustaining change, the internal factors play a necessary and sometimes sufficient role in creating change (DiClemente, 2003; DiClemente & Prochaska, 1998). Investigators also noted that many of the approaches families, friends, and even health care providers took to encourage change in patients often appeared to make patients more steadfast in their behavior. Arguing, lecturing, and particularly confronting often appeared to create resistance in the patient (W. R. Miller, Benefield, & Tonigan, 1993; W. R. Miller & Rollnick, 2002). Gradually, theorists gained a better understanding of those conditions under which change occurs naturally and without struggle.

An important theoretical foundation to understanding intentional human behavior change is the transtheoretical model (TTM; DiClemente & Prochaska, 1985, 1998; Prochaska & DiClemente, 1983; Prochaska et al., 1994). Prochaska and DiClemente theorized that, with change, people pass through a series of stages. They viewed change as a beginning with an initial precontemplation stage, where the person is not considering change. This progresses to contemplation, where the individual undertakes a serious evaluation of considerations for and against change. In preparation, the next stage, planning and commitment are secured. In the action stage, specific behavioral steps are taken. Finally, successful action leads to the fifth and final stage, maintenance, in which the person works to maintain and sustain long-term change. Research has isolated such stages of change among a wide variety of behavior, including cessation of smoking, alcohol, and drugs; medical screening; and birth control (Carney & Kivlahan, 1995; DiClemente & Hughes, 1990; DiClemente & Prochaska, 1998; DiClemente, Story, & Murray, 2000; Glanz et al., 1994; Grimley, Riley, Bellis, & Prochaska, 1993; Isenhart, 1994; Marcus, Rossi, Selby, Niaura, & Abrams, 1992; N. D. Weinstein, Rothman, & Sutton, 1998; Werch & DiClemente, 1994; Willoughby & Edens, 1996). It should be noted, however, that in more recent writing, DiClemente (2003; see also Carbonari & DiClemente, 2000) suggested that the stages are best considered as a heuristic for understanding client movement toward change and not truly discrete stages.

Despite this new perspective, the stages of change remain useful for clinicians as they evaluate individuals' readiness to change. Understanding the degree of readiness to change moment to moment can guide clinical interventions in real time. If someone is in the precontemplation stage, for example, it will seldom be useful for the clinician to provide interventions that work with people in the action stage, such as referral to a psychosocial pain management program. In fact, providing suggestions for change to someone who is not actively considering it can actually increase resistance to change. Understanding where an individual is in this cycle of change can often enable the clinician to interact with the patient in a way that facilitates forward movement rather than provokes resistance.

MI has been described as a cousin to the TTM (W. R. Miller & Rollnick, 2009). Although they grew up together, they are not the same. The TTM provides a heuristic description of how change occurs across multiple behaviors, whereas MI is a clinical method that helps increase readiness to change. While MI does not prescribe specific intervention methods for each stage of change, it is designed to help patients move through such stages of change with a minimum of effort, confrontation, and resistance—more quickly than they might do on their own. W. R. Miller and Rollnick (2002) defined MI as "a client-centered, directive method for enhancing intrinsic motivation to change by exploring and resolving ambivalence" (p. 25). They credited Carl Rogers and other client-centered therapists with generating the type of therapeutic work from which MI evolved. However, unlike the work of Rogers, Miller and Rollnick regarded MI as "consciously directive." Therapists work to resolve ambivalence and reduce resistance to unusual change. The authors regarded MI as a method of communication with a relational and technical component (Rosengren, 2009) rather than a set of techniques, and they saw the focus of therapy as eliciting a person's intrinsic motivation for change. Finally, MI seeks to resolve ambivalence in a way that is consistent with the person's own values and beliefs.

Although MI was largely developed for working with people who have addiction problems, it has been applied well beyond these origins, including extension to basic health care issues (Rollnick, Miller, & Butler, 2008). As is realized more and more with biopsychosocial models, the most effective means of preventing and managing chronic diseases is often through active patient involvement in behavior change (e.g., diet, smoking cessation, increased exercise, dental care). Frequently, patients are ambivalent about such changes. Their values and beliefs are consistent with being healthy, but they are reluctant to give up habits or endure the discipline necessary for healthy behavior; this is particularly relevant to chronic pain management.

A recurring theme of this book is that effective management of chronic pain involves a number of disciplined behavior changes such as increasing exercise, complying with physical therapy recommendations, and altering negative cognitions. Pain researchers such as Jensen and colleagues (Douaihy, Jensen, & Jou, 2005; M. P. Jensen, 1996, 2000, 2002, 2006; M. P. Jensen & Karoly, 1991; M. P. Jensen, Nielson, & Kerns, 2003; Molton, Jensen, Nielson, Cardenas, & Ehde, 2008) have long argued for the benefits of using an MI paradigm when working with patients who have chronic pain. The remainder of this chapter introduces parallels between MI and Ericksonian hypnosis and describes possible synergistic effects, which may enable patients to manage chronic pain more effectively.

COMMONALITIES BETWEEN MOTIVATIONAL INTERVIEWING AND ERICKSONIAN HYPNOSIS

There are a number of commonalities between MI and Ericksonian hypnosis. Interestingly, both approaches developed atheoretically. Rather than a theory of human behavior driving development, instead it was observation (and empirical study in the case of MI) of what led to behavior change that led to the development of the appearances. What evolved is a useful collection of interventions for behavior change. However, both approaches adhere to a number of underlying assumptions. It is remarkable how much concordance there is with some of these principles.

Humanistic Assumptions

MI largely has its roots in humanistic psychology. Humans are seen as innately good, and when provided with the proper conditions, it is assumed that they will grow. Therapy is often seen as a process of removing barriers to growth or providing the proper conditions to change. Under the proper conditions, it is assumed that humans will show growth independently. Rogers, as early as the 1950s, was describing these conditions (i.e., unconditional positive regard, genuineness, and acceptance; Rogers, 1957). These assumptions undergird the relational aspect of MI, which W. R. Miller and Rollnick (2002; see also Rollnick et al., 2008) described as the MI spirit and to which they ascribed three qualities: evocation, collaboration, and autonomy. The importance of these qualities will become apparent below. With respect to Ericksonian hypnosis, humanistic assumptions apply largely to the role of the unconscious. Unlike psychoanalytic theory in which the unconscious might be assumed to contain destructive urges, its role in Ericksonian approaches is regarded as much more of a resource. Intertwined in Erickson's work is the notion that the unconscious and a patient's inner resources are not only to be trusted but also potential sources of growth that are ideally elicited through hypnosis.

Collaborative Process

MI is viewed as a collaborative process between the therapist and client. Often, the therapist is seen as having a consulting or guiding role in the process of behavior change (Rollnick et al., 2008). Although advice might be given, it is done so sparingly and typically with the permission of the client. MI therapists high in collaboration "actively foster and encourage power sharing in the interaction in such a way that the client's ideas substantially influence the nature of the session" (Moyers, Martin, Manuel, & Miller, 2004). Ericksonian hypnosis has been termed the cooperative approach (Gilligan,

1987). Establishing a hypnotic state is regarded as a collaboration between the therapist and client. The notion of having the power reside with the therapist is discouraged because, in addition to contributing to resistance, it is seen as preventing patients from generating their own solutions.

Autonomy

Within MI, the therapist believes the patient is ultimately responsible for deciding when and if change will occur. The approach encourages patients to be active participants in the change process and to recognize their responsibility for choosing the timing and direction of change. The MI therapist seeks to "markedly expand the client's experience of control and choice" (Moyers et al., 2004). While Ericksonian hypnosis may circumvent some of the mechanisms of control that patients use to maintain the status quo, it ultimately encourages patients to rely on internal resources and make choices consistent with their beliefs and values.

Conceptualizing and Addressing Resistance

In both MI and Ericksonian hypnosis, resistance is often seen as an issue of the therapist rather than the client. That is, if the client resists behavior changes, then the problem likely lies with the therapist, not the client (W. R. Miller & Rollnick, 2002), and is regarded often as an issue of the therapist trying to push his or her agenda on the client. Ericksonian and MI therapists alike are encouraged to examine their own behavior when a patient demonstrates resistance; it is a cue that the therapist is not working in consonance with the patient. This tendency is often expressed as the righting reflex in current MI thinking (Rollnick et al., 2008). Similarly, if patients are not following the hypnotic suggestions in an Ericksonian approach, the therapist is encouraged to follow the patient rather than continue to push an agenda that is not welcomed by the patient.

Evocative

Both MI and Ericksonian approaches are viewed as being evocative. The role of the therapist in both approaches is to create the circumstances through which patients can generate their own solutions. Rather than suggest to patients the reason to change or how to change, the role of the therapist is to create the conditions in which patients are able to do that for themselves. The MI therapist high in evocation "works proactively to evoke the client's own reasons for change and ideas about how change should happen" (Moyers et al., 2004). This client language has been termed *change talk*

(Amrhein, Miller, Yahne, Knupsky, & Hochstein, 2004; Amrhein, Miller, Yahne, Palmer, & Fulcher, 2003), has been demonstrated to predict outcomes (e.g., Moyers et al., 2008; Moyers & Martin, 2006; Moyers et al., 2007), and is actively attended to and elicited in the course of an MI session (Arkowitz, Westra, Miller, & Rollnick, 2008; Rosengren, 2009). Ericksonian approaches might accomplish this by the use of indirect suggestions. As discussed in Chapter 4 of this volume, indirect suggestions are largely used to generate unconscious searches in patients and the ability for them to generate their own solutions to problems.

Following the Patient

Both MI and Ericksonian hypnosis rely heavily on following the patient's lead. A cornerstone of MI is reflective listening, in which statements are designed to reflect the patient's affect, as well generate more verbal output and reflection. Reflective listening requires that the therapist attends to client cues and responds to where the client leads. Rather than follow the client aimlessly, the MI therapist follows the client to acquire a deep understanding of his or her point of view (Moyers et al., 2004). Within MI, as with Ericksonian hypnosis, the clinician will move fluidly between following the patient's lead and at times directing the interaction toward productive directions. Ericksonian hypnosis, in turn, encourages the therapist to observe and listen carefully, and then follow the patient in hypnosis. Rather than the therapist simply providing the patient with suggestions, the therapist is encouraged to observe the patient and reinforce where the patient is with respect to considering change. The therapist is also encouraged to move slightly ahead of patients at times to direct the hypnotic process (e.g., pacing).

Providing Choices

MI writers (e.g., Rosengren, 2009) note that there are problems inherent in giving the client only one option for changing behavior. It does not respect the client's wisdom and experience with regard to change. Also, it creates a dynamic where therapists suggest solutions and clients reject them one at a time. So, an MI therapist typically avoids giving clients *the* approach to changing behavior and instead attempts to have clients generate the solution themselves. Further, MI therapists—when they offer solutions—do so in the context of a menu where patients can choose that which suits them best. Ericksonian approaches also emphasize the importance of providing choice for the patients. Indirect hypnotic suggestions are thought to potentially reduce resistance by providing options to the patient as to how he or she will experience hypnosis. As another example, one of the techniques from

Erickson that is particularly relied on in this book is the multiple-choice format for providing suggestions. Rather than being given one suggestion for pain reduction during hypnosis, patients are given the choice of several options.

INTEGRATING MOTIVATIONAL INTERVIEWING AND ERICKSONIAN HYPNOSIS

I hope it has been made clear that there are a number of compelling parallels between MI and Ericksonian hypnosis. However, the two clearly remain different approaches to behavior change. MI is a quiet and eliciting style, relying largely on few strategic questions, many reflections, and summaries of the patient's views to increase verbalization from the patient in favor of change. Ericksonian approaches, of course, rely heavily on giving patients hypnotic suggestion. Although patient verbalization is certainly encouraged prior to inductions, during hypnosis patients are encouraged far more to explore internal resources than to verbalize. Another clear difference is that notions of unconscious behavior discussed in Ericksonian hypnosis are for the most part not addressed in MI, which neither endorses nor refutes the unconscious, trusting simply that all parts of the person will strive for health under the right conditions.

At the same time, these two approaches can work in concert, with one picking up where the other leaves off. As a simple example, a patient may refuse to consider hypnosis for pain control, not because he or she has any inherent concerns with this approach, but because considering hypnosis may represent abandonment of a quest for a medical cure; this is particularly the case with patients who have an illness conviction. An MI therapist would seek and acknowledge the patient's strengths that may be driving this rigid quest for a medical cure (determination? not giving up? wanting to get more from life?) as a way to enlist the patient's energy toward healthy change. MI represents one of the most efficient methods for allowing patients to consider alternative treatments to their pain, be they hypnosis, physical therapy, yoga, or another nonmedical approach.

Conversely, hypnosis can be useful for a patient who is engaged in an MI approach to change addictive behavior or as an approach to chronic pain management. An example that comes to mind is with a patient who is actively engaged in behavior change but is struggling to sustain it. Hypnosis can be an effective means to generate creatively a menu of options for behavior change, and it can also be useful in allowing the patient to "try them out" through rehearsal.

The integration of MI and hypnosis is an area of conceptualization that is ripe for research. For example, a simple question is whether hypnosis is useful in eliciting more change talk from patients in favor of assuming psychosocial responsibility for their pain management. Similarly, it would be useful to determine empirically whether a preparatory session of MI may increase patient willingness and susceptibility to hypnotic suggestion. The following section provides some examples of how hypnosis can be integrated with MI not only for the purpose of research but also in practical clinical situations. In guiding this discussion, the FRAMES model (W. R. Miller & Rollnick, 1991) is used to describe the components of brief psychotherapies for behavior change (Bien, Miller, & Tonigan, 1993).

FRAMES is an acronym representing six common motivational components found in successful behavioral counseling interventions (Bien, Miller, & Boroughs, 1993). The elements of FRAMES are feedback, responsibility, advice, menu of options, empathy, and self-efficacy. The order in which these components are presented is not one suggested for treatment; the effective clinician will move fluidly from one to another. In some cases, discussion of these principles will be primarily useful for understanding how MI can be applied to pain management in itself; in others, the potential combination with Ericksonian hypnosis will be more relevant.

Feedback and Giving Information

Much of what underlies considerations of applying MI is the behaviors or strategies in which patients are engaged that are not working for them, if not outright destructive. Giving patients feedback about the nature of their behavior and how it is affecting them can be one of the most effective means of eliciting change. As an example, much of the early work done in this area was done in the area of problem drinking. Feedback from family and friends about the impact of drinking (Johnson, 1973) and medical checkups that provide information about how long-term use of substances can harm patients have both been found to reduce alcohol intake (Kristenson, Ohlin, Hulten-Nosslin, Trell, & Hood, 1983; W. R. Miller & Sovereign, 1989). Similarly, keeping a self-monitoring record of drinks taken can have an effect (W. R. Miller & Munoz, 2005), as can simply stepping on scales for reducing weight (W. R. Miller & Rollnick, 1991). Recent studies support that feedback alone can be a powerful intervention (Carey, Henson, Carey, & Maisto, 2009; Walters, Vader, Harris, Field, & Jouriles, 2009). These are examples of personalized, normative feedback, from which patients cannot distance themselves, as opposed to "health pamphlet" information about risky behaviors. Patients with chronic pain are most eager to learn their assessment when those results pertain to them personally. For example, a less effective message would be, "Patients with chronic pain often experience secondary suffering if they believe that their pain can be completely removed." A more effective message might be, "Compared with other patients with chronic pain, your answers on this family questionnaire suggest that your chronic pain causes you more conflict with your family than it does with most other chronic pain patients."

Similarly, giving patients information about their pain can be made more effective when it follows a thorough assessment, which should be a component of any type of pain treatment. What is known about MI would suggest that thorough feedback from an interview is enough to change pain behavior in itself. However, an edict throughout this literature is that such feedback be provided in a nonjudgmental, nonthreatening manner. Such feedback to a person with lower back pain might be put as follows: "You injured your back some time ago and have every reason to be feeling pain. I wonder what you know about how pain works in the body." Allow the patient time to describe his or her understanding, then reflect it back and add to it as follows:

> Would it be OK if I shared a few additional bits of information? Initially, the source of this pain was a slipped disk that was sending you pain signals. These signals told you that if you moved, your back would spasm and you would experience tremendous pain. Over time you began to adapt to this by moving less and less. You also started taking medications that might have made you feel better but did not really address the pain. After several months of not moving, you have begun to experience some atrophy in your muscles, so that when you try to move now, that very atrophy causes your pain. Further, you have begun to hold your body differently in a biomechanical sense. If you move like you used to, it will hurt, but because of your body mechanics, not because of your back injury. What do you make of that information?

Again, allow time for the patient's perspective. Reflect or summarize those concerns, then add an additional chunk of information.

> Here is a little more information you might find interesting. There is something called neuroplasticity that is often important for patients like yourself. After you've been in pain for so long, your mind can become imprinted to feel pain even though the lesion in your back that was causing the problem has long since healed. So the pain and suffering you are experiencing is very real; it is just that the fix for this is not to go and mess surgically with your back. We have ways to make you feel better that will be more effective but will take more time and discipline than a surgical fix. This will involve regular visits with specialists that will help you move more and differently. How does that sound to you?

Again, listen and reflect.

> I have seen this work well with many different patients and they have been able to avoid the trauma of another surgery. However, you must be the person who decides which way to go. I am curious about how this sounds to you.

Rollnick et al. (2008) called this process *information exchange* because it involves not just providing information to clients but also engaging in a dialogue in which both parties come to understand better the situation and the important issues at play. Because the concept of feedback is simply a matter of providing information, the parallels between it and Ericksonian hypnosis are not as apparent as are other elements of the FRAMES components. However, some associations can be found with the use of truisms. As has been discussed earlier, truisms are simple statements of what is. They can be used as a means to facilitate induction: "You are sitting in the chair, you are listening to my voice, you are breathing in and out." They can also be an effective means of providing suggestions: "Isn't it interesting that your unconscious mind can respond by allowing your right arm to float upward while your conscious mind can allow your left arm to remain in place."

In applying this concept to pain control, the therapist might say the following, whether or not the patient is in a hypnotic state:

> You have been in pain for a long amount of time. You have tried to do several things about it, but nothing seems to have been working. Yet you keep showing the motivation and effort to improve your situation, just as you have by coming in to see me today.

This statement, within an MI perspective, contains reflective listening and an affirmation of the client's strength and motivation, two key skills used in this approach.

Responsibility for Change

A central tenet of MI and other such brief strategies is that the responsibility of behavior change is with the patient. In this respect, MI and theories about motivation for change (Prochaska & DiClemente, 1982) have emphasized that confronting the patient and arguing for behavior change is more likely to increase resistance rather than facilitate behavior change. W. R. Miller and Rollnick (1991) argued that arguments are counterproductive, defending breeds defensiveness, and resistance is a signal to change strategies. Further, labeling an addictive behavior (e.g., "alcoholism") is generally not useful. Certainly, concerns about labeling also apply to chronic pain management, because it has long been known that telling patients that their pain is psychogenic or "all in their head" is one of the more pernicious communications that can be made. Rather than argue with the patient or label the problem behavior, MI therapists make it clear that responsibility for behavior change lies squarely with the patient. As G. Edwards and Orford (1977) and others in this field have emphasized, it is up to patients to decide what to do with the information that is provided to them. Nobody can decide for them, and no one can change their drinking if they do not want to change. It is the patient's choice, and if change is going to happen, the patient is the one who has to do it.

Similarly, effective clinicians using hypnosis will never claim that hypnosis is something they have done to the patient. Rather, they will stress that they have only provided guidance and that the patient is to be credited with hypnotically based changes. Some clinicians will argue that all hypnosis is essentially self-hypnosis. It is clear that having patients perceive that they are responsible for the effects of hypnosis is desirable, particularly with respect to chronic pain management.

When it comes to dealing with resistance, there are a number of clear parallels between MI and Ericksonian hypnosis in particular. MI teaches us to roll with resistance. If a patient shouts, "I am not an alcoholic!" it not is for the therapist to argue that his drinking caused multiple DWIs or his family to leave him. The therapist might instead reflect back, "You don't seem to think that your drinking has caused serious problems." Similarly, a patient may state, "My pain is caused by a problem in my back that only surgery can fix." Rather than arguing this, the therapist might state, "Yes. I absolutely agree there is a physical cause for your pain, which makes you wonder how these other factors might be making the pain worse and whether you might be able to do something about them." This statement is an example of an agreement with a twist that moves in a new direction by reframing the client statement.

This approach is consistent with the Ericksonian approach of using natural patient behaviors to move the process forward rather than meeting them with force. The Ericksonian approach teaches us that resistance is a problem of the therapist rather than the patient. If a patient shows a behavior that is different from that suggested by the Ericksonian therapist, the therapist is taught to follow the patient's lead. Most seasoned therapists have had the experience of patients generating their own strategies for pain control under hypnosis, and such initiative on the patient's part is almost always encouraged. In both MI and Ericksonian hypnosis, if a patient is not having a good experience with the process, the therapist is encouraged to examine his or her own behavior, often in terms of being less directive or being careful not to push an agenda unwittingly.

That the patient is ultimately responsible for change is an underlying assumption with both MI and Ericksonian hypnosis. However, there are specific examples of how responsibility for change can be integrated directly into hypnotic language. For example, the therapist might say, "And I can't really make you change how you might decide to cope with your pain, can I?" Or, "I wonder who it really is that can make you want to change?"

Advice

Giving clear advice has been identified as one of the factors that creates behavior change, particularly when given by the right health professional at the proper time. W. R. Miller and Rollnick (1991) recommended that the advice should "1) clearly identify the problem or risk area, 2) explain why change is important and 3) advocate specific change" (p. 21). There is substantial evidence that advice from a physician can have an impact on behaviors such as smoking and drinking reduction (Chick, Lloyd, & Crombie, 1985; Elvy, Wells, & Baird, 1988; W. R. Miller & Rollnick, 2002). In the context of pain, advice would be most applicable again to the patient with chronic pain, with the message being that the patient should engage in different treatment strategies, often ones that supplement or replace a medically focused regimen: "You have tried a medical approach several times without much success. My advice is for you to try something completely different." To keep this MI consistent, and to minimize push-back, one might also add, "Of course, you will have to decide if you're ready to do that. I couldn't decide that for you."

Giving advice in the literal sense seldom fits well with hypnosis. Hypnosis usually targets perceptual changes and/or urges and desires, and the cognition required to weigh advice is seldom compatible with the processing that occurs with this type of treatment. Although a patient will not be advised to stop drinking or smoking in hypnosis, suggestions can certainly target the urges or perceptions that go with behaviors. There is now reasonably good literature on the impact that hypnosis has on weight loss and some evidence of its potential impact on smoking cessation (Green & Lynn, 2000; Green, Lynn, & Montgomery, 2006, 2008). Certainly much of this book—particularly Chapters 5, 6, and 7—is about how hypnosis can create perceptual changes in a patient's pain level.

There are some instances in which advice can be integrated into hypnosis, but again, this will not be a matter of providing direct advice to the patient. Instead, advice might be given in the context of a metaphor. As an example, a goal of chronic pain management may be for patients to change their lifestyle. The effective clinician attempts to draw the motivation for change out of the patient. Metaphors and stories have the ability to generate a search process by essentially providing an indirect hypnotic suggestion. So again, rather than advising directly that the patient adopt a new strategy for pain control, the clinician might say,

> You might have had the experience of trying to solve a problem. Maybe it was a math problem or perhaps it was a different type of problem altogether. In any case, you tried and tried to solve the problem using a particular approach. Then, maybe even after you gave up, the solution seemed to come to you so quickly and easily.

As another example, even though the issue at hand may be to change a patient's approach to pain management, this can be addressed indirectly by dealing with a different, but parallel, health issue. In this case, the clinician might say,

> One thing we have learned about people quitting drinking is that most of them do it themselves, when they decide to do so. Isn't it interesting that when someone sat down and compared all of the approaches there are to alcohol reduction that ultimately they found most people give up drinking when they one day make up their mind to just do something different?

A final example of how advice might be integrated into hypnosis is when the patient is given suggestions either to seek advice from an inner observer or to provide advice to someone else for the target issue while in hypnosis. This serves the purpose of having the patient generate solutions without the complications inherent in the hypnotist providing advice.

Menu of Options

MI writers recommend offering a patient a variety of options rather than just one alternative. With one alternative, there is a greater chance that what is being offered to the patient is not a desirable or acceptable choice. Further, offering the patient only a single option for change is thought to potentially increase resistance. In providing a menu of options, an MI therapist may offer the patient a piece of paper with a series of circles written on it. In each circle, the therapist or patient then writes another potential option for changing behavior. The way this might sound with an MI therapist providing a series of options for controlling pain might be as follows:

> There are a number of things you might consider doing to make yourself more comfortable. It may be an increase in your therapy frequency from one to two times a week. You might start working in a gym with a personal trainer. Listening to deep relaxation tapes a minimum of once a day would very likely increase your pain tolerance. Finally, if you are able to work on altering your automatic thoughts about pain once a day, this would also likely have an impact on how much discomfort you experience.

The patient and therapist typically generate such a menu of options jointly. Working with a menu of options is particularly consistent with Ericksonian hypnosis and is the basis for several of the inductions included in this book. As discussed earlier, the clinician using hypnosis seldom knows what type of hypnotic suggestion for pain relief is going to work with a given patient at a particular time. It is consequently desirable to provide a range of options to the patient and let him or her choose which to instigate. Moreover, not only can clinicians provide different suggestions for pain reduction (e.g., amnesia or displacement of pain), but they can also affect different levels of processing, so that one or two hypnotic suggestions target analgesia whereas others may focus on lifestyle and/or activity changes. A clinician providing a menu of options in hypnosis might say to the patient,

> You might feel that you reach a level of such deep comfort that you do not seem to notice any other feelings. Or, maybe you will become so absorbed with playing with your children that you will increasingly forget about everything else. You may find that it suddenly not only becomes easy, but desirable to see your physical therapist. Perhaps it will simply be a matter that you just feel like walking. I am curious about how your mind does indeed allow you to become more comfortable.

Empathy

Empathy is a cornerstone of MI, and although it may appear simple, it can be one of the most difficult for clinicians to grasp and implement. As discussed earlier, MI and many other brief therapies are rooted in the humanistic approaches developed by Carl Rogers (1961) and others, and empathic listening, in turn, is a central component to such therapeutic approaches. Acceptance is a principal attitude underlying empathy, and reflective listening is central to this concept. Reflective listening involves carefully hearing what the patient says and mirroring the content and feeling of statements without judging, criticizing, or blaming. This does not mean that the clinician agrees with or approves of the patient's statement; it is more a matter of respectful listening with an attempt to understand the patient's perspective. W. R. Miller and Rollnick (1991) argued that approaching patients in this manner often frees them up for change, perhaps as much or more than any other component of brief therapies, because they no longer have to defend their old views.

If empathy is one of the most difficult concepts to grasp in MI, then reflective listening is certainly one of the more challenging skills to develop. Reflective listening is not simply a matter of mirroring back what the patient has just stated but rather a wholehearted effort to grasp and to communicate back what the patient means. Language is often far from perfect in allowing a patient to express his or her thoughts, feelings, or message. Reflective statements are designed to hold up a patient's statement for scrutiny so that both the patient and the therapist can begin to decode its meaning. To achieve this, the therapist must be trained to think empathically, to search constantly for the meaning behind the words, and then to reflect that to the patient. If a patient states, "I am feeling anxious," the potential range for what he or she actually means is extensive. It may be that the patient is worried about the future, scared, chronically nervous, or experiencing heart palpitations. Reflective listening discerns the patient's meaning, not by asking questions but by making statements that help the therapist truly understand the meaning behind the statement.

Although reflective statements may not come into play in actual inductions (particularly because patients seldom talk during hypnosis), there may be nothing more important than therapist empathy in facilitating truly effective results though hypnosis. Certainly, this is the case in the therapy leading up to the hypnotic work. The more patients can teach the therapist about who they are and how they function, the more effective the hypnosis will likely be. Empathy and reflective listening are the most efficient means to reach that understanding of the patient. To the degree that a therapist comes into a hypnotic session having established rapport through empathy, unconditional positive regard, and reflective listening, the potential therapeutic impact will almost certainly be maximized. Moreover, once an empathic relationship is established with a patient, the effects unquestionably carry into hypnosis itself.

Empathy comes into play in actual hypnotic inductions, particularly those from an individualized Ericksonian approach. Effective Ericksonian hypnosis is often a matter of following the patient, and as such cannot be done without diligent and empathic listening and observation. Hypnosis often takes this one step further since, during inductions, an understanding of what the patient is feeling and experiencing has to come from no verbal cues and even more of the "guessing" that W. R. Miller and Rollnick (1991) discussed. The masterful clinician using hypnosis is constantly scrutinizing the patient and hypothesizing about how subtle behaviors may be reflecting internal affective and/or cognitive states. Although prehypnosis interviewing can help the clinician gain a preliminary understanding of the patient, the effective clinician using hypnosis will learn to be empathic even when the only cues during hypnosis are nonverbal ones.

Self-Efficacy

Self-efficacy is the final component of the FRAMES acronym for effective brief counseling. Self-efficacy was a concept promoted by Bandura (1982; Bandura, Cioffi, Taylor, & Brouillard, 1988) and has to do with to what degree a patient predicts that he or she will be successful in carrying out a certain task. In terms of MI, this concept reflects the belief in the ability to engage in a specific act supportive of behavior change. Often, an MI therapist will have patients rate not only how important change is to them but also how likely they feel they will succeed at change. The therapist then works to identify specific acts that will support that endeavor. The concept of self-efficacy is well established in the literature and is associated with both positive mental health and physical outcomes (Frank & Frank, 1991). It is certainly an influential variable in determining how well patients respond to brief counseling techniques.

Self-efficacy has a close corollary in hypnosis with the concept of expectancy. A powerful variable in the health literature is the degree to which positive expectancies predict positive outcome. Certainly this is true with respect to the hypnosis literature in general (Kirsch & Lynn, 1995) as well as studies on hypnosis for pain control (Patterson & Jensen, 2003). It is interesting that treatment outcome is strongly influenced not only as a function of the patient's expectations for treatment but also from those of the health professional. In fact, expectations of treating professionals may be an even more powerful predictor of outcome than those of the patient (Turner & Jensen, 1993; Turner & Romano, 2001).

In terms of hypnosis, we as clinicians are constantly challenged to raise the expectations of our patients, as well as maintain our enthusiasm about treatment in a way that respects what we know scientifically. It is important to communicate to patients that some amount of clinical improvement not only is reasonable but is the norm. Montgomery DuHamel, and Redd's (2000) meta-analysis suggested that 75% of patients entering clinical or laboratory situations can expect to experience some pain reduction. Erickson advised us to be content with small gains in pain reduction over specific treatment situations. As discussed in Chapter 5, he argued that clinicians should be satisfied with 15% reductions in pain rather than expecting to eliminate it totally; the latter is indeed an unrealistic expectation in most clinical situations. Clinicians can take heart in knowing that the better the quality of studies on hypnotic pain control, in terms of randomized controlled studies, the more convincing the evidence for hypnotic analgesia (Patterson & Jensen, 2003).

Other Elements of Motivational Interviewing

Apart from the FRAMES components for understanding the effective elements of brief counseling, there are a number of other useful concepts associated with understanding how people change that can be related to pain control and hypnosis.

Core Values

MI theorists maintain that critical behavioral changes often occur when a problematic habit of behavior conflicts with a patient's core value(s). In other words, when a person gains insight into how much a behavior is in contrast to an important self-concept or dearly held worldview, it can often be sufficient to instigate behavior change. W. R. Miller and Rollnick (2002) provided a compelling example of this in a man who was a smoker. At one point, the man went to pick up his children from school. As he approached the school, his children began to walk out of school and were becoming soaked by a sudden rainstorm. At that instant, the man realized he was out of cigarettes and drove past the school in order to get to a store, thereby leaving his children in the rain. It was at this moment when he realized that his need for cigarettes was so strong that it conflicted with a core value: his sense of being a good father and putting his children's best interests first. The man immediately turned around and reportedly stopped smoking from that day on.

The notion of core values is equally important in hypnotic suggestion. Finding out the patient's core values and how problems with pain control may conflict with them may lead to the most powerful suggestions that a clinician can offer in an induction. Almost any patient in chronic pain will go through losses as a result of their pain. In some instances, the pain will lead to losses that a patient will have to accept and grieve. A gymnast with enough damage and musculoskeletal problems may very well have to give up the sport. However, at other times, restrictions from chronic pain may conflict with core values. A grandparent may find that lack of movement prevents her from being able to spend the time she would like with her grandchildren. People who thrive on travel may find that chronic pain prevents them from being able to live this valuable part of their life. The wording of such suggestions is done so that the strength of the core value drives the effectiveness. As an example, the value that one places on being a parent can be paired with a suggestion for amnesia for pain:

> And wouldn't it be interesting if you seemed to become lost in the sheer joy of playing with your daughter? That when you're playing with her, you become so absorbed in the experience that you seem to forget about everything else?

Often hypnotic suggestions may target several levels of the patient's awareness and function, perhaps with some addressing analgesia and other addressing core values.

Ambivalence About Behavior Change

MI is particularly applicable to people who are ambivalent about changing their approach to pain management. If people are highly motivated to change and open to considering lifestyle alternatives, change can happen quite easily and MI interventions are not necessary. When MI is working at its best, it is often because it enables patients to resolve their ambivalence about changing behavior. Through such techniques as reflective listening and amplifying the patients' position, MI therapists are able to help patients generate reasons why they should change or not change. A therapist using this approach may ask a patient in chronic pain to describe what the "good things" about his or her approach to pain management approach are, as well as the "not so good things." Again, the object is not to try to convince patients to change their position; rather, it is a matter of allowing them to explore their ambivalence in a therapeutic environment.

An important implication of this in terms of hypnosis is that if a patient is highly ambivalent about behavior change, then providing too strong of a direct suggestion in one direction or another may further entrench a patient in his or her position rather than facilitating any type of behavior change. It is likely that Erickson recognized this when he developed indirect hypnotic suggestions, although his rationale for such techniques certainly extended beyond addressing ambivalence in patients. When provided with indirect suggestions, it is far more difficult for an ambivalent patient to become further entrenched in a position. To illustrate, patients with chronic pain are often ambivalent about giving up the notion of a surgical cure for their pain. Contrast a suggestion of "You will abandon your desire to undergo surgery" with "Wouldn't it be interesting if the course of action that will truly benefit you in the long run just seems to come to you easily and naturally?" Indirect suggestions provide the patient with more choice and less direction; interacting with the patient in this manner decreases the probability that hypnosis therapists unwittingly entrench the patient in an undesirable stance.

INTEGRATING MOTIVATIONAL INTERVIEWING AND HYPNOSIS: A DIALOGUE AND AN INDUCTION

What follows is an example of an MI-based therapeutic dialogue with a patient who has illness conviction about the cause of his chronic pain and is almost hostile to alternative approaches such as hypnosis. An example of a hypnotic induction that integrates MI principles is provided after the dialogue.

Induction Dialogue (Based on a Motivational Interviewing Approach)

Therapist: Thanks for coming in. Tell me what brings you here today?

Client: The doctors made me come see you for the pain in my back.

Therapist: It sounds like it was not your idea to come see me.

Client: No, the doctor seems to think that my pain is all in my head and so I should get my head shrunk.

Therapist: OK, so you don't agree with your doctor about the cause of your pain. Tell me what *you* believe is causing your pain? In other words, what is your model for what is making you hurt?

Client: I have a damaged disk in my back and the only thing that is going to help me is a surgery that fixes it.

Therapist: The way you see it, it is definitely *not* all in your head, because you have an injured disk. You see your pain as caused by an injury and further, the only way to feel better is for you to undergo surgery. What type of message have you been getting from your doctors?

Client: I have been to five different doctors. They all tell me that I have abnormalities in my MRI [magnetic resonance imaging], but none of them think that surgery will do me any good. They say it might even make the problem worse.

Therapist: This sounds very frustrating. You are experiencing bad pain, and none of the doctors are willing to take the surgical approach that you feel is the only solution to you at this point. I would think this disagreement would only add to your pain. I wonder how this pain is having an impact on your life

Client: It is horrible. I can't do anything. My wife is mad at me all the time. I don't get to do any sports with my kids.

Therapist: So it has a very large impact. And what makes the pain better?

Client: The only things that help me are lying flat on my back and taking Vicodin.

Therapist: Let me see if I'm understanding you correctly. You injured your back a year ago and have been on disability ever since. Many of the things in your life make it hurt, and you are afraid that the pain is going to become worse. This is straining your marriage and preventing you from doing many things that you enjoy like spending time with your kids. Your doctors are frustrating you because none of them seem to agree to do the surgery that you feel is the only thing that will do the trick.

Client: Yeah, I just want the pain to go away.

Therapist: And, through your eyes, surgery is the only thing that will make it go away.

Client: Well . . . I don't know if it is the *only* thing. I'm no doctor.

Therapist: Neither am I; at least I am not a neurosurgeon. So I can't say whether surgery can make the pain better. But I do know of some nonsurgical approaches that might make you feel more comfortable.

Client: Now you are saying it is all in my head too.

Therapist: Is it OK if I give you some information?

Client: Sure.

Therapist: Actually, there is no way the pain is all in your head. You have had an injury and there is some damage to your back. There is more evidence now that this type of pain becomes imprinted in your brain, so you are feeling real pain; I just don't know if surgery is going to fix it.

Client: If I try other approaches, then I will never get the surgery I need.

Therapist: Actually, I am not suggesting anything that competes with surgery. That will always be an option. The types of approaches I wanted to discuss work in concert with surgery.

Client: What do you have in mind?

Therapist: Well, there are actually a number of things you can consider, but it's of course up to you whether you decide to try anything new at this point. Physical therapy can address some of biomechanical problems that you are experiencing. A personal trainer can address some of the atrophy you have undergone. What I have to offer in particular is hypnosis.

Client: Hypnosis? You'll have me quacking like a duck.

Therapist: I am hearing an age-old concern. That a doctor doing hypnosis can make you do things you don't want to do. Actually, the scientific evidence is the opposite.

Client: If you are talking about hypnosis, then you are saying the pain really is in my head.

Therapist: Actually, hypnosis is useful for the most severe types of pain you can imagine. We developed it here to help our patients who had burn injuries. As I said, there is no question that the sufferings you have experienced are real.

Client: How would you use it with me today?

Therapist: Actually, today I was more interested in using hypnosis to explore some of the issues we have been talking about. One of the most valuable applications of hypnosis is to help people explore alternatives to a problem they are experiencing. I am not convinced that you want to try to reduce your pain through hypnosis yet. However, what is really clear to me is how motivated you are to reduce your pain. You have approached many health care professionals and you are willing to subject yourself to an invasive surgery, and you were even willing to come in here today, despite misgivings. So today I am suggesting that we do not even try to reduce the pain itself with hypnosis; I am rather suggesting that we use it to explore your relationship with a terrible problem in your life, as well as what you can do about it. How does that sound?

Example of an MI-Integrated Hypnotic Induction

I am going to take you to a state of mind where you can hold your thoughts and perceptions in front of you and examine them in a different way. I am not going to do the old-fashioned type of hypnotic induction where I will swing a watch. Rather, I am going to just talk and would like you to drift comfortably along. Sometimes you may find yourself right here, other times you may find your mind wandering, it may be that you get a sense of yourself drifting, anything is fine, as long as you begin to feel more comfortable. I think that you will be pleasantly surprised to notice that wherever your mind seems to go, that part of you is able to pick up and remember those things that are useful to you (*emphasizes autonomy*).

Let's start by having you put yourself in as a relaxed state as possible. Any way you do that is fine (*emphasizes autonomy*). You may sink into relaxation by slowing down your breathing, taking deep comfortable breaths. You may find yourself turning yourself inward (*offers menu of options of what to experience*). By sensing what is going on in your body or in your mind; it really doesn't matter. Anything you do to make yourself comfortable is absolutely fine (*emphasizes autonomy*).

This type of unstructured induction continues by following the patient's lead. The therapist observes the patient and guides him with indirect suggestions for deepening and attention. Given the nature of the suggestions that follow, it is better that the induction be less rather than more structured. In the interest of space, let us assume that the clinician has spent several minutes longer establishing a state of relaxation that is described here.

And as you drift comfortably along, let's talk more about your relationship with your pain. We know that your back is hurting you a lot. You have been to many doctors trying to find a solution for your problem; it hurts for you to move and you have been moving less and less as a result. The pain is interfering more and more with your life. You are not getting a chance to do the things that you enjoy and, particular, you do not get nearly the quality time for with your children (*reflecting patient's story*).

This constitutes the feedback portion of the FRAMES model. It is critical that this information be given back to the patient only after a careful interview with the patient in which his agenda is pulled out using reflective listening, summarizing, and so on. The clinician would like to get to the point where these statements are as close to accurate reflections of the patient's dilemma as they can be; in other words, for these statements to be more truisms than guesses or hypotheses. To put it another way, the clinician is aiming here for deeper reflection that mirrors implicit truths within client statements, but about which they may not have full awareness. In MI, this is often how "stuck" clients are able to move forward. At this point, the therapist is acting as a mirror by holding up the patient's pain dilemma in front of him.

> Your pain is presenting a challenge to you and sometimes it seems like there is no way out. However, something is happening that you may not have realized. You keep doing something that you may not be aware of. Specifically, no matter how bad the pain gets, you keep doing something to try to make it better. You continue to go through all the trouble to see yet another doctor. You have made the investment of time and effort to come see me. What is clear is that there is a force within you that makes you feel better that you cannot ignore. This force will not be ignored and will not leave the problem alone. There is something very powerful within you that cannot help but continue to push for your best interests (*affirming patient's strengths*).

Although the feedback portion highlights the struggles the patient is having with his pain issues, pointing out his actions highlights resources that he may not have been aware of and provides hope for change. It also sets the state for tapping into these resources later in the induction.

> Another thing that I have learned about you is how much you hate for people to tell you what to do. From what I hear, your doctor is telling you to do things differently, your therapist is telling you to do things differently, and your wife is telling you to do things differently. Yet you are a man who has spent most of his life in the army where your job has been to tell other people what to do. There is one thing I can tell you for sure: No one can make you change (*autonomy*). And the other thing I have learned after doing this for 20 years is that when someone makes up their mind that they want to change, that change can come so much more quickly and easily than they might have expected. It becomes a matter much like turning on a light switch. I don't know when it happens or why it happens but I have seen it time and time again: When everything lines up properly and that internal drive is strong enough, change can come effortlessly (*self-efficacy*).

This section reinforces the important concept that the responsibility for change lies within the patient and no one will make him change. However, it also introduces self-efficacy for change and pulls for the drive for change that the patient has shown. One of the things that can happen in hypnosis is that patients can be given suggestions for ease with which change can occur. Such perceptual suggestions may not have as much impact if provided in a normal conversation rather than the context of hypnosis.

> Yes, as I mentioned, you are the type of man who will change only when he wants to, and no one is going to make you change. We have also seen that there is a powerful part of you, deep within, that is driving for change. Just continue to relax, to drift along, and to just let thoughts and feelings come and go, just drifting along and noticing anything that is happening, letting thoughts come and go but not necessarily thinking them. And while you drift along, I would like to talk to that force that wants to change deep within you. What I would like to say to you is that there are many, many options for you, if you decide you want to do things differently. For example, you might find that you start walking far more often than you might have expected and that with every walk it seems to get easier. You might find that you start doing your therapy exercises without thinking about them, that you finish each day knowing you have done them but you don't even remember having willed yourself to do them. Or perhaps you will start finding yourself so absorbed in activities with your children that you will begin to forget about everything else (*menu of options*). Indeed, is there anything more important to you than your children at this point? I don't know how but I do know that this force within you is going to allow you to begin taking care of yourself in ways that you might never have imagined (*self-efficacy*).

As mentioned, giving advice does not fit in well with many forms of hypnosis, but a menu of options does. Basically, this part of the induction involves providing a menu of options in the sense of hypnotic suggestions. This is very similar to the multiple-choice method of giving suggestions that Erickson discussed (see Chapter 4, this volume). Suggestions are also tied to the internal drive to change that is brought up earlier in the induction. Finally, the core value, the patient's relationship with his children, is also integrated into the suggestions.

The example demonstrates how MI might be blended into a hypnotic induction. For ease of illustration, this was provided in chunks that might correspond to the parts of the FRAMES approach. However, an actual induction could be far more integrated and elaborate. Needless to say, the induction would also be tailored to the individual needs of the patient. It is important to emphasize that, when it comes to doing hypnosis, a logical, sequential presentation of the information will likely not have the maximal impact. As illustrated at the end of Chapter 4, Ericksonian hypnosis is often presented in a linear manner. So, whereas an MI therapist may do a summary in an organized, logical manner, the style is much more free-flowing when this is done in a hypnotic fashion. If patients cannot grasp the logical sequence of information presented in a hypnotic context, it is far more difficult for them to show resistance to the process.

SUMMARY

The greatest challenge in managing chronic pain may be to enable patients to entertain alternative models for their suffering and to engage in the associated health-related behaviors. MI is a powerful way to enable patients to change their behavior not only in an efficient manner but also in a way that tends to be pleasant for both the clinician and patient. Very often, patients with chronic pain are entrenched in models of understanding their pain that do no lead readily to change. Often, they have received negative information that their pain is "psychosomatic" or "all in their head" that has made them more entrenched in their position. An MI approach can gently allow patients to adapt a new strategy toward their pain and disability. This, in turn, can open them up for hypnotic interventions that can help relieve their pain or possibly alter their lifestyle.

I am not aware of any attempts in the literature to integrate MI and hypnosis, as potentially fruitful at this area is. Many MI techniques have a number of compelling parallels with hypnosis, particularly that done through Ericksonian approaches. What is perhaps most striking is that in both approaches a high value is placed on having the patient being the source of generating behavioral change. Rather than pushing the patient to change, the goal is to create the conditions through which the behavior change comes naturally and easily from the patient.

SUMMARY AND CONCLUSIONS

The field of pain control is in need of exciting developments, both in terms of any approaches that will reduce patient suffering and within the realm of psychology. Hypnosis is certainly not a new treatment, but the groundswell of scientific evidence that supports its effectiveness with both acute and chronic pain is a new phenomenon. This growth in scientific evidence is also good for the field of hypnosis in general. Few, if any, clinical applications of hypnosis in the area have this type of empirical support. This fits in nicely with societal demands for medical approaches that are natural, that are devoid of potential side effects, and that can complement conventional medicine. We are only scratching the surface of the issue of cost-effectiveness of hypnosis. The evidence for cost offsetting is dramatic when investigated with respect to the use of hypnosis with interventional radiological procedure and cancer pain and will likely only increase as more effective and efficient ways are found to apply hypnosis to pain control. As medical treatment for suffering increases in society and biological treatments are emphasized, there will always be a place for safe, empirically supported alternatives. For all of these reasons, it is a particularly opportune time to make hypnosis more prominent as a treatment for clinical pain.

Many, if not most treatments for pain, particularly that from chronic etiologies, use a biopsychosocial model of treatment. With this model, the potential contributions of medical, psychological, and social components are all considered in pain assessment. When pain is viewed in such a comprehensive fashion, a number of relationships among relevant variables can be observed that are important to treatment. For example, it is difficult to determine, on the basis of the nature, severity, or location of a wound or injury, how much a patient will suffer. Similarly, we have learned that through such mechanisms as neuroplasticity and classical and operant conditioning, patients can respond as if they are in pain, even if an injury or tissue damage is no longer present. By understanding such relationships, as well as the interaction between anxiety or depression and pain, clinicians can use psychological approaches to produce a substantially beneficial impact on pain reduction. Examples of successful approaches used over the past few decades include information, education, classical conditioning, operant conditioning, cognitive–behavioral interventions, and relaxation training. The successful clinician using hypnosis will often build on these approaches. In fact, clinicians might be doing the patient a disservice if they do not have a foundation of psychological approaches to pain.

The degree to which hypnosis has a solid theoretical basis may escape many clinicians. Analogue or laboratory studies do not translate well into treatment for some psychological disorders, but such is not the case with hypnosis. Numerous laboratory studies have helped elucidate variables that mediate and moderate hypnotic analgesia. The role of hypnotizability, dissociated control concepts (e.g., effortless strategies), and sociocognitive variables (e.g., expectancy) all can help clinicians understand how to reduce pain. Further, there is now a rich body of literature on physiological correlates of hypnotic analgesia. It is now known that hypnosis brings about a series of changes in the mind and body. Not only do hypnotic suggestions for pain relief result in measurable brain activity, but the nature of the suggestion for pain reduction also influences which parts of the brain show activity.

Hypnosis has a strong body of theoretical and physiological studies to support its application to pain control, and it now enjoys the strong backing of clinical research. Up until roughly 2 decades ago, the only empirical support for clinical hypnotic pain reduction was a rich and compelling series of anecdotal studies. Now, however, there are dozens of controlled and randomized controlled trials that demonstrate hypnotic pain reduction over control conditions or other types of treatment. Such studies have been reported with acute pain (invasive medical procedures, burn injuries, labor and delivery, bone marrow aspirations, women's health issues) and chronic pain (headaches, low back pain, arthritis, temporomandibular, sickle cell, disability, irritable bowel, chest pain). Hypnotizability has proved to be an influential variable with patient populations, just as it has in laboratory studies. There are still many questions to be answered through such controlled studies, such as the number of sessions needed, additive effects (e.g., what happens when hypnosis is added to a multidisciplinary chronic pain program), and how one can best design control groups to address completing explanations for study findings.

In addressing practical applications of hypnosis for pain control, this book largely followed a model that is based on the work of Milton Erickson. Although Ericksonian hypnosis is a mainly atheoretical approach, there is a surprising amount of empirical support for the building blocks of his approach, particularly from the social–psychological literature. Erickson viewed hypnosis as a cooperative endeavor between the patient and the clinician. He also promoted the concept of utilization, in which the clinician takes whatever the patient offers, and resistance is viewed as a problem of the therapist rather than the patient. By treating each patient uniquely and focusing on the concept of utilization, Erickson introduced a number of elaborate techniques to the field of hypnosis that came to define much of his work. Examples of these approaches include indirect suggestions, multiple-choice formats for suggestions, truisms, double binds, and metaphors. Erickson did devote a couple of chapters and several case examples in his writing to the treatment of pain. Some of the suggestions for analgesia with which he was largely credited included permissive indirect suggestions, amnesia, symptom substitution/replacement, pain displacement, body distortion, time distortion, and reinterpretation of pain. The approaches he discussed are highly creative as well as effective with patients.

Acute pain is typically intense, short-lived, unpleasant, and confounded by anxiety. One of the more useful applications of hypnosis is to treat acute pain and the anxiety that goes with it. The hospital environment is one that can be a constant threat to patients and a factor that enhances their pain and anxiety. Hypnosis can be extremely useful to hospitalized patients, but the clinician must be aware of the challenges presented by the hospital environment, the effects of medications, and cognitive changes in the patient. The most common type of acute pain addressed with hypnosis is that from medical procedures such as surgery, dentistry, wound care, invasive procedures, and labor and delivery. This type of pain is often ideal for hypnosis because the procedures are often scheduled and allow the clinician and patient time to prepare with hypnosis. For such procedures, hypnosis often works by providing posthypnotic suggestions that are tied to the stimuli that might otherwise elicit anxiety. Thus, the insertion of an intravenous needle before surgery can be the cue for a patient to enter a hypnotic state.

Chronic pain is a much more difficult problem to treat than that from acute etiologies. With acute pain, hypnotic suggestions can often be geared to reduce pain and increase comfort. With chronic pain, hypnotic suggestions often must focus on a myriad of accompanying problems, such as low activity, poor sleep, catastrophizing, and poor coping techniques. In some instances, more comfort may not be a goal of chronic pain treatment, and in other instances, suggesting pain control may not even be in the patient's best interest. Nevertheless, there are many instances when hypnotic suggestions for increased pain control fit well into a chronic pain treatment plan. The assessment of the patient with chronic pain is particularly important for hypnosis to be successful. It should be clear to the patient and the clinician that simple medical treatments are often not viable for chronic pain. The impact of the pain on patients and their families also needs to be carefully assessed, as well as whether the patient does well (or not so well) to cope with it. Clinicians who understand a biopsychosocial approach to chronic pain and are able to embed hypnosis within it stand a good chance of reducing a patient's suffering.

The final chapter of this book discussed a somewhat unusual blend of Ericksonian hypnosis and motivational interviewing (MI), a form of brief therapy focused on changing difficult habits. A theme throughout this volume is that treating chronic pain is often a difficult clinical challenge that involves helping patients change their philosophy of health care as well as lifestyles. MI represents a promising, relatively new approach to stimulating the patient's intrinsic motivation for performing behaviors useful to chronic pain management. There are a number of striking parallels between MI and Ericksonian hypnosis. The parallels of these approaches are discussed largely with the hope that this discussion will engender creativity from clinicians with respect to combining hypnosis and brief therapies. Chapter 8 ended with a discussion of how MI concepts might be integrated into hypnosis, although it should be noted that this is a departure from the true spirit of MI, a conversational approach designed to engender change-related statements from the patient.

Clinicians who are not experienced in hypnosis often feel more comfortable using hypnosis if they are provided with a script. In the spirit of doing what is necessary for hypnosis to be used more widely for pain control, an appendix at the end of this book provides a list of sample scripts for pain problems (burn injuries, headaches, cancer, fibromyalgia, and neuropathy). The clinician should be warned that using generic scripts will seldom be a replacement for tailoring interventions to individual needs of a patient. That said, any of the scripts provided can be altered in whatever manner the clinician feels is best.

Hypnosis is an empirically supported, often profoundly effective approach to managing acute and chronic pain with the majority of people faced with this difficult problem. It is my hope that this book will stimulate the increased use of clinical hypnosis, particularly in concert with other therapeutic approaches. A hypnotic induction used by one who is not familiar with health care or pain control theory will seldom have lasting effects. In contrast, if clinicians combine hypnosis with a sophisticated understanding of the factors that create and maintain pain, the probability that they will have a powerful effect on reducing patient suffering will be greatly enhanced. This book has been written for both the scientist and the practical clinician. The intent is to stimulate scientists to add to an already substantial body of research on the theory and clinical application of analgesia. For clinicians, the hope is that this volume will revive the wonderful creativity and range of opportunities made available through those familiar with Ericksonian approaches. I hope this was accomplished by descriptions of some of Erickson's theoretical approaches, as well as a number of examples of the language that might be used with patients in pain. Hypnosis, with few or no downsides, offers a wonderful window for the clinician to enable patients to use their own internal resources to reduce their most profound suffering.

APPENDIX: EXAMPLES OF INDUCTIONS FOR SPECIFIC PAIN PROBLEMS

This appendix provides scripts of hypnotic inductions for some of the more common and problematic types of pain. Some caveats are warranted. First, there are hundreds of etiologies for pain; space allows for discussion of only a few. At the same time, many of the etiologies of pain will generalize to others. For example, treatment for burn pain generalizes easily to that from other sorts of trauma.

As has been repeatedly emphasized throughout this book, hypnotic pain interventions should be based on the patient's specific complaints, cognitive and interpersonal style, and history. In other words, each intervention should be individual to the patient. This is particularly the case with chronic pain. It is important that clinicians avoid cookbook approaches when treating pain with hypnosis.

Having said that, it is still useful to give examples of how hypnosis can be applied to exemplary pain syndromes. The following are some examples of potential scripts for pain from headaches, fibromyalgia, burn injuries, cancer, and neuropathy. The scripts for headaches and fibromyalgia include initial inductions for relaxation and deepening; for burn, cancer, and neuropathic pain, only the specific suggestions are provided (with the understanding that the clinician will substitute in an initial induction). Space limitations do not allow a discussion of the pain syndromes. Although the inductions below are based on a literature review, it is the clinician's responsibility to familiarize themselves with the specific syndromes addressed.

Hypnotic Induction for Headaches

Right now I would like you to start by taking a nice, deep comfortable breath. Go ahead and get the sense of what it feels for air to come into your body, and for air to leave your body as you exhale. Just inhaling and exhaling. We often don't think about the experience of breathing, what the sensation is like, to feel the air coming in and your bellybutton leaving your spine, and then for the sensation of the air to leave your body, and the relaxation that comes with it. And now, as you listen more and more carefully to the sounds of my voice, I would like you to notice that with every breath you become deeper and deeper relaxed. And while this deep relaxation begins to develop, I would just like you to imagine yourself in a tropical forest now. It is a very warm day, and you are standing in the forest and you are surrounded by lush, green tropical trees and plants. Above you, you can see the sky, and all around you are thick, tropical, thriving green plants. Looking ahead of you, you can see a path that begins to wind down and you cannot see where the path goes. You find that you are at the top of a hill in this forest, and that this path winds down the hill in a direction that you cannot see. You find yourself moving to that path, and you start walking down it. On the path is lush, green moss. Your feet are bare and you can feel them bouncing up and down in the spongy moss. Now, as you continue down this path, you will see a series of rocks. Each rock will have a number painted on it. As you pass each rock, I will say the number and you will find that you become more deeply relaxed. So, the larger the number on the rock, the deeper relaxed you will become. When you reach the 10th rock, you will be at the bottom of the hill and profoundly and utterly relaxed.

We begin to go down this path even further. And 1 . . . you see the first rock and come to it, and already you begin to notice relaxation on the top of your head beginning to spread downward, spreading and flowing all over every hair follicle in the top of your head, spreading down to your forehead, your cheeks, your mouth and jaw. Deep, comfortable, relaxation allowing your mouth and jaw to just let go.

You continue to move downward toward the comfortable path. There's a brilliant blue sky above you. There's a sun above, and the sun is shining down on you, on the top of your head, making your entire body warm and relaxed. On either side of you, there continues to be lush, green tropical plants. Ferns, palm trees, all different types of flowering plants. You can even smell the flowers as you comfortably walk down.

And 2 . . . you come to the second rock, and that relaxation continues to spread down through your body, down through your neck, into your shoulders, allowing your neck and shoulders to become comfortably relaxed. Continuing to move downward.

And now, 3 . . . you pass the third rock. Relaxation spreads down from your shoulders into your arms, into your forearms, into your hands. Deep, comfortable, relaxation. Noticing how easy it is to focus on the sound of my voice, how clear the words I'm saying are, as you continue to move down the path.

And 4 . . . relaxation goes down into your chest now, slowing down your breathing, even more deeply, even more completely. Just beginning to get the sense of drifting, not a care in the world, nothing to worry about, nothing even to think about as this sense of drifting and absolute well-being continues more and more. You continue to move further down the path.

And 5 . . . you reach the fifth rock, and you're halfway to the bottom. Relaxation moves down into your waist now, down into your legs, into your feet. Your entire body now, deeply and profoundly relaxed. And yet, only halfway to the bottom. You move downward, down the path, blue sky above you, plants all around you.

And 6 . . . you see the sixth rock, profoundly, comfortably relaxed. Almost beginning to get a sense of drifting, almost a sense of floating as the sun makes your entire body feel profoundly comfortable, profoundly relaxed.

And 7 . . . you pass the seventh rock. You find it is easier and easier to focus on the sound of my voice. Clearly hearing everything that I say and moving everything else into the background of your mind. Totally focused on my voice now, total relaxation, total well-being.

8 . . . you pass the eighth rock, knowing that you're almost at the bottom of the path, and yet not knowing what you might experience at the bottom of the path, interested in what that may be. And yet at the same time, profoundly, comfortably, deeply relaxed. A sense of drifting, closer to the bottom now.

And 9 . . . you pass the ninth rock and a sense of complete, utter calmness has filled your entire body. Profound relaxation, still able to hear my voice, yet experiencing a pleasant sense of drifting without a care in the world. Deeply and comfortably relaxed.

And now, 10 . . . you pass the 10th rock. You're profoundly relaxed and able to follow any instructions that your mind finds are useful to you. You find yourself wandering in an even more beautiful, lush forest. And looking ahead of you, you see some rocklike structures. Beautiful, flat rocks, like a granite quarry. Smooth, shiny rocks that reflect the sun shining against them and radiate multiple colors, reds, blues, yellow, greens. You walk over to those rocks, and there is a shallow pool with a waterfall.

Now, this pool is only about a foot and a half deep, and the interesting thing about this water is that you find you can lie on your back, float in it, and yet still touch the bottom of the pool. It is an absolutely stunning, blue-colored pool, surrounded by multicolored, flat beautiful rocks, and those, in turn, are surrounded by the forest. Lying there in the water, you see the blue sky above you, you see some clouds moving through that are fascinating to you. You find that you are able to lie in the water and that your body floats very easily in the shallow water. Every bit of your body is supported, and you can just let your body go. You begin to get the sense of drifting like you are just floating in mid-air. The water can be any temperature that you like and you can change it. If you want it to be slightly cool, that's fine; if you want it to be slightly warm, that's fine, as long as it's at a temperature that's comfortable for you, that's perfectly fine.

In the prehypnosis interview, it is helpful to gain a sense of what will be useful for patients in terms of coolness or warmness; often they will prefer cool imagery, but there is no universal rule.

And as you float in the water, profoundly relaxed, focusing on my voice, you will begin to notice that things that are very useful to you, thoughts, images, and feelings begin to float in and out of your mind. Just drifting and floating in and out. You realize that you have a very powerful part of your mind that can be a great friend to you. And so, while part of your mind is floating comfortably in the pool and just noticing what the sky looks like and wondering how you could be so profoundly comfortable, another part of your mind starts having images that are profoundly useful to you.

The next suggestions have to be adjusted to whether the patient has headache pain at the time of the session.

And one thing I'd like you to notice now is that if you can actually notice, in a comfortable way, strangely enough, what it's like to have the headache pain. What the pain looks like in your head. What color is it? How much does it weigh? What shape is it? How much water would it hold? Just beginning to form an image of the headache within your head. Looking at it from a distance and being fascinated with that. And as you watch your headache, you begin to watch it gently flow out of your head, into the water around you. Certainly not all at once, but slowly, just flowing out like a balloon filled with water, and the water squeezing out.

I don't know exactly how your mind is going to make you more comfortable. Your mind may serve you now by noticing that in the future, that when you begin to get the aura before a headache, when you begin to get the signs of a headache, that that will become a signal to you from your mind. A signal to become utterly, comfortably, deeply relaxed, more relaxed than you are now. You'll still be able to function, to walk around, to talk to people, to do what you're doing. But you'll have an immediate rush of well-being and comfort as soon as you begin to get the early signs. And maybe once you get those early signs, you'll become so profoundly relaxed, that maybe the headache will never appear at all. If it does appear, perhaps you will find that you are watching the headache from a distance. Just noticing that it's there but yet not being bothered by it anymore. And maybe you'll find too that the headache will disappear far faster than you would have ever imagined. Perhaps you won't remember whether or not you had ever been in any type of discomfort.

It may be that you are able to picture the blood vessels in your head. Further, they may appear to be large and swollen. Yet as you observe them, they begin to shrink and return to normal. However it happens, you find that a normal, comfortable amount of blood flow now travels through your brain.

I don't know exactly how it will seem as one part of your mind remains floating in this comfortable pool, sun shining on you, not a care in the world, thoughts coming in and out of your mind. And one thought that you may have, or one image, is a time in your past that you didn't have any headaches at all. How did it feel at this earlier time in your life not to have any headaches? Maybe you were even a child. Or perhaps your mind goes back to pleasant images in the past, perhaps when you were far younger. Any images that come up are fine as long as they are enjoyable. Just noticing that image, memory, or symbol from the past, as long as it is a happy one.

And now some more images start coming to mind, and those are pleasant images in the future where you don't have any pain at all. Just noticing what you're doing, who you're with, what it looks like to be absolutely, profoundly comfortable. And also you begin to notice that the time between the past and the future begins to become blended, and so that time begins to have no meaning. I don't know exactly how your mind will allow you to feel more comfortable. I do know that your mind is a very powerful ally, and it can do many things to make you feel more comfortable. It may be that in the future that just closing your eyes and counting from 1 to 10 will allow you to reach an even more profound state of relaxation. It may be that periods of discomfort seem to go into fast-motion, and what might have seemed like 10 minutes or half an hour or 2 hours, all of a sudden seems like 6 minutes, or 3 minutes, or maybe 1 and a half minutes. And perhaps you will suddenly be looking back and being surprised by all the comfort that you've been remembering.

I don't know how your mind will serve as a resource for you, but I do know that it is a powerful resource and will continue to serve you. And as you lie in the pool now, drifting along, knowing that you'll remember everything that is useful, and that you'll forget anything that wasn't particularly useful. I'd like you to begin to get ready to end this particular journey down the path and head back up the path. Only this time, when you do reach the top of the path it will be quite a different experience from when you were there before. This time when you return back up the path, you'll find yourself alert, oriented, but profoundly comfortable. It'll be as if you've had a nice, comfortable nap, but alert, awake, and refreshed.

You feel yourself getting up out of the water now, walking back toward the path. You see the 10th rock, and as we head up the path together, I'll begin to count up the path. And as you know, as I count each number, you'll start to feel more and more alert, more and more awake, more and more comfortable.

10 . . . you pass the 10th rock, start moving up and slowly feel yourself returning to an awakened state.

9 . . . more and more awake, more and more refreshed.

8 . . . 7 . . . beginning to move around now, beginning to notice the sensations in your body in a different way.

6 and 5 . . . halfway back up to the top and already feeling more and more awake. Still remaining comfortable of course, but more and more awake.

4 . . . that's right, beginning to orient yourself now.

3 . . . really waking up now.

2, and 1. Alert. Awake and refreshed.

Hypnotic Induction for Fibromyalgia

The first thing I'd like you to do is just go ahead and take a deep comfortable breath. Experience the sensation of air going into your body as you inhale and then of air leaving your body as you exhale. Just continue now to take deep, slow comfortable breaths. And with each breath you take, begin to notice how much more comfortable you can feel. Also, notice how as you attend to your breathing, your direction of attention becomes inward. That everything in the outside world starts to fade away as you turn comfortably inside. Now as you continue breathing, slowing and deeply and comfortably, I would like you to picture a staircase with 10 stairs. You're at the top of the staircase looking down. In a moment, I will begin to start counting from 1 to 10. With each count, you'll find yourself taking a step down the staircase. The larger the number, the farther down the staircase. The farther down the staircase, the more comfortable and relaxed you can feel. OK, now we're going to begin.

1 . . . one step down the staircase, and feeling now relaxation at the top of your head that seems to enter every hair follicle in your head. You feel that relaxation moving down to your forehead, your eyes, your cheeks, your mouth and jaw, deep, warm, comfortable relaxation.

And 2 . . . two steps down the staircase feeling the relaxation spread down into your neck and shoulders and already perhaps noticing that many of your thoughts seem to be moving away, that you seem to be able to listen to my voice in a much easier fashion.

3 . . . three steps down the staircase, relaxation moving down to your shoulders, into your arms, down into your forearms and into both hands. Both hands and arms now feeling heavy, comfortable, and relaxed.

4 . . . relaxation moves into your chest now, slowing down your breathing even more deeply and comfortably. Relaxation now down into your stomach.

And 5 . . . halfway to the bottom of the staircase and now noticing relaxation spreading down into your thighs, down into your calves, and down into your feet.

6 . . . six steps down the staircase, your entire body now is deeply and comfortably relaxed. You find that the words that I say are very clear, that you can easily understand everything I'm saying. You begin to pay more and more attention to my voice as everything else moves into the background.

7 . . . seven steps down the staircase. Becoming so relaxed now that perhaps you are getting a sense of drifting, not a care in the world, everything seems to be coming so easy now.

8 . . . closer and closer to the bottom, more and more comfortable. Deeper and deeper relaxed. Drifting, comfortable, and relaxed.

9 . . . you've now reached a profound state of relaxation and at the same time find it very easy to focus on the sound of my voice. Deeper and deeper relaxed, more and more comfortable, and now . . .

10 . . . ten steps down the staircase, deeply and profoundly relaxed, and you find yourself in a dark room and looking in front of you see a door with a bright gold doorknob. You walk over to the door and put your

hand on the doorknob, turn the doorknob, pull open the door, walk in the room, and pull the door closed behind you. When you pull the door closed behind you, everything that is negative becomes shut out of the special new room.

And now you find yourself in a new room, and it can be any type of room that you'd like, as long as it is a place of profound comfort and safety for you. It may be that your room is something that is inside a house, or it may be a place on the beach, or it may be in the forest. However you see your room is absolutely fine. As a matter of fact, it may be that as you return down here the room can change at times. Just notice what it looks like to be here. What you can see, what you can hear, how you feel. And now that you're in your room, you can find yourself sitting down or lying down and being very comfortable with any suggestions that you experience.

What becomes obvious to you now is that your mind can serve you in a variety of different ways. That you have a special part of your mind that allows you to breathe, that allows your heart to beat and is always there for you. When called upon, this part of your mind can be a tremendous resource. So, as you remain in your comfortable room, even though one part of you might only be noticing how comfortable you feel and how nice it is and how much you're enjoying yourself, another part of you is aware of that special friend your mind can be. And how it can serve you. I'm not sure exactly how your mind will indeed make you far more comfortable, long after your eyes open.

It may be that your mind now allows you to have the experience of your entire body being filled with a comfortable blue liquid. It can start from the top of your head and just flow down. And when this blue liquid makes contact with areas of your body where there was once discomfort, they just become numb, cool, and comfortable. It may also be a sense of warmth. Only your mind knows what can make you feel the most comfortable. Just a blue liquid, spreading out through your entire body, making you feel comfortable and relaxed. Maybe that is how your mind will serve you. Or perhaps your mind will serve you just by noticing that you begin to forget about the times that you're in pain. That with time, you begin to look back and realize that you've only been in pain for a few minutes, whereas it might have felt like hours before. Your mind can serve you in other ways too. It may be that your mind serves you by making you realize how easy it has become to move. That you find yourself motivated to exercise, to be active, I don't know how. I don't know where or when. I just know that movement will come so easily. Now, it doesn't matter how your mind makes you more comfortable. It really only matters that you do feel more comfortable. It may be that your mind serves you by having you gain an incredible sense of energy when your eyes eventually open, an energy that can last for hours, days, or weeks. But perhaps your mind will serve you just by allowing you to begin to ignore the pain. To put it in the background of your perceptions, that your mind will serve you by knowing that you are beginning to gain so much joy from being with your friends or your family or in activities that you really like, that you begin to forget about the discomfort.

I don't know what it is that your mind is going to do to serve you, I only know that you're going to be so much more comfortable and more relaxed than you ever would have dreamed of. Perhaps your mind will serve you by allowing the tension in your life to decrease. That suddenly your world will be as it was once when you were a child: fun, entertaining, not a care in the world. All the tension moving away. It may be that your mind serves you by allowing you to have the sensation of coolness and numbness in any areas where there is discomfort. But perhaps your mind will serve you by allowing you to fall into profoundly deep sleep whenever your head hits a pillow at bedtime.

Again, it really doesn't matter the route that your mind takes as long as you feel more comfortable. And it may be that you find that your mind serves you by greatly reducing the time that you spend in pain. It may be that you discover an internal switch in your body that can turn down the pain, just as a dimmer switch would turn down the lights. It may be that you just feel more comfortable and relaxed with life, that everything seems to come more easily. I don't know how it is that your mind will serve you, I only know that you will be profoundly more comfortable, profoundly more energetic, and profoundly more content than you would have imagined.

And I want you to notice how good you feel right now in your special room. And in awhile, we're going to head back up the stairs. But I want to remind you that you can return to your room any time you want. And wouldn't it be interesting if each time you returned, your ability to make yourself comfortable quickly increases dramatically, so that the more you go into your room, the more comfortable you feel? Now before we go up, I'm going to give you 30 seconds of time to yourself to allow you to give any suggestions that you would like to yourself. Anything that you'd like to suggest to yourself or anything that you would like to do to complete your experience; 30 seconds of silence starting now.

(Pause)

OK, now, as you know, we're going to leave the room. You close the door behind you and start walking toward the stairs. As you see the 10th stair, you know that as I count each number, you'll start to become more and more alert, awake, and refreshed.

10 . . . you step on the 10th stair and already you begin to feel yourself wake up.

9 . . . feeling more and more awake, more and more refreshed.

8 . . . just beginning to return to a waking state, knowing that you'll bring all the comfort and all the benefits with you.

7, 6, 5 . . . halfway up now, feeling more and more awake, more and more alert, more and more refreshed, energetic and rested.

4 . . . that's right, more and more awake, more and more refreshed.

3 . . . perhaps amazed at how rested you could feel in a short amount of time.

2 . . . almost there now.

And 1 . . . wide awake, alert, energetic and refreshed, comfortable and relaxed, but also energetic and alert.

Hypnotic Suggestions for Burn Pain

A hypnotic induction, typically with deepening relaxation, should precede the suggestions given here.

It is interesting to realize how life can throw unexpected surprises in our direction. Suddenly you are on a burn unit. Did you ever take a course in school about how to handle being on a burn unit? I know I didn't. That is an interesting thing about all of this, nothing in life really can prepare us for what to expect when you end up here. One nice thing I can tell you is that the people who work up here do a lot of this. Every day, we take care of people with bad burn injuries, and every day we send some of them home, back to their families and their lives. The good news is that you have gotten over the hard part, you have survived, and now it is time to get you back to your life. *(This presumes that there is good clinical evidence that the patient will survive, which is usually the case once a patient has moved through the intensive care stage.)*

Now it is time to do what we need to get you out of here and back to what you enjoy doing. Even though you have done a lot of things well in your life, you have not learned how to take care of burn injuries; that is what we do here for a living, and we do it very well. But in doing what we do, we make patients do all sorts of things that they may have not expected. In some cases we might ask our patients to do things that hurt for awhile, but what I can tell you is that we will never do any harm. Every day, our patients walk out of here, and they do it sooner when they are able to understand that everything we ask them to do is part of making them better.

The important thing is that you understand that nothing that we ask you to do is going to make you worse, only better, and once our patients understand that at a very deep level, they seem to be able to just let go. There are some things that I turn over to experts. I am not good at fixing the inside of a computer. I turned this over to the experts. I also let doctors fix my knee when I was asleep. I had no idea what they were doing, because I was asleep, but I trusted that they would do the right thing, and one thing that I can tell you is that you can trust the doctors, nurses, and therapists taking care of you. Most of them have dedicated their lives to helping people recover from burn injuries.

Maybe what I am saying is that you can take a vacation during this part of your care and leave everything to us. Your doctors and nurses are not going to make anything worse. Many of our patients just choose to go somewhere else in their minds. Maybe they find themselves at the beach, maybe relaxing in the woods, or it may even be a comfortable chair at home. What is important is that they just seem to drift off to another world. Wouldn't it be interesting if, even as I am talking to you, one part of your mind seems to hear what I am saying while another part is drifting comfortably off? And also noticing how slow and comfortable your breathing is, how clear the words I am saying are. Totally absorbed and yet drifting, not a care in the world right now. It is all coming so easily, and with an incredible sense of safety.

Yes, isn't it nice to feel the sense of utter profound, deep relaxation, not a care in the world, knowing that you can be wherever you want as long as it is safe and positive, and knowing that you can return to this state of profound relaxation whenever you want. And there will be cues for this. Signs for you to return to a deep, deep state of comfort. I know for example that, from now on, whenever you go in for your dressing changes and you feel the nurses pulling off your bandages, that that will be a signal for the relaxation to return. And, at the same time, you will find that any areas where you are burned are becoming cool and numb. Nothing but coolness, numbness, comfort, and relaxation in any of those areas, but you may not even notice because maybe it will just be more fun for your mind to be somewhere else all together. Or maybe the comfort will be when you go in for physical therapy. When the therapist is ranging your joints, profound relaxation instead, coolness and warmth at the same time. Numbness. Smiling, not what you had expected. The mind is so profoundly powerful that you may not even remember, not even remember you are there.

Wouldn't it be interesting if you could now imagine some point in the future, a point in the future when you are out of the hospital, your wounds are healed, and you are happy, satisfied, content. So easy to picture, such a happy thought. Everything has become so easy, and the time between now and then just seems to disappear, to move so quickly, to move so easily. And you move calmly and easily through the time between now and that special time in the future.

Alerting occurs now at a pace appropriate to the patient.

Hypnotic Suggestions for Cancer Pain

These suggestions for cancer pain are divided into pain from cancer *procedures* (in this example, chemotherapy) and more general *background pain* and anxiety from this disease. It usually useful to combine the inductions with the more general, background pain induction presented first (see next section, Hypnotic Induction for Chronic Cancer Pain). The suggestions below are contingent on the therapist first providing some sort of initial induction.

And now that you are in a profoundly relaxed state, I want to remind you of what a powerful resource your mind is, how it will serve you in some remarkable ways as you continue to recover. There is something that is very interesting about how our minds work. When we experience a very compelling smell, perhaps that of bread baking, it can cause instant reactions, such as feeling hungry, or maybe if we hear a bell ringing, it reminds us that is time to go back to class or to turn off the alarm clock. Wouldn't it be interesting if certain cues that you experienced in your environment signaled your brain to be profoundly relaxed, if all of the deep relaxation you are currently feeling came quickly and automatically flooding back just because of a signal? And why not have that signal be something that is part of what you are doing to recover? For example, it may be that whenever you experience yourself entering the cancer treatment, that that will be the signal, a signal for the comfort you are feeling now to come rushing back, a signal for you to become even more comfortable and relaxed than you even feel now. But that experience will become even more profound when you enter the treatment room *(any stimuli here have to be adjusted to what the patient will be experiencing)*, deep relaxation, comfort, not a care in the world. Yet perhaps the most profound experience of relaxation will occur when you feel the nurse or technician insert the IV in your arm. Yes, wouldn't that be interesting? To understand deeply that the very process that is allowing you to recover also becomes the most profound signal for you to relax, and that anything that follows the placement of the needle comes with ease and calmness. So profoundly relaxed then that you might lose all sense of time, maybe not even remembering what is occurring until you're awake from what feels like a deep, relaxing sleep.

Hypnotic Induction for Chronic Cancer Pain

As you lay in a profoundly relaxed state, drifting comfortably and listening to my voice, you may find how interesting it is to know that your mind can function on many different levels. One part of your mind can listen to my voice, while another part is allowing you to breathe slowly and deeply. It may be that still another part of you goes to a special place where you like to relax, perhaps the beach, maybe in the woods, or perhaps in a comfortable chair at home. Yes, your mind can hold several thoughts and images at once, but I want to address one part of your mind in particular. This is a very special part of your mind that can be a great friend and resource to you. It is the part of your mind that allows you to breathe slowly and comfortably without even thinking about it. It is also the part of your mind that can bring about tremendous resources when you need them the most, and while one part of your mind is listening to my voice, it becomes the special part of your mind that seems to be able to hear me the best, and it is that part of your mind that we want to address now. Because that part of your mind is a friend, a special resource that can serve you in a variety of different ways.

I wonder how your mind will serve you as you go through this journey with your health. Wouldn't it be interesting if you gained the sense that you are doing everything you need for your health and, if you are not, you will start doing it soon? Because once that happens, you can just begin to start letting go of any worries or concerns. So that you are able to learn which types of discomfort you are supposed to tell your doctor about, but also begin to ignore that pain which is useless.

Yes, your mind can help you feel more comfortable in a variety of different ways. Perhaps you will experience a sense of coolness and numbness in any areas of your body that were once bothering you. Perhaps you will just notice that you have stopped thinking about it all together, that you will begin to look back in time in the future and be so pleasantly surprised that the amount of time that you have remained comfortable has increased without your even thinking about it. Where you were once comfortable for a few minutes, this will extend for several hours. The mind truly is a remarkable resource, and I don't know how it will serve you. It may be that you discover that there is a dial inside your body that can turn down any pain, that just as you can slide or turn a dimmer switch to slowly turn down your lights, you will be able to turn down your pain. I don't know exactly how your mind will do it, I just know you will indeed feel more comfortable. It may be that your mind makes you more comfortable automatically, through means that we don't even understand.

But now you are drifting, relaxed, experiencing profound relaxation, and maybe even going deeper if that is what is useful to you at this point. Not even thinking, not even caring, just listening to my voice and attending to those things that are useful to you. And wouldn't it be interesting if, as you drift along, you begin to have some extremely pleasant and positive images of yourself in the future. You are content and comfortable. I don't know how far ahead this is in the future but I do know that the manner in which you experience yourself is happy and content, and maybe it is not an actual image but is rather a feeling, or a symbol, or a vision. Just notice where you are, who is there, and how you feel, or maybe it will be more than one image, or symbol, or thought, or nice feeling. I just know that no matter what, you will indeed be satisfied and content, relaxed, comfortable, and that the time between now and that point in the future will move so much more quickly than you might have expected. In fact, it may be as if you seem to forget about everything else between now and that magical time in the future.

Hypnotic Suggestions for Neuropathic Pain

The following suggestions are given after the basic induction has been performed. The beginning of the headache and fibromyalgia inductions are potential examples.

And now that you are profoundly relaxed, listening to my voice, and maybe experiencing the sense of comfortable drifting, wouldn't it be interesting if you discovered that your mind can allow things to happen to you, as long as they are in your best interest? Right now when you feel pain, your brain may think that it is because a certain part of your body is hurting. But what is the really interesting thing is that what you are feeling is because of the signals being broken rather than that part of your body being damaged. If I called you from Walla Walla, Washington, but told you I was calling from Singapore, you wouldn't be able to tell the difference, would you? I could be telling you I was calling from China, but maybe I would be in the house next door. You don't really know where the signal is coming from, but the point is that the telephone line is damaged, not your phone. You have done everything you need to do to make yourself better medically (*this is presuming that the patient has gone through the appropriate medical workups, which is a prerequisite for hypnosis*), now you are just getting some signals that you can just learn to ignore. You can still get the phone call when you need it, but you can ignore the ringing if it is a nuisance.

There is a very interesting psychology experiment that has been done: People are given eyeglasses that not only turn their world upside down, they also reverse the world that they see. The interesting thing is that after people wear these glasses for several hours, the brain is able to adapt to these changes. The brain is able to see the world normally; it is really fascinating how much the brain can adapt when the mind tells it to.

And so, if you really do not need to experience a sensation, your mind can do some very interesting things. I am wondering if you have ever had the experience of camping near a rushing river or stream, or perhaps it could be a memory of staying in a hotel above a busy street. At first it seems like all you can hear is the rushing of the water or the sound of the cars. Gradually, without even thinking about it, your mind begins to focus on other things. Ultimately, you do not even think about the sound of the water or the cars. Although it is there, it just seems to have moved into the background, and, without even realizing it, you have started to focus your attention on other things. You don't think about how you move things out of your attention, you just naturally begin to focus on the things you enjoy in life. You don't know how you do it, it just seems to happen comfortably and naturally.

Your mind is a very powerful friend to you and can serve you in a variety of different ways. I don't know quite how it will help reduce those signals and move them to a level where they just don't bother you anymore. It may be that you find a dimmer switch in your body, just like you have seen with lights in houses, and when you turn the dial the sensations decrease. It might be that you find yourself looking back and realizing that the times you have experienced the sensations become less intense and less strong, days become hours, hours become minutes, minutes become seconds, a 10 becomes an 8, a 6 becomes a 4, a 2 becomes a 1. It just seems to have happened even if you don't know how it did. Or maybe it will be as if that part of your body is immersed in a stream of water at whatever temperature is useful to you; maybe it is a cool stream that makes you feel numb and comfortable. Or maybe you prefer a warm stream; it really doesn't matter how your mind decides to dim the signals and make you feel more comfortable; all that matters is that you will begin to notice how much more comfortable you feel.

And I also wonder if you are now able to see a picture of yourself in the future, a clear image of you enjoying doing something that you love. I don't know if it is a few hours from now, a few days, or a few weeks, but whenever it is, isn't it interesting to see how content you look? Doing what you want, feeling as you want, no longer bothered.

At this point the suggestion phase is completed, and the patient is alerted.

REFERENCES

Alladin, A. (2008). *Cognitive hypnotherapy: An integrated approach to the treatment of emotional disorders*. West Sussex, England: Wiley.

American Psychiatric Association. (2000). *Diagnostic and statistical manual of mental disorders* (4th ed., text rev.). Washington, DC: Author.

Amrhein, P. C., Miller, M. R., Yahne, C. E., Knupsky, A., & Hochstein, D. (2004). Strength of client commitment language improves with training in motivational interviewing. *Alcoholism: Clinical and Experimental Research, 28*(5), 74A.

Amrhein, P. C., Miller, W. R., Yahne, C. E., Palmer, M., & Fulcher, L. (2003). Client commitment language during motivational interviewing predicts drug use outcomes. *Journal of Consulting and Clinical Psychology, 71*, 862–878.

Anderson, J. A., Basker, M. A., & Dalton, R. (1975). Migraine and hypnotherapy. *International Journal of Clinical and Experimental Hypnosis, 23*, 48–58.

Andreychuk, T., & Skriver, C. (1975). Hypnosis and biofeedback in the treatment of migraine headache. *International Journal of Clinical and Experimental Hypnosis, 23*, 172–183.

Appel, P. R. (1992). The use of hypnosis in physical medicine and rehabilitation. *Psychiatric Medicine, 10*, 133–148.

Appel, P. R., & Bleiberg, J. (2005). Pain reduction is related to hypnotizability but not to relaxation or to reduction in suffering: A preliminary investigation. *American Journal of Clinical Hypnosis, 48*, 153–161.

Arena, J. G., & Blanchard, E. B. (1996). Biofeedback and relaxation therapy for chronic pain disorders. In R. J. Gatchel & D. C. Turk (Eds.), *Psychological approaches to pain management: A practitioner's handbook* (pp. 179–230). New York, NY: Guilford Press.

Arendt-Nielsen, L., Zachariae, R., & Bjerring, P. (1990). Quantitative evaluation of hypnotically suggested hyperaesthesia and analgesia by painful laser stimulation. *Pain, 42*, 243–251.

Arkowitz, H., Westra, H. A., Miller, W. R., & Rollnick, S. (2008). *Motivational interviewing in the treatment of psychological problems*. New York, NY: Guilford Press.

Baker, E. L., & Nash, M. R. (2008). Psychoanalytic approaches to clinical hypnosis. In M. R. Nash & A. J. Barnier (Eds.), *The Oxford handbook of hypnosis: Theory, research, and practice* (pp. 439–456). New York, NY: Oxford University Press.

Bandura, A. (1982). The assessment and predictive generality of self-percepts of efficacy. *Journal of Behavior Therapy and Experimental Psychiatry, 13*, 195–199.

Bandura, A., Cioffi, D., Taylor, C. B., & Brouillard, M. E. (1988). Perceived self-efficacy in coping with cognitive stressors and opioid activation. *Journal of Personality and Social Psychology, 55*, 479–488.

Banyai, E. I., & Hilgard, E. R. (1976). A comparison of active-alert hypnotic induction with traditional relaxation induction. *Journal of Abnormal Psychology, 85,* 218–224.

Barabasz, A. F. (1982). Restricted environmental stimulation and the enhancement of hypnotizability: Pain, EEG alpha, skin conductance and temperature responses. *International Journal of Clinical and Experimental Hypnosis, 30,* 147–166.

Barabasz, A. F., & Barabasz, M. (1989). Effects of restricted environmental stimulation: enhancement of hypnotizability for experimental and chronic pain control. *International Journal of Clinical and Experimental Hypnosis, 37,* 217–231.

Barabasz, A. F., & Barabasz, M. (2006). Effects of tailored and manualized hypnotic inductions for complicated irritable bowel syndrome patients. *International Journal of Clinical and Experimental Hypnosis, 54,* 100–112.

Barabasz, A. F., Barabasz, M., Jensen, S., Calvin, S., Trevisan, M., & Warner, D. (1999). Cortical event-related potentials show the structure of hypnotic suggestions is crucial. *International Journal of Clinical and Experimental Hypnosis, 47,* 5–22.

Barabasz, A. F., & Christensen, C. (2006). Age regression: Tailored versus scripted inductions. *American Journal of Clinical Hypnosis, 48,* 251–261.

Barabasz, A. F., & Lonsdale, C. (1983). Effects of hypnosis on P300 olfactory evoked potential amplitudes. *Journal of Abnormal Psychology, 92,* 520–523.

Barabasz, A. F., Olness, K., Boland, R., & Kahn, S. (2006). *Evidence based medical hypnosis: A primer for health care practitioners* (Vol. 1). New York, NY: Routledge.

Barabasz, A. F., & Watkins, J. G. (2005). *Hypnotherapeutic techniques* (2nd ed.). New York, NY: Brunner/Routledge-Taylor & Francis.

Barber, J. (1977). Rapid induction analgesia: A clinical report. *American Journal of Clinical Hypnosis, 19,* 138–147.

Barber, J., & Mayer, D. (1977). Evaluation of the efficacy and neural mechanism of a hypnotic analgesia procedure in experimental and clinical dental pain. *Pain, 4,* 41–48.

Barber, J. E. (1996). *Hypnosis and suggestion in the treatment of pain: A clinical guide.* New York, NY: Norton.

Barber, T. X., & Hahn, K. W. J. (1962). Physiological and subjective responses to pain-producing stimulation under hypnotically suggested and waking-imagined "analgesia." *Journal of Abnormal and Social Psychology, 65,* 411–415.

Barber, T. X., Spanos, N. P., & Chaves, J. F. (1974). *Hypnotism: Imagination and human potentialities.* Elmsford, NY: Pergamon Press.

Barnier, A. J., & Nash, M. R. (2008). A roadmap for explanation, a working definition. In M. R. Nash & A. J. Barnier (Eds.), *The Oxford handbook of hypnosis: Theory, research and practice* (pp. 1–18). New York, NY: Oxford University Press.

Bayer, T. L., Coverdale, J. H., Chiang, E., & Bangs, M. (1998). The role of prior pain experience and expectancy in psychologically and physically induced pain. *Pain, 74,* 327–331.

Beck, A. (1976). *Cognitive therapy and the emotional disorders*. New York, NY: International Universities Press.

Beck, A. (1979). *Cognitive therapy and the emotional disorders*. New York, NY: Plume.

Beecher, H. K. (1959). *Measurement of subjective responses: Quantitative effects of drugs*. New York, NY: Oxford University Press.

Bellack, A. (1973). Reciprocal inhibition of a laboratory conditioned fear. *Behaviour Research and Therapy, 11*, 11–18.

Ben-Zvi, Z., Spohn, W. A., Young, S. H., & Kattan, M. (1982). Hypnosis for exercise-induced asthma. *American Review of Respiratory Disease, 125*, 392–395.

Benham, G., Woody, E. Z., Wilson, K. S., & Nash, M. R. (2006). Expect the unexpected: Ability, attitude, and responsiveness to hypnosis. *Journal of Personality and Social Psychology, 91*, 342–350.

Bennett, H. (1993). Preparing for surgery and medical procedures. In D. Goleman & J. Gurin (Eds.), *Mind–body medicine* (pp. 401–427). Yonkers, NY: Consumer Reports Books.

Berne, E. (1975). *Transactional analysis in psychotherapy*. London, England: Souvenir Press.

Bien, T. H., Miller, W. R., & Boroughs, J. M. (1993). Motivational interviewing with alcohol outpatients. *Behavioral and Cognitive Psychotherapy, 21*, 347–356.

Bien, T. H., Miller, W. R., & Tonigan, J. S. (1993). Brief interventions for alcohol problems: A review. *Addiction, 88*, 315–336.

Bone, R. C., Hayden, W. R., Levine, R. L., McCartney, J. R., Barkin, R. L., Clark, S., . . . Guerrero, M. (1995). Recognition, assessment, and treatment of anxiety in the critical care patient: Consensus guidelines from a working party. *Disease-a-Month, 41*, 293–360.

Bonica, J. J. (Ed.). (1990). *The management of pain* (2nd ed., Vol. 1–2). Philadelphia, PA: Lea & Febiger.

Boothby, J. L., Thorn, B. E., Stroud, M. W., & Jensen, M. P. (1999). Coping with pain. In R. J. Gatchel & D. C. Turk (Eds.), *Psychosocial factors in pain* (pp. 343–359). New York, NY: Guilford Press.

Borckardt, J. J., & Nash, M. R. (2002). How practitioners (and others) can make scientifically viable contributions to clinical-outcome research using the single-case time-series design. *International Journal of Clinical and Experimental Hypnosis, 50*, 114–148.

Bortz, W. (1984). The disuse syndrome. *Western Journal of Medicine, 141*, 691–694.

Bowers, K. S. (1990). Unconscious influences and hypnosis. In J. L. Singer (Ed.), *Repression and dissociation: Implications for personality theory, psychopathology, and health* (pp. 143–178). Chicago, IL: University of Chicago Press.

Bowers, K. S. (1992). Imagination and dissociation in hypnotic responding. *International Journal of Clinical and Experimental Hypnosis, 40*, 253–275.

Bowers, K. S., & Brennenman, H. A. (1981). Hypnotic dissociation, dichotic listening, and active versus passive modes of attention. *Journal of Abnormal Psychology*, 90, 55–67.

Bowers, K. S., & Davidson, T. M. (1991). A neodissociative critique of Spanos's social-psychological model of hypnosis. In S. J. Lynn & J. W. Rhue (Eds.), *Theories of hypnosis: Current models and perspectives* (pp. 105–143). New York, NY: Guilford Press.

Bradley, L. A. (1996). Cognitive–behavioral therapy for chronic pain. In R. J. Gatchel & D. C. Turk (Eds.), *Psychological approaches to pain management: A practitioner's handbook* (pp. 131–147). New York, NY: Guilford Press.

Brown, C., Albrecht, R., Pettit, H., McFadden, T., & Schermer, C. (2000). Opioid and benzodiazepine withdrawal syndrome in adult burn patients. *American Surgeon*, 66, 367–370.

Brown, D. C., & Hammond, D. C. (2007). Evidence-based clinical hypnosis for obstetrics, labor and delivery, and preterm labor. *International Journal of Clinical and Experimental Hypnosis*, 55, 355–371.

Carbonari, J. P., & DiClemente, C. C. (2000). Using transtheoretical model profiles to differentiate levels of alcohol abstinence success. *Journal of Consulting Clinical Psychology*, 68, 810–817.

Carey, K. B., Henson, J. M., Carey, M. P., & Maisto, S. A. (2009). Computer versus in-person intervention for students violating campus alcohol policy. *Journal of Consulting and Clinical Psychology*, 77, 74–87.

Carney, M. M., & Kivlahan, D. R. (1995). Motivational subtypes among veterans seeking substance abuse treatment: Profiles based on stages of change. *Psychology of Addictive Behaviors*, 9, 1135–1142.

Casiglia, E., Schiavon, L., Tikhonoff, V., Haxhi Nasto, H., Azzi, M., Rempelou, P., . . . Rossi, A. M. (2007). Hypnosis prevents the cardiovascular response to cold pressor test. *American Journal of Clinical Hypnosis*, 49, 255–266.

Castel, A., Perez, M., Sala, J., Padrol, A., & Rull, M. (2007). Effect of hypnotic suggestion on fibromyalgic pain: Comparison between hypnosis and relaxation. *European Journal of Pain*, 11, 463–468.

Chance, W. T. (1980). Autoanalgesia: Opiate and non-opiate mechanisms. *Neuroscience and Biobehavioral Reviews*, 4, 55–67.

Chapman, C. R. (1985). Psychological factors in postoperative pain and their treatment. In G. Smith & B. G. Covino (Eds.), *Acute pain* (pp. 22–41). London, England: Butterworths.

Chapman, C. R., & Bonica, J. J. (1983). Acute pain. In *Current concepts* (p. 44). Kalamazoo, MI: Upjohn Company.

Chapman, C. R., & Nakamura, Y. (1999). A passion of the soul: An introduction to pain for consciousness researchers. *Consciousness and Cognition*, 8, 391–422.

Chapman, C. R., Nakamura, Y., & Flores, L. Y. (1999). Chronic pain and consciousness: A constructivist perspective. In R. J. Gatchel & D. C. Turk (Eds.),

Psychosocial factors in pain: Critical perspectives (pp. 35–55). New York, NY: Guilford Press.

Chapman, C. R., & Turner, J. A. (1986). Psychological control of acute pain in medical settings. *Journal of Pain and Symptom Management, 1*, 9–20.

Chaves, J. F. (1986). Hypnosis in the management of phantom limb pain. In E. Dowd & J. Healy (Eds.), *Case studies in hypnotherapy* (pp. 198–209). New York, NY: Guilford Press.

Chaves, J. F. (1989). Hypnotic control of clinical pain. In N. P. Spanos & J. F. Chaves (Eds.), *Hypnosis: The cognitive–behavioral perspective*. Buffalo, NY: Prometheus Books.

Chaves, J. F. (1993). Hypnosis in pain management. In J. W. Rhue, S. J. Lynn, & I. Kirsch (Eds.), *Handbook of clinical hypnosis* (pp. 511–532). Washington, DC: American Psychological Association.

Chaves, J. F. (1994). Recent advances in the application of hypnosis to pain management. *American Journal of Clinical Hypnosis, 37*, 117–129.

Chaves, J. F., & Barber, T. X. (1974). Acupuncture analgesia: A six factor theory. *Psychoenergetic Systems, 1*, 11–21.

Chaves, J. F., & Barber, T. X. (1976). Hypnotic procedures and surgery: A critical analysis with applications to acupuncture analgesia. *American Journal of Clinical Hypnosis, 18*, 217–236.

Chaves, J. F., & Brown, J.M. (1987). Spontaneous coping strategies for pain. *Journal of Behavioral Medicine, 10*, 263–276.

Chaves, J. F., & Dworkin, S. F. (1997). Hypnotic control of pain: Historical perspectives and future prospects. *International Journal of Clinical and Experimental Hypnosis, 45*, 356–376.

Chen, A. C. N., Chapman, C. R., & Harkins, S. W. (1979). Brain evoked potentials are functional correlates of induced pain in man. *Pain, 6*, 305–314.

Cherny, N., Ripamonti, C., Pereira, J., Davis, C., Fallon, M., McQuay, H., . . . Ventafridda, V. (2001). Strategies to manage the adverse effects of oral morphine: An evidence-based report. *Journal of Clinical Oncology, 19*, 2542–2554.

Chick, J., Lloyd, G., & Crombie, E. (1985). Counselling problem drinkers in medical wards: A controlled study. *British Medical Journal (Clinical Research Edition), 290*, 965–967.

Chou, R., & Huffman, L. H. (2007). Nonpharmacologic therapies for acute and chronic low back pain: A review of the evidence for an American Pain Society/American College of Physicians clinical practice guideline. *Annals of Internal Medicine, 147*, 492–504.

Cleeland, C. S., & Ryan, K. M. (1994). Pain assessment: Global use of the Brief Pain Inventory. *Annals Academy of Medicine Singapore, 23*, 129–138.

Cohen, L. L., Blout, R. L., & Panopoulos, G. (1997). Nurse coaching and cartoon distraction: An effective and practical intervention to reduce child, parent and nurse distress during immunizations. *Journal of Pediatric Psychology, 22*, 355–370.

Cooper, L. F., & Erickson, M. H. (1959). *Time distortion in hypnosis: An experimental and clinical investigation.* Bancyfelin, Carmarthen, Wales: Crown House.

Covino, N. A. (2008). Medical illnesses, conditions and procedures. In M. R. Nash & A. J. Barnier (Eds.), *The Oxford handbook of hypnosis: Theory, research and practice* (pp. 611–624). New York, NY: Oxford University Press.

Crasilneck, H. B. (1979). Hypnosis in the control of chronic low back pain. *American Journal of Clinical Hypnosis, 22,* 71–78.

Crasilneck, H. B. (1995). The use of the Crasilneck bombardment technique in problems of intractable organic pain. *American Journal of Clinical Hypnosis, 37,* 255–266.

Crasilneck, H. B., Stirman, J. A., & Wilson, B. J. (1955). Use of hypnosis in the management of patients with burns. *Journal of the American Medical Association, 158,* 103–106.

Crawford, H. J. (1990). Cognitive and psychophysiological correlates of hypnotic responsiveness and hypnosis. In M. L. Mass & D. Brown (Eds.), *Creative mastery in hypnosis and hypnoanalysis: A festschrift for Erika Fromm* (pp. 47–54). Hillsdale, NJ: Erlbaum.

Crawford, H. J. (1994). Brain dynamics and hypnosis: Attentional and disattentional processes. *International Journal of Clinical and Experimental Hypnosis, 42,* 204–232.

Crawford, H. J., Knebel, T., Kaplan, L., Vendemia, J. M., Xie, M., Jamison, S., & Pribram, K. H. (1998). Hypnotic analgesia: 1. Somatosensory event-related potential changes to noxious stimuli. 2. Transfer learning to reduce chronic low back pain. *International Journal of Clinical and Experimental Hypnosis, 46,* 92–132.

Curry, S., Wagner, E. H., & Grothaus, L. C. (1990). Intrinsic and extrinsic motivation for smoking cessation. *Journal of Consulting and Clinical Psychology, 58,* 310–316.

Cyna, A. M., McAuliffe, G. L., & Andrew, M. I. (2004). Hypnosis for pain relief in labour and childbirth: A systematic review. *British Journal of Anaesthesia, 93,* 505–511.

Dahl, J. C., Wilson, K. G., Luciano, C., & Hayes, S. C. (2005). *Acceptance and commitment therapy for chronic pain.* Reno, NV: Context Press.

Dahl, J. C., Wilson, K. G., & Nilsson, A. (2004). Acceptance and commitment therapy and the treatment of persons at risk for long-term disability resulting from stress and pain symptoms: A preliminary randomized trial. *Behavior Therapy, 35,* 785–801.

Dane, J. R. (1996). Hypnosis for pain and neuromuscular rehabilitation with multiple sclerosis: Case summary, literature review, and analysis of outcomes. *International Journal of Clinical and Experimental Hypnosis, 44,* 208–231.

Danziger, N., Fournier, E., Bouhassira, D., Michaud, D., De Broucker, T., Santarcangelo, E., . . . Willer, J. C. (1998). Different strategies of modulation can be operative during hypnotic analgesia: A neurophysiological study. *Pain, 75,* 85–92.

Das, D., Grimmer, K., Sparnon, A., McRae, S., & Thomas, B. (2005). The efficacy of playing a virtual reality game in modulating pain for children with acute burn injuries: A randomized controlled trial. *BMC Pediatric, 5*(1), 1.

Daut, R. L., Cleeland, C. S., & Flanery, R. C. (1983). Development of the Wisconsin Brief Pain Questionnaire to assess pain in cancer and other diseases. *Pain, 17,* 197–210.

Davidson, J. (1962). An assessment of the value of hypnosis in pregnancy and labour. *British Medical Journal,* 951–952.

Davidson, R. J., Kabat-Zinn, J., Schumacher, J., Rosenkranz, M., Muller, D., Santorelli, S., . . . Sheridan, J. (2003). Alterations in brain and immune function produced by mindfulness meditation. *Psychosomatic Medicine, 65,* 564–570.

Davies, K. A., Macfarlane, G. J., Nicholl, B. I., Dickens, C., Morriss, R., Ray, D., & McBeth, J. (2008). Restorative sleep predicts the resolution of chronic widespread pain: Results from the EPIFUND study. *Rheumatology (Oxford), 47,* 1809–1813.

De Jong, J. R., Vangronsveld, K., Peters, M. L., Goossens, M. E., Onghena, P., Bulte, I., & Vlaeyen, J. W. (2008). Reduction of pain-related fear and disability in post-traumatic neck pain: A replicated single-case experimental study of exposure in vivo. *Journal of Pain, 9,* 1123–1134.

De Pascalis, V., Bellusci, A., Gallo, C., Magurano, M. R., & Chen, A. C. (2004). Pain-reduction strategies in hypnotic context and hypnosis: ERPs and SCRs during a secondary auditory task. *International Journal of Clinical and Experimental Hypnosis, 52,* 343–363.

De Pascalis, V., Cacace, I., & Massicolle, F. (2004). Perception and modulation of pain in waking and hypnosis: Functional significance of phase-ordered gamma oscillations. *Pain, 112,* 27–36.

De Pascalis, V., Cacace, I., & Massicolle, F. (2008). Focused analgesia in waking and hypnosis: Effects on pain, memory, and somatosensory event-related potentials. *Pain, 134,* 197–208.

De Pascalis, V., Magurano, M. R., & Bellusci, A. (1999). Pain perception, somatosensory event-related potentials and skin conductance responses to painful stimuli in high, mid, and low hypnotizable subjects: Effects of differential pain reduction strategies. *Pain, 83,* 499–508.

De Pascalis, V., Magurano, M. R., Bellusci, A., & Chen, A. C. (2001). Somatosensory event-related potential and autonomic activity to varying pain reduction cognitive strategies in hypnosis. *Clinical Neurophysiology, 112,* 1475–1485.

De Pascalis, V., & Perrone, M. (1996). EEG asymmetry and heart rate during experience of hypnotic analgesia in high and low hypnotizables. *International Journal of Psychophysiology, 21,* 163–175.

DiClemente, C. C. (1999). Motivation for change: Implications for substance abuse. *Psychological Science, 10,* 209–213.

DiClemente, C. C. (2003). *Addiction and change: How addictions develop and addicted people recover.* New York, NY: Guilford Press.

DiClemente, C. C., & Hughes, S. O. (1990). Stages of change profiles in outpatient alcoholism treatment. *Journal of Substance Abuse, 2,* 217–235.

DiClemente, C. C., & Prochaska, J. O. (1985). Processes and stages of change: Coping and competence in smoking behavior change. In S. Shiffman & T. A. Wills (Eds.), *Coping and substance abuse* (pp. 319–343). New York, NY: Academic Press.

DiClemente, C. C., & Prochaska, J. O. (1998). Toward a comprehensive, transtheoretical model of change: Stages of change and addictive behaviors. In W. R. Miller & N. Heather (Eds.), *Treating addictive behaviors* (2nd ed., pp. 3–24). New York, NY: Plenum Press.

DiClemente, C. C., Story, M., & Murray, K. (2000). On a roll: The process of initiation and cessation of problem gambling among adolescents. *Journal of Gambling Studies, 16,* 289–313.

Difede, J., Ptacek, J. T., Roberts, J., Barocas, D., Rives, W., Apfeldorf, W., & Yurt, R. (2002). Acute stress disorder after burn injury: A predictor of posttraumatic stress disorder? *Psychosomatic Medicine, 64,* 826–834.

Dinges, D. F., Whitehouse, W. G., Orne, E. C., Bloom, P. B., Carlin, M. M., Bauer, N. K., . . . Orne, M. T. (1997). Self-hypnosis training as an adjunctive treatment in the management of pain associated with sickle cell disease. *International Journal of Clinical and Experimental Hypnosis, 45,* 417–432.

Dixon, M., & Laurence, J. (1992). Two hundred years of hypnosis research: Questions resolved? Questions unanswered! In E. Fromm & M. R. Nash (Eds.), *Contemporary hypnosis research* (pp. 34–66). New York, NY: Guilford Press.

Douaihy, A., Jensen, M. P., & Jou, R. J. (2005). Motivating behavior change in persons with chronic pain. In B. McCarberg & S. Passik (Eds.), *Expert guide to pain management* (pp. 217–231). Philadelphia, PA: American College of Physicians.

Dougher, M. J. (Ed.). (2002). *Clinical behavior analysis.* Reno, NV: Context Press.

Dunn, C., Deroo, L., & Rivara, F. P. (2001). The use of brief interventions adapted from motivational interviewing across behavioral domains: A systematic review. *Addiction, 96,* 1725–1742.

Dworkin, R. H., O'Connor, A. B., Backonja, M., Farrar, J. T., Finnerup, N. B., Jensen, T. S., . . . Wallace, W. S. (2007). Pharmacologic management of neuropathic pain: Evidence-based recommendations. *Pain, 132,* 237–251.

Dynes, J. B. (1947). Objective method for distinguishing sleep from the hypnotic trance. *Neurological Psychiatry, 57,* 84–93.

Eastwood, J. D., Gaskovski, P., & Bowers, K. S. (1998). The folly of effort: Ironic effects in the mental control of pain. *International Journal of Clinical and Experimental Hypnosis, 46,* 77–91.

Eccleston, C., & Crombez, G. (1999). Pain demands attention: A cognitive–affective model of the interruptive function of pain. *Psychological Bulletin, 125,* 356–366.

Edelson, J., & Fitzpatrick, J. L. (1989). A comparison of cognitive–behavioral and hypnotic treatments of chronic pain. *Journal of Clinical Psychology, 45,* 316–323.

Edmonston, W. E., Jr. (1991). Anesis. In S. J. Lynn & J. W. Rhue (Eds.), *Theories of hypnosis: Current models and perspectives* (pp. 197–237). New York, NY: Guilford Press.

Edwards, G., & Orford, J. (1977). A plain treatment for alcoholism. *Proceedings of the Royal Society of Medicine, 70,* 344–348.

Edwards, R. R., & Fillingim, R. B. (1999). Ethnic differences in thermal pain responses. *Psychosomatic Medicine, 61,* 346–354.

Eisenberg, D. M., Kessler, R. C., Foster, C., Norlock, F. E., Calkins, D. R., & Delbanco, T. L. (1993). Unconventional medicine in the United States: Prevalence, costs, and patterns of use. *New England Journal of Medicine, 328,* 246–252.

Elkins, G., Jensen, M. P., & Patterson, D. R. (2007). Hypnotherapy for the management of chronic pain. *International Journal of Clinical and Experimental Hypnosis, 55,* 275–287.

Elkins, G., Marcus, J., Palamara, L., & Stearns, V. (2004). Can hypnosis reduce hot flashes in breast cancer survivors? A literature review. *American Journal of Clinical Hypnosis, 47,* 29–42.

Ellermeier, W., & Westphal, W. (1995). Gender differences in pain ratings and pupil reactions to painful pressure stimuli. *Pain, 61,* 435–439.

Ellis, A. (1961). *A new guide to rational living:* Hollywood, CA: Wehman Brothers.

Ellis, A. (1980). Rational-emotive therapy and cognitive behavior therapy: Similarities and differences. *Cognitive Therapy and Research, 4,* 325–340.

Ellis, A. (1995). *Better, deeper, and more enduring brief therapy: The rational emotive behavior therapy approach.* New York, NY: Routledge.

Ellis, J. A., & Spanos, N. P. (1994). Cognitive–behavioral interventions for children's distress during bone marrow aspirations and lumbar punctures: A critical review. *Journal of Pain and Symptom Management, 9,* 96–108.

Elvy, G. A., Wells, J. E., & Baird, K. A. (1988). Attempted referral as intervention for problem drinking in the general hospital. *British Journal of Addiction, 83,* 83–89.

Erickson, M. H. (1967). *Advanced techniques of hypnosis and therapy: Selected papers of Milton H. Erickson.* Boston, MA: Allyn & Bacon.

Erickson, M. H. (1980a). Hypnotic psychotherapy. In E. L. Rossi (Ed.), *The collected papers of Milton H. Erickson on hypnosis: IV. Innovative hypnotherapy* (pp. 35–48). New York, NY: Irvington. (Original work published 1948)

Erickson, M. H. (1980b). *The collected papers of Milton Erickson on hypnosis: Vol. IV. Innovative hypnotherapy* (E. L. Rossi, Ed.). New York, NY: Irvington.

Erickson, M. H. (1983). *Healing in hypnosis.* New York, NY: Irvington.

Erickson, M. H., & Rossi, E. L. (1979). *Hypnotherapy, an exploratory casebook.* New York, NY: Irvington.

Erickson, M. H., & Rossi, E. L. (1980). Autohypnotic experiences of Milton Erickson. In E. L. Rossi (Ed.), *The nature of hypnosis and suggestion by Milton Erickson: The collected papers of Milton H. Erickson on hypnosis* (Vol. 1, pp. 108–132). New York, NY: Irvington.

Erickson, M. H., & Rossi, E. L. (1981). *Experiencing hypnosis: Therapeutic approaches to altered states*. New York, NY: Irvington.

Erickson, M. H., Rossi, E. L., & Rossi, S. (1976). *Hypnotic realities: The induction of clinical hypnosis and forms of indirect suggestion*. New York, NY: Irvington.

Esdaile, J. (1957). *Hypnosis in medicine and surgery*. New York, NY: Julian Press.

Evans, F. J. (1989). Hypnosis and chronic pain: Two contrasting case studies. *Clinical Journal of Pain, 5*, 169–176.

Everett, J. J., Patterson, D. R., Burns, G. L., Montgomery, B. K., & Heimbach, D. M. (1994). Adjunctive interventions for burn pain control: Comparison of hypnosis and Ativan. *Journal of Burn Care and Rehabilitation, 14*, 676–683.

Everett, J. J., Patterson, D. R., & Chen, A. C. (1990). Cognitive and behavioral treatments for burn pain. *The Pain Clinic, 3*, 133–145.

Ewer, T. C., & Stewart, D. E. (1986). Improvement in bronchial hyper-responsiveness in patients with moderate asthma after treatment with a hypnotic technique: A randomised controlled trial. *British Medical Journal (Clinical Research Edition), 293*, 1129–1132.

Ewin, D. M. (1983). Emergency room hypnosis for the burned patient. *American Journal of Clinical Hypnosis, 26*, 5–8.

Ewin, D. M. (1984). Hypnosis in surgery and anesthesia. In W. C. Wester II & A. H. Smith Jr. (Eds.), *Clinical hypnosis: A multidisciplinary approach* (pp. 210–235). Philadelphia, PA: Lippincott.

Ewin, D. M. (1986). Emergency room hypnosis for the burned patient. *American Journal of Clinical Hypnosis, 29*, 7–12.

Faymonville, M. E., Boly, M., & Laureys, S. (2006). Functional neuroanatomy of the hypnotic state. *Journal of Physiology (Paris), 99*, 463–469.

Faymonville, M. E., Mambourg, P. H., Joris, J., Vrijens, B., Fissette, J., Albert, A., & Lamy, M. (1997). Psychological approaches during conscious sedation— Hypnosis versus stress reducing strategies: A prospective randomized study. *Pain, 73*, 361–367.

Feldman, J. B. (2009). Expanding hypnotic pain management to the affective dimension of pain. *American Journal of Clinical Hypnosis, 51*, 235–254.

Fernandez, E., & Turk, D. C. (1989). The utility of cognitive coping strategies for altering pain perception: A meta-analysis. *Pain, 38*, 123–135.

Finer, B., & Graf, K. (1968). Circulatory changes accompanying hypnotic imagination of hyperalgesia and hypoalgesia in causalgic limbs. *Zeitschrift fur die Gesamte Experimentelle Medizin, 146*, 97–114.

Finer, B. L., & Nylen, B. O. (1961). Cardiac arrest in the treatment of burns, and report on hypnosis as a substitute for anesthesia. *Plastic and Reconstructive Surgery, 27*, 49–55.

Flor, H. (2003). Cortical reorganisation and chronic pain: Implications for rehabilitation. *Journal of Rehabilitation Medicine, 41* (Suppl.), 66–72.

Flor, H., Kerns, R. D., & Turk, D. C. (1987). The role of spouse reinforcement, perceived pain, and activity levels of chronic pain patients. *Journal of Psychosomatic Research, 31,* 251–259.

Flor, H., Knost, B., & Birbaumer, N. (2002). The role of operant conditioning in chronic pain: An experimental investigation. *Pain, 95,* 111–118.

Flor, H., Turk, D. C., & Rudy, T. E. (1989). Relationship of pain impact and significant other reinforcement of pain behaviors: The mediating role of gender, marital status and marital satisfaction. *Pain, 38,* 45–50.

Flowers, C. E., Littlejohn, T. W., & Wells, H. B. (1960). Pharmacologic and hypnoid analgesia: Effect upon labor and the infant response. *Obstetrics and Gynecology, 16,* 210–221.

Fordyce, W. E. (1976). *Behavioral methods for chronic pain and illness.* St. Louis, MO: Mosby Year Book.

Fordyce, W. E. (1988). Pain and suffering. *American Psychologist, 43,* 276–283.

France, R. D., Krishnan, K. R. R., & Houpt, J. L. (1988). Overview. In R. D. France & K. R. R. Krishnan (Eds.), *Chronic pain* (pp. 3–15). Washington, DC: American Psychiatric Press.

Frank, J. D., & Frank, J. B. (1991). *Persuasion and healing: A comparative study of psychotherapy* (3rd ed.). Baltimore, MD: Johns Hopkins University Press.

Freeman, R., Barabasz, A., Barabasz, M., & Warner, D. (2000). Hypnosis and distraction differ in their effects on cold pressor pain. *American Journal of Clinical Hypnosis, 43,* 137–148.

Freeman, R. M., Macaulay, A. J., Eve, L., Chamberlain, G. V., & Bhat, A. V. (1986). Randomised trial of self hypnosis for analgesia in labour. *British Medical Journal (Clinical Research Edition), 292,* 657–658.

Friedman, H., & Taub, H. A. (1984). Brief psychological training procedures in migraine treatment. *American Journal of Clinical Hypnosis, 26,* 187–200.

Frischholz, E. J. (2007). Hypnosis, hypnotizability, and placebo. *American Journal of Clinical Hypnosis, 50,* 49.

Frischholz, E. J., Blumstein, R., & Spiegel, D. (1982). Comparative efficacy of hypnotic behavioral training and sleep/trance hypnotic induction: Comment on Katz. *Journal of Consulting and Clinical Psychology, 50,* 766–769.

Gainer, M. J. (1992). Hypnotherapy for reflex sympathetic dystrophy. *American Journal of Clinical Hypnosis, 34,* 227–232.

Galer, B. S., Schwartz, L., & Turner, J. A. (1997). Do patient and physician expectations predict response to pain-relieving procedures? *Clinical Journal of Pain, 13,* 348–351.

Gasma, A. (1994). The role of psychological factors in chronic pain: I. A half century study. *Pain, 57,* 5–15.

Gatchel, R. J., & Epker, J. (1999). Psychosocial predictors of chronic pain and response to treatment. In R. J. Gatchel & D. C. Turk (Eds.), *Psychosocial factors in pain: Clinical perspectives* (pp. 412–434). New York, NY: Guilford Press.

Gatchel, R. J., & Turk, D. C. (Eds.). (1996). *Psychological approaches to pain management: A practitioner's handbook*. New York, NY: Guilford Press.

Gay, M. C., Philippot, P., & Luminet, O. (2002). Differential effectiveness of psychological interventions for reducing osteoarthritis pain: A comparison of Erickson hypnosis and Jacobson relaxation. *European Journal of Pain, 6*, 1–16.

Gholamrezaei, A., Ardestani, S. K., & Emami, M. H. (2006). Where does hypnotherapy stand in the management of irritable bowel syndrome? A systematic review. *Journal of Alternative and Complementary Medicine, 12*, 517–527.

Gilboa, D., Borenstein, A., Seidman, D., & Tsur, H. (1990). Burn patients' use of autohypnosis: Making a painful experience bearable. *Burns, 16*, 441–444.

Gillett, P. L., & Coe, W. C. (1984). The effects of rapid induction analgesia (RIA), hypnotic susceptibility and the severity of discomfort on reducing dental pain. *American Journal of Clinical Hypnosis, 27*, 81–90.

Gilligan, S. G. (1985). Generative autonomy: Principles for an Ericksonian hypnotherapy. In J. K. Zeig (Ed.), *Ericksonian psychotherapy: I. Structures*. New York, NY: Brunner/Mazel.

Gilligan, S. G. (1987). *Therapeutic trances*. New York, NY: Brunner/Mazel.

Glanz, K., Patterson, R. E., Kristal, A. R., DiClemente, C. C., Heimendinger, J., Linnan, L., & McLerran, D. F. (1994). Stages of change in adopting healthy diets: Fat, fiber, and correlates of nutrient intake. *Health Education Quarterly, 21*, 499–519.

Goldenberg, D. L., Burckhardt, C., & Crofford, L. (2004). Management of fibromyalgia syndrome. *Journal of the American Medical Association, 292*, 2388–2395.

Goldstein, A., & Hilgard, E. R. (1975). Lack of influence of the morphine antagonist naloxone on hypnotic analgesia. *Proceedings of the National Academy of Sciences, 72*, 2041–2043.

Gonsalkorale, W. M., Miller, V., Afzal, A., & Whorwell, P. J. (2003). Long term benefits of hypnotherapy for irritable bowel syndrome. *Gut, 52*, 1623–1629.

Green, J. P., & Lynn, S. J. (2000). Hypnosis and suggestion-based approaches to smoking cessation: An examination of the evidence. *International Journal of Clinical and Experimental Hypnosis, 48*, 195–224.

Green, J. P., Lynn, S. J., & Montgomery, G. H. (2006). A meta-analysis of gender, smoking cessation, and hypnosis: A brief communication. *International Journal of Clinical and Experimental Hypnosis, 54*, 224–233.

Green, J. P., Lynn, S. J., & Montgomery, G. H. (2008). Gender-related differences in hypnosis-based treatments for smoking: A follow-up meta-analysis. *American Journal of Clinical Hypnosis, 50*, 259–271.

Greene, R. J., & Reyher, J. (1972). Pain tolerance in hypnotic analgesic and imagination states. *Journal of Abnormal Psychology, 79*, 29–38.

Grimley, D. M., Riley, G. E., Bellis, J. M., & Prochaska, J. O. (1993). Assessing the stages of change and decision-making for contraceptive use for the prevention of pregnancy, sexually transmitted diseases, and acquired immunodeficiency syndrome. *Health Education Quarterly, 20,* 455–470.

Gruzelier, J., Allison, J., & Conway, A. (1988). A psychophysiological differentiation between hypnotic behaviour and simulation. *International Journal of Psychophysiology, 6,* 331–338.

Grzesiak, R. C., Ury, G. M., & Dworkin, R. H. (1996). Psychodynamic psychotherapy with chronic pain patients. In R. J. Gatchel & D. C. Turk (Eds.), *Psychological approaches to pain management: A practitioner's handbook* (pp. 148–178). New York, NY: Guilford Press.

Haanen, H. C., Hoenderdos, H. T., van Romunde, L. K., Hop, W. C., Mallee, C., Terwiel, J. P., & Hekster, G. B. (1991). Controlled trial of hypnotherapy in the treatment of refractory fibromyalgia. *Journal of Rheumatology, 18,* 72–75.

Halliday, A. M., & Mason, A. A. (1964). Cortical evoked potentials during hypnotic anaesthesia. *Electroencephalography and Clinical Neurophysiology, 16,* 312–314.

Hammond, D. C. (1988). Will the real Milton Erickson please stand up? *International Journal of Clinical and Experimental Hypnosis, 36,* 173–181.

Hammond, D. C. (2007). Review of the efficacy of clinical hypnosis with headaches and migraines. *International Journal of Clinical and Experimental Hypnosis, 55,* 207–219.

Hammond, D. C. (2008). Hypnosis as sole anesthesia for major surgeries: Historical and contemporary perspectives. *American Journal of Clinical Hypnosis, 51,* 101–121.

Hargadon, R., Bowers, K. S., & Woody, E. Z. (1995). Does counterpain imagery mediate hypnotic analgesia? *Journal of Abnormal Psychology, 104,* 508–516.

Harmon, T. M., Hynan, M. T., & Tyre, T. E. (1990). Improved obstetric outcomes using hypnotic analgesia and skill mastery combined with childbirth education. *Journal of Consulting and Clinical Psychology, 58,* 525–530.

Hartland, J. (1971). *Medical and dental hypnosis.* Baltimore, MD: Williams & Wilkins.

Henchoz, Y., & Kai-Lik So, A. (2008). Exercise and nonspecific low back pain: A literature review. *Joint Bone Spine, 75,* 533–539.

Hendrix, C., & Barfield, W. (1995, March). *Presence in virtual environments as a function of visual and auditory cues.* Paper presented at the Virtual Reality Annual International Symposium, Research Triangle Park, NC.

Hernandez-Peon, R., Dittborn, J., Borlone, M., & Davidovich, A. (1960). Modifications of a forearm skin reflex during hypnotically induced anesthesia and hyperesthisia. *Acta Neurologica Latinoamericana, 6,* 32–42.

Hettema, J., Steele, J., & Miller, W. R. (2005). Motivational interviewing. *Annual Review of Clinical Psychology, 1,* 91–111.

Hilgard, E. R. (1967). A quantitative study of pain and its reduction through hypnotic suggestion. *Proceedings of the National Academy of Sciences, 57,* 1581–1586.

Hilgard, E. R. (1969). Pain as a puzzle for psychology and physiology. *American Psychologist, 24,* 103–113.

Hilgard, E. R. (1992). Dissociation and theories of hypnosis. In E. Fromm & M. R. Nash (Eds.), *Contemporary perspectives in hypnosis research* (pp. 69–101). New York, NY: Guilford Press.

Hilgard, E. R., & Hilgard, J. R. (1975). *Hypnosis in the relief of pain*. Los Altos, CA: William Kaufmann.

Hilgard, E. R., & Morgan, A. H. (1975). Heart rate and blood pressure in the study of laboratory pain in man under normal conditions and as influenced by hypnosis. *Acta Neurobiologiae Experimentalis, 35*, 741–759.

Hilgard, J. R., & LeBaron, S. (1984). *Hypnotherapy of pain in children with cancer*. Los Altos, CA: William Kaufman.

Hofbauer, R., Rainville, P., Duncan, G., & Bushnell, M. (2001). Cortical representation of the sensory dimension of pain. *Journal of Neurophysiology, 86*, 402–411.

Hoffman, H. G. (2004, August). Virtual reality therapy. *Scientific American, 291*(2), 58–65.

Hoffman, H. G., Doctor, J. N., Patterson, D. R., Carrougher, G. J., & Furness, T. A., III. (2000). Use of virtual reality as an adjunctive treatment of adolescent burn pain during wound care: A case report. *Pain, 85*, 305–309.

Hoffman, H. G., Garcia-Palacios, A., Carlin, C., Furness, T. I., & Botella-Arbona, C. (2003). Interfaces that heal: Coupling real and virtual objects to cure spider phobia. *International Journal of Human-Computer Interaction, 16*, 283–300.

Hoffman, H. G., Patterson, D. R., & Carrougher, G. J. (2000). Use of virtual reality for adjunctive treatment of adult burn pain during physical therapy: A controlled study. *Clinical Journal of Pain, 16*, 244–250.

Hoffman, H. G., Patterson, D. R., Carrougher, G. J., Nakamura, D., Moore, M., Garcia-Palacios, A., & Furness, T. A., III. (2001). The effectiveness of virtual reality pain control with multiple treatments of longer durations: A case study. *International Journal of Human-Computer Interaction, 13*, 1–12.

Hoffman, H. G., Patterson, D. R., Carrougher, G. J., & Sharar, S. R. (2001). Effectiveness of virtual reality-based pain control with multiple treatments. *Clinical Journal of Pain, 17*, 229–235.

Hoffman, H. G., Patterson, D. R., Magula, J., Carrougher, G., Zeltzer, K., & Sharar, S. (2004). Water-friendly virtual reality pain control during wound care. *Journal of Clinical Psychology, 60*, 189–195.

Hoffman, H. G., Sharar, S., Coda, B., Everett, J., Ciol, M., Richards, T., & Patterson, D. R. (2004). Manipulating presence influences the magnitude of virtual reality analgesia. *Pain, 111*, 162–168.

Holroyd, J. (1996). Hypnosis treatment of clinical pain: Understanding why hypnosis is useful. *International Journal of Clinical and Experimental Hypnosis, 44*, 33–51.

Holroyd, K. A., & Penzien, D. B. (1990). Pharmacological versus non-pharmacological prophylaxis of recurrent migraine headache: A meta-analytic review of clinical trials. *Pain, 42*, 1–13.

Holzman, A. D., Turk, D. C., & Kerns, R. D. (1986). The cognitive–behavioral approach to the management of chronic pain. In A. D. Holzman & D. C. Turk (Eds.), *Pain management: A handbook of psychological treatment approaches* (pp. 31–50). New York, NY: Pergamon Press.

Isenberg, S. A., Lehrer, P. M., & Hochron, S. (1992). The effects of suggestion on airways of asthmatic subjects breathing room air as a suggested bronchoconstrictor and bronchodilator. *Journal of Psychosomatic Research, 36,* 769–776.

Isenhart, C. E. (1994). Motivational subtypes in an inpatient sample of substance abusers. *Addictive Behaviors, 19,* 463–475.

Iserson, K. V. (1999). Hypnosis for pediatric fracture reduction. *Journal of Emergency Medicine, 17,* 53–56.

Jack, M. S. (1999). The use of hypnosis for a patient with chronic pain. *Contemporary Hypnosis, 16,* 231–237.

Jacobson, E. (1938). *Progressive relaxation.* Chicago, IL: University of Chicago Press.

Jacobson, L., & Mariano, A. J. (2001). General considerations of chronic pain. In J. D. Loeser, S. H. Butler, C. R. Chapman, & D. C. Turk (Eds.), *Bonica's management of pain* (pp. 241–254). Philadelphia, PA: Lippincott Williams & Wilkins.

Jaffe, S. E., & Patterson, D. R. (2004). Treating sleep problems in patients with burn injuries: Practical considerations. *Journal of Burn Care Rehabilitation, 25,* 294–305.

Jensen, M. P. (1996). Enhancing motivation to change in pain treatment. In R. J. Gatchel & D. C. Turk (Eds.), *Psychological approaches to pain management: A practitioner's handbook* (pp. 78–111). New York, NY: Guilford Press.

Jensen, M. P. (2000). Motivating the pain patient for behavior change. In J. D. Loeser, D. C. Turk, C. R. Chapman, & S. Butler (Eds.), *Bonica's management of pain* (3rd ed., pp. 1796–1804). Media, PA: Williams & Wilkins.

Jensen, M. P. (2002). Enhancing motivation to change in pain treatment. In D. C. Turk & R. J. Gatchel (Eds.), *Psychological treatment for pain: A practitioner's handbook* (2nd ed., pp. 71–93). New York, NY: Guilford Press.

Jensen, M. P. (2006). Motivational aspects of pain. In R. F. Schmidt & W. D. Willis (Eds.), *Encyclopedia of pain* (Vol. 2, pp. 371–373). Heidelberg, Germany: Springer.

Jensen, M. P. (2008). The neurophysiology of pain perception and hypnotic analgesia: Implications for clinical practice. *American Journal of Clinical Hypnosis, 51,* 123–148.

Jensen, M. P., & Barber, J. (2000). Hypnotic analgesia of spinal cord injury pain. *Australian Journal of Clinical and Experimental Hypnosis, 28,* 150–168.

Jensen, M. P., Barber, J., Romano, J. M., Hanley, M. A., Raichle, K. A., Molton, I. R., . . . Patterson, D. R. (2009). Effects of self-hypnosis training and EMG biofeedback relaxation training on chronic pain in persons with spinal cord injury. *International Journal of Clinical and Experimental Hypnosis, 57,* 239–268.

Jensen, M. P., Barber, J., Romano, J. M., Molton, I. R., Raichle, K. A., Osborne, T. L., . . . Patterson, D. R. (2009). A comparison of self-hypnosis versus progressive muscle relaxation in patients with multiple sclerosis and chronic pain. *International Journal of Clinical and Experimental Hypnosis, 57,* 198–221.

Jensen, M. P., Ehde, D. M., Hoffman, A. J., Patterson, D. R., Czerniecki, J. M., & Robinson, L. R. (2002). Cognitions, coping and social environment predict adjustment to phantom limb pain. *Pain, 95,* 133–142.

Jensen, M. P., Hanley, M. A., Engel, J. M., Romano, J. M., Barber, J., Cardenas, D. D., . . . Patterson, D. R. (2005). Hypnotic analgesia for chronic pain in persons with disabilities: A case series. *International Journal of Clinical and Experimental Hypnosis, 53,* 198–228.

Jensen, M. P., & Karoly, P. (1991). Motivation and expectancy factors in symptom perception: A laboratory study of the placebo effect. *Psychosomatic Medicine, 53,* 144–152.

Jensen, M. P., McArthur, K. D., Barber, J., Hanley, M. A., Engel, J. M., Romano, J. M., . . . Patterson, D. R. (2006). Satisfaction with, and the beneficial side effects of, hypnotic analgesia. *International Journal of Clinical and Experimental Hypnosis, 54,* 432–447.

Jensen, M. P., Nielson, W. R., & Kerns, R. D. (2003). Toward the development of a motivational model of pain self-management. *Journal of Pain, 4,* 477–492.

Jensen, M. P., & Patterson, D. (2005). Control conditions in hypnotic analgesia clinical trials: Challenges and recommendations. *International Journal of Clinical and Experimental Hypnosis, 53,* 170–198.

Jensen, M. P., & Patterson, D. R. (2006). Hypnotic treatment of chronic pain. *Journal of Behavioral Medicine, 29,* 95–124.

Jensen, M. P., & Patterson, D. (2008). Hypnosis and the relief of pain and pain disorders. In M. Nash & A. Barnier (Eds.), *The Oxford handbook of hypnosis* (pp. 503–533). New York, NY: Oxford University Press.

Jensen, S. M., Barabasz, A., Barabasz, M., & Warner, D. (2001). EEG P300 event-related markers of hypnosis. *American Journal of Clinical Hypnosis, 44,* 127–139.

Johnson, V. (1973). *I'll quit tomorrow: A practical guide to alcoholism treatment.* New York, NY: Harper & Row.

Jones, H., Cooper, P., Miller, V., Brooks, N., & Whorwell, P. J. (2006). Treatment of non-cardiac chest pain: A controlled trial of hypnotherapy. *Gut, 55,* 1403–1408.

Kabat-Zinn, J. (1982). An outpatient program in behavioral medicine for chronic pain patients based on the practice of mindfulness meditation: Theoretical considerations and preliminary results. *General Hospital Psychiatry, 4,* 33–47.

Kabat-Zinn, J., Massion, A. O., Kristeller, J., Peterson, L. G., Fletcher, K., Pbert, L., . . . Santorelli, S. F. (1992). Effectiveness of a meditation-based stress reduction program in the treatment of anxiety disorders. *American Journal of Psychiatry, 149,* 936–943.

Karoly, P., & Jensen, M. P. (1987). *Multimethod assessment of chronic pain.* New York, NY: Pergamon.

Katz, E. R., Kellerman, J., & Ellenberg, L. (1987). Hypnosis in the reduction of acute pain and distress in children with cancer. *Journal of Pediatric Psychology, 12,* 379–394.

Kazdin, A. E. (1979). Nonspecific treatment factors in psychotherapy outcome research. *Journal of Consulting and Clinical Psychology, 47,* 846–851.

Kerns, R. D., Rosenberg, R., & Otis, J. D. (2002). Self-appraised problem solving and pain-relevant social support as predictors of the experience of chronic pain. *Annals of Behavioral Medicine, 24,* 100–105.

Kiernan, B., Dane, J., Phillips, L., & Price, D. (1995). Hypnotic analgesia reduces R-III nociceptive reflex: Further evidence concerning the multifactorial nature of hypnotic analgesia. *Pain, 60,* 39–47.

Kihlstrom, J. F. (1992). Hypnosis: A sesquicentennial essay. *International Journal of Clinical and Experimental Hypnosis, 50,* 301–314.

Kihlstrom, J. F. (2008). The domain of hypnosis, revisited. In M. R. Nash & A. J. Barnier (Eds.), *The Oxford handbook of hypnosis: Theory, research, and practice* (pp. 21–52). New York, NY: Oxford University Press.

Killeen, P. R., & Nash, M. R. (2003). The four causes of hypnosis. *International Journal of Clinical and Experimental Hypnosis, 51,* 195–231.

Kirsch, I. (1996). Hypnotic enhancement of cognitive–behavioral weight loss treatments: Another meta-reanalysis. *Journal of Consulting and Clinical Psychology, 64,* 517–519.

Kirsch, I., & Lynn, S. J. (1995). The altered state of hypnosis. *American Psychologist, 50,* 846–858.

Kirsch, I., Montgomery, G., & Sapirstein, G. (1995). Hypnosis as an adjunct to cognitive–behavioral psychotherapy: A meta-analysis. *Journal of Consulting and Clinical Psychology, 63,* 214–220.

Knox, V. J., Morgan, A. H., & Hilgard, E. R. (1974). Pain and suffering in ischemia: The paradox of hypnotically suggested anesthesia as contradicted by reports from the "hidden observer." *Archives of General Psychiatry, 30,* 840–847.

Kosambi, D. D. (1967). Living prehistory in India. *Scientific American, 216,* 105.

Kozarek, R. K., Raltz, S. L., Neal, L., Wilbur, P., Stewart, S., & Ragsdale, J. (1997). Prospective trial using Virtual Vision as a distraction technique in patients undergoing gastric laboratory procedures. *Gastroenterology Nursing, 20,* 12–14.

Kristenson, H., Ohlin, H., Hulten-Nosslin, M. B., Trell, E., & Hood, B. (1983). Identification and intervention of heavy drinking in middle-aged men: Results and follow-up of 24–60 months of long-term study with randomized controls. *Alcoholism: Clinical and Experimental Research, 7,* 203–209.

Kroeber, A. L. (1948). *Anthropology.* New York, NY: Harcourt.

Kübler-Ross, E. (1969). *On death and dying.* New York, NY: Macmillan.

Kuttner, L. (1988). Favorite stories: A hypnotic pain-reduction technique for children in acute pain. *American Journal of Clinical Hypnosis, 30,* 289–295.

Lambert, S. (1996). The effects of hypnosis/guided imagery on the postoperative course of children. *Developmental and Behavioral Pediatrics, 17,* 307–310.

Lang, E. V. (in press). Procedural hypnosis. In A. Barabasz, K. Olness, R. Boland, & S. Kahn (Eds.), *Evidence based medical hypnosis: A primer for health care practitioners.* New York, NY: Routledge.

Lang, E. V., Benotsch, E. G., Fick, L. J., Lutgendorf, S., Berbaum, M. L., Berbaum, K. S., . . . Spiegel, D. (2000). Adjunctive non-pharmacological analgesia for invasive medical procedures: A randomised trial. *Lancet, 355,* 1486–1490.

Lang, E. V., Berbaum, K. S., Faintuch, S., Hatsiopoulou, O., Halsey, N., Li, X., . . . Baum, J. (2006). Adjunctive self-hypnotic relaxation for outpatient medical procedures: A prospective randomized trial with women undergoing large core breast biopsy. *Pain, 126,* 155–164.

Lang, E. V., Berbaum, K. S., Pauker, S. G., Faintuch, S., Salazar, G. M., Lutgendorf, S., . . . Spiegel, D. (2008). Beneficial effects of hypnosis and adverse effects of empathic attention during percutaneous tumor treatment: When being nice does not suffice. *Journal of Vascular and Interventional Radiology, 19,* 897–905.

Lang, E. V., Joyce, J. S., Spiegel, D., Hamilton, D., & Lee, K. K. (1996). Self-hypnotic relaxation during interventional radiological procedures: Effects on pain perception and intravenous drug use. *International Journal of Clinical and Experimental Hypnosis, 44,* 106–119.

Lang, E. V., & Rosen, M. (2002). Cost analysis of adjunct hypnosis with sedation during outpatient interventional radiologic procedures. *Radiology, 222,* 375–382.

Lankton, S. (2008). An Ericksonian approach to clinical hypnosis. In M. R. Nash & A. J. Barnier (Eds.), *The Oxford handbook of hypnosis: Theory, research and practice* (pp. 467–486). New York, NY: Oxford University Press.

Lazaro, C., Bosch, F., Torrubia, R., & Banos, J. E. (1994). The development of a Spanish Questionnaire for assessing pain: Preliminary data concerning reliability and validity. *European Journal of Psychological Assessment, 10,* 145–151.

Leeuw, M., Goossens, M. E., van Breukelen, G. J., de Jong, J. R., Heuts, P. H., Smeets, R. J., . . . Vlaeyen, J. W. (2008). Exposure in vivo versus operant graded activity in chronic low back pain patients: Results of a randomized controlled trial. *Pain, 138,* 192–207.

Lenox, J. R. (1970). Effect of hypnotic analgesia on verbal report and cardiovascular responses to ischemic pain. *Journal of Abnormal Psychology, 75,* 199–206.

Lichstein, K. L. (1988). *Clinical relaxation therapies.* New York, NY: Wiley.

Linehan, M. (1993). *Cognitive–behavioral treatment of borderline personality disorder.* New York, NY: Guilford Press.

Linton, S. J., Boersma, K., Jansson, M., Overmeer, T., Lindblom, K., & Vlaeyen, J. W. (2008). A randomized controlled trial of exposure in vivo for patients with spinal pain reporting fear of work-related activities. *European Journal of Pain, 12,* 722–730.

Liossi, C., & Hatira, P. (1999). Clinical hypnosis versus cognitive behavioral training for pain management with pediatric cancer patients undergoing bone marrow aspirations. *International Journal of Clinical and Experimental Hypnosis, 47,* 104–116.

Liossi, C., White, P., & Hatira, P. (2009). A randomized clinical trial of a brief hypnosis intervention to control venepuncture-related pain of paediatric cancer patients. *Pain, 142,* 255–263.

Loeser, J. D. (1980). Perspectives on pain. In P. Turner (Ed.), *Clinical pharmacology and therapeutics* (pp. 313–316). London, England: Macmillan

Loeser, J. D. (Ed.). (2001a). *Bonica's management of pain* (3rd ed.). Philadelphia, PA: Lippincott, Williams & Wilkins.

Loeser, J. D. (2001b). Evaluation of the pain patient. In J. D. Loeser (Ed.), *Bonica's management of pain* (3rd ed.). Philadelphia, PA: Lippincott, Williams & Wilkins.

Lopez-Martinez, A. E., Esteve-Zarazaga, R., & Ramirez-Maestre, C. (2008). Perceived social support and coping responses are independent variables explaining pain adjustment among chronic pain patients. *Journal of Pain, 9,* 373–379.

Ludwig, D. S., & Kabat-Zinn, J. (2008). Mindfulness in medicine. *Journal of the American Medical Association, 300,* 1350–1352.

Luthe, W. (Ed.). (1969–1973). *Autogenic therapy* (6 vols.). New York, NY: Grune & Stratton.

Lynn, S. J., Kirsch, I., & Hallquist, M. N. (2008). Social cognitive theories of hypnosis. In M. R. Nash & A. J. Barnier (Eds.), *The Oxford handbook of hypnosis: Theory, research and practice* (pp. 111–140). New York, NY: Oxford University Press.

Lynn, S. J., & Rhue, J. W. (1991). *Theories of hypnosis: Current models and perspectives.* New York, NY: Guilford Press.

Mackersie, R. C., & Karagianes, T. G. (1990). Pain management following trauma and burns. *Anesthesiology Clinics of North America, 7,* 433–449.

Maher-Loughnan, G. P., Mason, A. A., Macdonald, N., & Fry, L. (1962). Controlled trial of hypnosis in the symptomatic treatment of asthma. *British Medical Journal, 2,* 371–376.

Malone, M. D., & Strube, M. J. (1988). Meta-analysis of non-medical treatments for chronic pain. *Pain, 34,* 231–244.

Marc, I., Rainville, P., Masse, B., Verreault, R., Vaillancourt, L., Vallee, E., & Dodin, S. (2008). Hypnotic analgesia intervention during first-trimester pregnancy termination: An open randomized trial. *American Journal of Obstetrics and Gynecology, 199,* 461–469.

Marcus, B. H., Rossi, J. S., Selby, V. C., Niaura, R. S., & Abrams, D. B. (1992). The stages and processes of exercise adoption and maintenance in a worksite sample. *Health Psychology, 11,* 386–395.

Martin-Herz, S. P., Patterson, D. R., Ptacek, J. T., Finch, C. P., & Heimbach, D. M. (1998, March). *Impact of inpatient pain on long term adjustment in adult burn patients: An update.* Paper presented at the meeting of the American Burn Association, Chicago, IL.

Mauer, M. H., Burnett, K. F., Ouellette, E. A., Ironson, G. H., & Dandes, H. M. (1999). Medical hypnosis and orthopedic hand surgery: Pain perception, postoperative recovery, and therapeutic comfort. *International Journal of Clinical and Experimental Hypnosis, 47,* 144–161.

McCarthy, P. (2001). Hypnosis in obstetrics and gynecology. In L. E. Fredericks (Ed.), *The use of hypnosis in surgery and anesthesiology* (pp. 163–211). Springfield, IL: Charles C Thomas.

McCauley, J. D., Thelen, M. H., Frank, R. G., Willard, R. R., & Callen, K. E. (1983). Hypnosis compared to relaxation in the outpatient management of chronic low back pain. *Archives of Physical Medicine and Rehabilitation, 64,* 548–552.

McCracken, L. M., Carson, J. W., Eccleston, C., & Keefe, F. J. (2004). Acceptance and change in the context of chronic pain. *Pain, 109,* 4–7.

McCracken, L. M., & Eccleston, C. (2003). Coping or acceptance: What to do about chronic pain? *Pain, 105,* 197–204.

McCracken, L. M., & Eccleston, C. (2005). A prospective study of acceptance of pain and patient functioning with chronic pain. *Pain, 118,* 164–169.

McCracken, L. M., Vowles, K. E., & Eccleston, C. (2004). Acceptance of chronic pain: Component analysis and a revised assessment method. *Pain, 107,* 159–166.

McGlashan, T. H., Evans, F. J., & Orne, M. T. (1969). The nature of hypnotic analgesia and placebo response to experimental pain. *Psychosomatic Medicine, 31,* 227–246.

McKibben, J. B., Bresnick, M. G., Wiechman Askay, S. A., & Fauerbach, J. A. (2008). Acute stress disorder and posttraumatic stress disorder: A prospective study of prevalence, course, and predictors in a sample with major burn injuries. *Journal of Burn Care Research, 29,* 22–35.

McMain, S., Korman, L. M., & Dimeff, L. (2001). Dialectical behavior therapy and the treatment of emotion dysregulation. *Journal of Clinical Psychology, 57,* 183–196.

Meier, W., Klucken, M., Soyka, D., & Bromm, B. (1993). Hypnotic hypo- and hyperalgesia: Divergent effects on pain ratings and pain-related cerebral potentials. *Pain, 53,* 175–181.

Melis, P. M., Rooimans, W., Spierings, E. L., & Hoogduin, C. A. (1991). Treatment of chronic tension-type headache with hypnotherapy: A single-blind time controlled study. *Headache, 31,* 686–689.

Melzack, R. (1973). *The puzzle of pain.* New York, NY: Basic Books.

Melzack, R. (1975). The McGill Pain Questionnaire: Major properties and scoring methods. *Pain, 1,* 277–299.

Melzack, R. (1990, February). The tragedy of needless pain. *Scientific American, 262,* 27–33.

Melzack, R. (1999). From the gate to the neuromatrix. *Pain, 6,* 121–126.

Melzack, R., & Perry, C. (1975). Self-regulation of pain: The use of alpha-feedback and hypnotic training for the control of chronic pain. *Experimental Neurology, 46,* 452–469.

Melzack, R., & Wall, P. D. (1965, November). Pain mechanisms: A new theory. *Science, 150,* 971–979.

Melzack, R., & Wall, P. D. (1973). *The challenge of pain.* New York, NY: Basic Books.

Meszaros, I., Banyai, E. I., & Greguss, A. C. (1980). Evoked potential, reflecting hypnotically altered state of consciousness. In G. Adam, I. Meszaros & E. I. Banyai (Eds.), *Advances in physiological sciences: Vol. 17. Brain behavior* (pp. 467–475). Oxford, England: Pergamon.

Miller, A. C., Hickman, L. C., & Lemasters, G. K. (1992). A distraction technique for control of burn pain. *Journal of Burn Care Rehabilitation, 13,* 576–580.

Miller, M. F., Barabasz, A. F., & Barabasz, M. (1991). Effects of active alert and relaxation hypnotic inductions on cold pressor pain. *Journal of Abnormal Psychology, 100,* 223–226.

Miller, W. R. (1983). Motivational interviewing with problem drinkers. *Behavioural Psychotherapy, 11,* 147–172.

Miller, W. R., Benefield, R., & Tonigan, S. (1993). Enhancing motivation in problem drinking: A controlled comparison of two therapist styles. *Journal of Consulting and Clinical Psychology, 61,* 455–461.

Miller, W. R., & Munoz, R. F. (2005). *Controlling your drinking: Tools to make moderation work for you.* New York, NY: Guilford Press.

Miller, W. R., & Rollnick, S. (1991). *Motivational interviewing: Preparing people to change addictive behavior.* New York, NY: Guilford Press.

Miller, W. R., & Rollnick, S. (2002). *Motivational interviewing: Preparing people for change* (2nd ed.). New York, NY: Guilford Press.

Miller, W. R., & Rollnick, S. (2009). Ten things that motivational interviewing is not. *Behavioural and Cognitive Psychotherapy, 37,* 129–140.

Miller, W. R., & Sovereign, R. G. (1989). Check-up: A model for early intervention in addictive behaviors. In T. Loberg, M. R. Miller, P. E. Nathan, & G. A. Marlatt (Eds.), *Addictive behaviors: Prevention and early intervention* (pp. 219–231). Amsterdam, the Netherlands: Swets & Zeitlinger.

Milling, L. S. (2008). Is high hypnotic suggestibility necessary for successful hypnotic pain intervention? *Current Pain and Headache Reports, 12,* 98–102.

Milling, L. S., Shores, J. S., Coursen, E. L., Menario, D. J., & Farris, C. D. (2007). Response expectancies, treatment credibility, and hypnotic suggestibility: Mediator and moderator effects in hypnotic and cognitive–behavioral pain interventions. *Annals of Behavioral Medicine, 33,* 167–178.

Molton, I. R., Jensen, M. P., Nielson, W., Cardenas, D., & Ehde, D. M. (2008). A preliminary evaluation of the motivational model of pain self-management in persons with spinal cord injury related pain. *Journal of Pain, 9,* 606–612.

Montgomery, G. H., Bovbjerg, D. H., Schnur, J. B., David, D., Goldfarb, A., Weltz, C. R., . . . Silverstein, J. H. (2007). A randomized clinical trial of a brief hypnosis intervention to control side effects in breast surgery patients. *Journal of National Cancer Institute, 99,* 1304–1312.

Montgomery, G. H., David, D., Winkel, G., Silverstein, J. H., & Bovbjerg, D. H. (2002). The effectiveness of adjunctive hypnosis with surgical patients: A meta-analysis. *Anesthesia and Analgesia, 94,* 1639–1645.

Montgomery, G. H., DuHamel, K. N., & Redd, W. H. (2000). A meta-analysis of hypnotically induced analgesia: How effective is hypnosis? *International Journal of Clinical and Experimental Hypnosis, 48,* 138–153.

Montgomery, G. H., Hallquist, M. N., Schnur, J. B., David, D., Silverstein, J. H., & Bovbjerg, D. H. (in press). Mediators of a brief hypnosis intervention to control side effects in breast surgery patients: Response expectancies and emotional distress. *Journal of Consulting and Clinical Psychology.*

Morgan, A. H., & Hilgard, J. (1978/1979). The Stanford Hypnotic Clinical Scale for Adults. *American Journal of Clinical Hypnosis, 21,* 134–147.

Morgan, A. H., Johnson, D. L., & Hilgard, E. R. (1974). The stability of hypnotic susceptibility: A longitudinal study. *International Journal of Clinical and Experimental Hypnosis, 22,* 249–257.

Moya, F., & James, L. S. (1960). Medical hypnosis for obstetrics. *Journal of the American Medical Association, 174,* 80–86.

Moyers, T. B., Manuel, J. K., Wilson, P. G., Hendrickson, S. M., Talcott, W., & Durand, P. (2008). A randomized trial investigating training in motivational interviewing for behavioral health providers. *Behavioural and Cognitive Psychotherapy, 36,* 149–162.

Moyers, T. B., & Martin, T. (2006). A conceptual framework for transferring research into practice. *Journal of Substance Abuse Treatment, 30,* 245–251.

Moyers, T. B., Martin, T., Christopher, P. J., Houck, J. M., Tonigan, J. S., & Amrhein, P. C. (2007). Client language as a mediator of motivational interviewing efficacy: Where is the evidence? *Alcoholism: Clinical and Experimental Research, 31*(Suppl.), 40s–47s.

Moyers, T. B., Martin, T., Manuel, J. K., & Miller, W. R. (2004). *Motivational Interviewing Treatment Integrity (MITI) coding system.* Retrieved from http://casaa-0031. unm/edu

Nash, M. R. (2001, July). The truth and the hype of hypnosis. *Scientific American, 285,* 46–49, 52–45.

Nash, M. R., & Barnier, A. J. (Eds.). (2008). *The Oxford handbook of hypnosis: Theory, research and practice.* New York, NY: Oxford University Press.

Neron, S., & Stephenson, R. (2007). Effectiveness of hypnotherapy with cancer patients' trajectory: Emesis, acute pain, and analgesia and anxiolysis in procedures. *International Journal of Clinical and Experimental Hypnosis, 55,* 336–354.

Ohrbach, R., Patterson, D. R., Carrougher, G., & Gibran, N. (1998). Hypnosis after an adverse response to opioids in an ICU burn patient. *Clinical Journal of Pain, 14,* 167–175.

Olness, K., & Kohen, D. P. (1996). *Hypnosis and hypnotherapy with children.* New York, NY: Guilford Press.

Oneal, B. J., Patterson, D. R., Soltani, M., Teeley, A., & Jensen, M. P. (2008). Virtual reality hypnosis in the treatment of chronic neuropathic pain: A case report. *International Journal of Clinical and Experimental Hypnosis, 56,* 451–462.

Palsson, O. S., Turner, M. J., Johnson, D. A., Burnelt, C. K., & Whitehead, W. E. (2002). Hypnosis treatment for severe irritable bowel syndrome: Investigation of mechanism and effects on symptoms. *Digestive Diseases and Sciences, 47,* 2605–2614.

Patterson, D. R. (1992). Practical applications of psychological techniques in controlling burn pain. *Journal of Burn Care and Rehabilitation, 13,* 13–18.

Patterson, D. R. (1996). Burn pain. In J. Barber (Ed.), *Hypnosis and suggestion in the treatment of pain* (pp. 267–302). New York, NY: Norton.

Patterson, D. R. (2001). Is hypnotic pain control effortless or effortful? *Hypnos, 28,* 132–134.

Patterson, D. R. (2004). Treating pain with hypnosis. *Current Directions in Psychological Science, 13,* 252–255.

Patterson, D. R. (2005). Behavioral methods for chronic pain and illness: A reconsideration and appreciation. *Rehabilitation Psychology, 50,* 312–315.

Patterson, D. R. (2009). Acute pain. In A. F. Barabasz, K. Olness, R. Boland, & S. Kahn (Eds.), *Medical hypnosis primer: Clinical and research evidence* (pp. 17–22). New York, NY: Routledge.

Patterson, D. R., Adcock, R. J., & Bombardier, C. H. (1997). Factors predicting hypnotic analgesia in clinical burn pain. *International Journal of Clinical and Experimental Hypnosis, 45,* 377–395.

Patterson D. R., Ehde, D. M., & Ptacek, J. T. (1994). Nonpharmacologic therapy for anxiety in the critical care setting. In R. C. Bone (Ed.), *Recognition, assessment and treatment of anxiety in the critical care patient: Proceedings of a consensus conference.* Yardley, PA: The Medicine Group.

Patterson, D. R., Everett, J. J., Bombardier, C. H., Questad, K. A., Lee, V. K., & Marvin, J. A. (1993). Psychological effects of severe burn injuries. *Psychological Bulletin, 113,* 362–378.

Patterson, D. R., Everett, J. J., Burns, G. L., & Marvin, J. A. (1992). Hypnosis for the treatment of burn pain. *Journal of Consulting and Clinical Psychology, 60,* 713–717.

Patterson, D. R., Hoffman, H. G., Palacios, A. G., & Jensen, M. J. (2006). Analgesic effects of posthypnotic suggestions and virtual reality distraction on thermal pain. *Journal of Abnormal Psychology, 115,* 834–841.

Patterson, D. R., & Jensen, M. (2003). Hypnosis and clinical pain. *Psychological Bulletin, 129*, 495–521.

Patterson, D. R., Jensen, M. P., Wiechman Askay, S. A., & Sharar, S. R. (in press). Virtual reality hypnosis for pain associated with recovery from physical trauma. *International Journal of Clinical and Experimental Hypnosis*.

Patterson, D. R., Miller-Perrin, C., McCormick, T. R., & Hudson, L. D. (1993). When life support is questioned early in the care of patients with cervical-level quadriplegia. *New England Journal of Medicine, 328*, 506–509.

Patterson, D. R., & Ptacek, J. T. (1997). Baseline pain as a moderator of hypnotic analgesia for burn injury treatment. *Journal of Consulting and Clinical Psychology, 65*, 60–67.

Patterson, D. R., Ptacek, J. T., Carrougher, G. J., & Sharar, S. (1997). Lorazepam as an adjunct to opioid analgesics in the treatment of burn pain. *Pain, 72*, 367–374.

Patterson, D. R., Ptacek, J. T., & Esselman, P. C. (1997). Management of suffering in patients with severe burn injury. *Western Journal of Medicine, 166*, 272–273.

Patterson, D. R., Questad, K. A., & Boltwood, M. D. (1987). Hypnotherapy as a treatment for pain in patients with burns: Research and clinical considerations. *Journal of Burn Care and Rehabilitation, 8*, 263–268.

Patterson, D. R., Questad, K. A., & DeLateur, B. J. (1989). Hypnotherapy as an adjunct to pharmacologies for the treatment of pain from burn debridement. *American Journal of Clinical Hypnosis, 31*, 156–163.

Patterson, D. R., & Sechrest, L. B. (1983). Non-reactive measures in psychotherapy outcome research. *Clinical Psychological Review, 3*, 391–416.

Patterson, D. R., & Sharar, S. R. (1997). Treating pain from severe burn injuries. *Advances in Medical Psychotherapy, 9*, 55–71.

Patterson, D. R., & Sharar, S. (2001). Burn pain. In J. Loeser (Ed.), *Bonica's management of pain* (3rd ed., pp. 780–787). Philadelphia, PA: Lippincott, Williams & Wilkins.

Patterson, D. R., Tininenko, J. R., Schmidt, A. E., & Sharar, S. (2004). Virtual reality hypnosis: A case report. *International Journal of Clinical and Experimental Hypnosis, 52*, 27–38.

Patterson, D. R., Wiechman, S. A., Jensen, M., & Sharar, S. R. (2006). Hypnosis delivered through immersive virtual reality for burn pain: A clinical case series. *International Journal of Clinical and Experimental Hypnosis, 54*, 130–142.

Piccione, C., Hilgard, E. R., & Zimbardo, P. G. (1989). On the degree of stability of measured hypnotizability over a 25-year period. *Journal of Personality and Social Psychology, 56*, 289–295.

Pincus, D., & Sheikh, A. A. (2009). *Imagery for pain relief: A scientifically grounded guidebook for clinicians*. New York, NY: Routledge.

Price, D. D., & Barber, J. (1987). An analysis of factors that contribute to the efficacy of hypnotic analgesia. *Journal of Abnormal Psychology, 96*, 46–51.

Price, D. D., & Barrell, J. J. (2000). Mechanisms of analgesia produced by hypnosis and placebo suggestions. In E. A. Mayer & C. B. Saper (Eds.), *Progress in brain research* (Vol. 122, pp. 255–271). New York, NY: Elsevier Science.

Price, D. D., & Bushnell, M. C. (Eds.). (2004). *Psychological methods of pain control: Basic science and clinical perspectives* (Vol. 29). Seattle, WA: IASP Press.

Price, D. D., Harkins, S. W., & Baker, C. (1987). Sensory–affective relationships among different types of clinical and experimental pain. *Pain, 28,* 297–307.

Prochaska, J. O., & DiClemente, C. C. (1982). Transtheoretical therapy: Toward a more integrative model of change. *Psychotherapy: Theory, Research, and Practice, 19,* 276–288.

Prochaska, J. O., & DiClemente, C. C. (1983). Stages and process of self-change of smoking: Toward an integrative model of change. *Journal of Consulting and Clinical Psychology, 51,* 390–395.

Prochaska, J. O., Velicer, W. F., Rossi, J. S., Goldstein, M. G., Marcus, B. H., Rakowski, W., . . . Rosenbloom, D. (1994). Stages of change and decisional balance for 12 problem behaviors. *Health Psychology, 13,* 39–46.

Prothero, J. D., & Hoffman, H. G. (1995). *Widening the field-of-view increases the sense of presence in immersive virtual environments* (Technical Report No. TR-95-2). Retrieved from http://www.hitl.washington.edu/publications/r-95-5/

Ptacek, J. T., Patterson, D. R., Montgomery, B. K., Ordonez, N. A., & Heimbach, D. M. (1995). Pain, coping, and adjustment in patients with severe burns: Preliminary findings from a prospective study. *Journal of Pain and Symptom Management, 10,* 446–455.

Rainville, P. (2004). Pain and emotions. In D. D. Price & M. C. Bushnell (Eds.), *Psychological methods of pain control: Basic science and clinical perspectives.* Seattle, WA: IASP Press.

Rainville, P., Carrier, B., Hofbauer, R. K., Bushnell, M. C., & Duncan, G. H. (1999). Dissociation of sensory and affective dimensions of pain using hypnotic modulation. *Pain, 82,* 159–171.

Rainville, P., Duncan, G. H., Price, D. D., Carrier, B., & Bushnell, M. C. (1997, August 15). Pain affect encoded in human anterior cingulate but not somatosensory cortex. *Science, 277,* 968–971.

Rainville, P., Hofbauer, R. K., Paus, T., Duncan, G. H., Bushnell, M. C., & Price, D. D. (1999). Cerebral mechanisms of hypnotic induction and suggestion. *Journal of Cognitive Neuroscience, 11,* 110–125.

Rainville, P., & Price, D. D. (2004). The neurophenomenology of hypnosis and hypnotic analgesia. In D. D. Price & M. C. Bushnell (Eds.), *Psychological methods of pain control: Basic science and clinical perspectives* (Vol. 29, pp. 235–267). Seattle, WA: IASP Press.

Rausch, V. (1980). Cholecystectomy with self-hypnosis. *American Journal of Clinical Hypnosis, 22,* 124–129.

Ray, W. J., & Tucker, D. M. (2003). Evolutionary approaches to understanding the hypnotic experience. *International Journal of Clinical and Experimental Hypnosis, 51*, 256–281.

Raz, A. (2005). Attention and hypnosis: Neural substrates and genetic associations of two converging processes. *International Journal of Clinical and Experimental Hypnosis, 53*, 237–258.

Raz, A. (2008). Genetics and neuroimaging of attention and hypnotizability may elucidate placebo. *International Journal of Clinical and Experimental Hypnosis, 56*, 99–116.

Raz, A., Fan, J., & Posner, M. I. (2005). Hypnotic suggestion reduces conflict in the human brain. *Proceedings of the National Academy of Sciences USA, 102*, 9978–9983.

Raz, A., Lamar, M., Buhle, J. T., Kane, M. J., & Peterson, B. S. (2007). Selective biasing of a specific bistable-figure percept involves fMRI signal changes in frontostriatal circuits: A step toward unlocking the neural correlates of top-down control and self-regulation. *American Journal of Clinical Hypnosis, 50*, 137–156.

Raz, A., & Shapiro, T. (2002). Hypnosis and neuroscience: A cross talk between clinical and cognitive research. *Archives of General Psychiatry, 59*, 85–90.

Richardson, A. (1969). *Mental imagery*. London, England: Routledge & Kegan Paul.

Richardson, J., Smith, J. E., McCall, G., & Pilkington, K. (2006). Hypnosis for procedure-related pain and distress in pediatric cancer patients: A systematic review of effectiveness and methodology related to hypnosis interventions. *Journal of Pain and Symptom Management, 31*, 70–84.

Roberts, L., Wilson, S., Singh, S., Roalfe, A., & Greenfield, S. (2006). Gut-directed hypnotherapy for irritable bowel syndrome: Piloting a primary care-based randomised controlled trial. *British Journal of General Practice, 56*, 115–121.

Rogers, C. R. (1957). The necessary and sufficient conditions of therapeutic personality change. *Journal of Consulting Psychology, 21*, 95–103.

Rogers, C. R. (1961). *On becoming a person: A therapist's view of psychotherapy*. Boston, MA: Houghton Mifflin.

Rollnick, S., Miller, M. R., & Butler, C. (2008). *Motivational interviewing in health care: Helping patients change behavior*. New York, NY: Guilford Press.

Romano, J. M., & Turner, J. A. (1985). Chronic pain and depression: Does the evidence support a relationship? *Psychological Bulletin, 97*, 18–34.

Rosengren, D. B. (2009). *Building motivational interviewing skills: A practitioner workbook*. New York, NY: Guilford Press.

Rossi, E. L. (Ed.). (1980). *The collected papers of Milton H. Erickson on hypnosis: Vol. IV. Innovative hypnotherapy*. New York, NY: Irvington.

Saadat, H., Drummond-Lewis, J., Maranets, I., Kaplan, D., Saadat, A., Wang, S. M., & Kain, Z. N. (2006). Hypnosis reduces preoperative anxiety in adult patients. *Anesthesia and Analgesia, 102*, 1394–1396.

Sacerdote, P. (1978). Teaching self-hypnosis to patients with chronic pain. *Journal of Human Stress, 4*(2), 18–21.

Sanders, S. H. (1996). Operant conditioning with chronic pain: Back to basics. In R. J. Gatchel & D. C. Turk (Eds.), *Psychological approaches to pain management: A practitioner's handbook* (pp. 112–130). New York, NY: Guilford Press.

Saxe, G., Stoddard, F., Courtney, D., Cunningham, K., Chawla, N., Sheridan, R., . . . King, L. (2001). Relationship between acute morphine and the course of PTSD in children with burns. *Journal of the American Academy of Child and Adolescent Psychiatry, 40,* 915–921.

Schlutter, L. C., Golden, C. J., & Blume, H. G. (1980). A comparison of treatments for prefrontal muscle contraction headache. *British Journal of Medical Psychology, 53,* 47–52.

Schneider, J. C., Holavanahalli, R., Helm, P., Goldstein, R., & Kowalske, K. (2006). Contractures in burn injury: Defining the problem. *Journal of Burn Care Research, 27,* 508–514.

Schnur, J. B., Bovbjerg, D. H., David, D., Tatrow, K., Goldfarb, A. B., Silverstein, J. H., . . . Montgomery, G. H. (2008). Hypnosis decreases presurgical distress in excisional breast biopsy patients. *Anesthesia and Analgesia, 106,* 440–444.

Schwartz, L., Jensen, M. P., & Romano, J. M. (2005). The development and psychometric evaluation of an instrument to assess spouse responses to pain and well behavior in patients with chronic pain: The Spouse Response Inventory. *Journal of Pain, 6,* 243–252.

Scott, E. L., Lagges, A., & LaClave, L. (2008). Treating children using hypnosis. In M. R. Nash & A. J. Barnier (Eds.), *The Oxford handbook of hypnosis: Theory, research and practice* (pp. 593–610). New York, NY: Oxford University Press.

Shakibaei, F., Harandi, A. A., Gholamrezaei, A., Samoei, R., & Salehi, P. (2008). Hypnotherapy in management of pain and reexperiencing of trauma in burn patients. *International Journal of Clinical and Experimental Hypnosis, 56,* 185–197.

Shapiro, S. L., & Carlson, L. E. (2009). *The art and science of mindfulness: Integrating mindfulness into psychology and the helping professions.* Washington, DC: American Psychological Association.

Shapiro, S. L., Oman, D., Thoresen, C., Plante, T., & Flinders, T. (2008). Cultivating mindfulness: Effects on well-being. *Journal of Clinical Psychology, 64:* 840–862.

Sharar, S., Patterson, D. R., & Wiechman Askay, S. A. (2007). Burn pain. In S. D. Waldman (Ed.), *Pain management* (Vol. 1, pp. 240–256). Philadelphia, PA: Saunders Elsevier.

Sharav, Y., & Tal, M. (1989). Masseter inhibitory periods and sensations evoked by electrical tooth-pulp stimulation in subjects under hypnotic anesthesia. *Brain Research, 479,* 247–254.

Sharav, Y., & Tal, M. (2006). Focused hypnotic analgesia: Local and remote effects. *Pain, 124,* 280–286.

Sherman, S. J., & Lynn, S. J. (1990). Social-psychological principles in Milton Erickson's psychotherapy. *British Journal of Experimental and Clinical Hypnosis, 7,* 37–46.

Shor, R. E. (1962). Physiological effects of painful stimulation during hypnotic analgesia under conditions designed to minimize anxiety. *International Journal of Clinical and Experimental Hypnosis, 10,* 183–202.

Siegel, E. F. (1979). Control of phantom limb pain by hypnosis. *American Journal of Clinical Hypnosis, 21,* 285–286.

Simon, E. P., & Lewis, D. M. (2000). Medical hypnosis for temporomandibular disorders: Treatment efficacy and medical utilization outcome. *Oral Surgery, Oral Medicine, Oral Pathology, Oral Radiology, and Endodontics, 90,* 54–63.

Simren, M., Ringstrom, G., Bjornsson, E. S., & Abrahamsson, H. (2004). Treatment with hypnotherapy reduces the sensory and motor component of the gastrocolonic response in irritable bowel syndrome. *Psychosomatic Medicine, 66,* 233–238.

Slack, D., Nelson, L., Patterson, D., Burns, S., Hakimi, K., & Robinson, L. (2009). The feasibility of hypnotic analgesia in ameliorating pain and anxiety among adults undergoing needle electromyography. *American Journal of Physical Medicine & Rehabilitation, 88,* 21–29.

Slater, M., & Wilbur, S. (1997). A framework for immersive virtual environments (FIVE): Speculations on the role of presence in virtual environments. *Presence: Teleoperators and Virtual Environments, 6,* 603–616.

Slifer, K. J. (1996). A video system to help children cooperate with motion control for radiation treatment without sedation. *Journal of Pediatric Oncology Nursing, 13,* 91–97.

Smith, G., & Covino, B. G. (1985). *Acute pain.* London, England: Butterworth.

Smith, J. T., Barabasz, A., & Barabasz, M. (1996). Comparison of hypnosis and distraction in severely ill children undergoing painful medical procedures. *Journal of Counseling Psychology, 42,* 187–195.

Smith, S. J., & Balaban, A. B. (1983). A multidimensional approach to pain relief: Case report of a patient with systemic lupus erythematosus. *International Journal of Clinical and Experimental Hypnosis, 31,* 72–81.

Smith, S. M., & Blankenship, S. E. (1991). Incubation and the persistence of fixation in problem solving. *American Journal of Psychology, 104,* 61–87.

Spanos, N. P., & Chaves, J. F. (1989a). The cognitive–behavioral alternative in hypnosis research. In N. P. Spanos & J. F. Chaves (Eds.), *Hypnosis: The cognitive–behavioral perspective* (pp. 9–16). Buffalo, NY: Prometheus Books.

Spanos, N. P., & Chaves, J. F. (1989b). Future prospects for the cognitive–behavioral perspective. In N. P. Spanos & J. F. Chaves (Eds.), *Hypnosis: The cognitive–behavioral perspective* (pp. 437–446). Buffalo, NY: Prometheus Books.

Spanos, N. P., & Chaves, J. F. (1989c). Hypnotic analgesia, surgery and reports of nonvolitional pain reduction. *British Journal of Experimental and Clinical Hypnosis, 6,* 131–139.

Spiegel, D., Bierre, P., & Rootenberg, J. (1989). Hypnotic alteration of somatosensory perception. *American Journal of Psychiatry, 146,* 749–754.

Spiegel, D., & Bloom, J. R. (1983). Group therapy and hypnosis reduce metastatic breast carcinoma pain. *Psychosomatic Medicine, 45,* 333–339.

Spiegel, H., & Bridger, A. A. (1970). *Manual for hypnotic induction profile: Eye-roll levitation method.* New York, NY: Soni Medica.

Spiegel, H., & Spiegel, D. (1978). *Trance and treatment.* Washington, DC: American Psychiatric Press.

Spinhoven, P. (1988). Similarities and dissimilarities in hypnotic and nonhypnotic procedures for headache control: A review. *American Journal of Clinical Hypnosis, 30,* 183–194.

Spinhoven, P., & Linssen, A. C. (1989). Education and self-hypnosis in the management of low back pain: A component analysis. *British Journal of Clinical Psychology, 28,* 145–153.

Spinhoven, P., Linssen, A. C., Van Dyck, R., & Zitman, F. G. (1992). Autogenic training and self-hypnosis in the control of tension headache. *General Hospital Psychiatry, 14,* 408–415.

Stanton, H. (1985). Permissive vs. authoritarian approaches in clinical and experimental settings. In J. K. Zeig (Ed.), *Ericksonian psychotherapy: Vol. 1: Structures* (pp. 293–304). New York, NY: Brunner/Mazel.

Stern, C. R. (1985). There's no theory like no theory: The Ericksonian approach in perspective. In J. K. Zeig (Ed.), *Ericksonian psychotherapy: Vol. 1. Structures.* New York, NY: Brunner/Mazel.

Stern, D. B., Spiegel, H., & Nee, J. C. (1979). The hypnotic induction profile: Normative observations, reliability, and validity. *American Journal of Clinical Hypnosis, 21,* 219–236.

Stoelb, B. L., Molton, I. R., Jensen, M. P., & Patterson, D. R. (2009). The efficacy of hypnotic analgesia in adults: A review of the literature. *Contemporary Hypnosis, 26,* 24–39.

Stowell, H. (1984). Event related brain potentials and human pain: A first objective overview. *International Journal of Psychophysiology, 1,* 137–151.

Sullivan, M. J., & D'Eon, J. L. (1990). Relation between catastrophizing and depression in chronic pain patients. *Journal of Abnormal Psychology, 99,* 260–263.

Sullivan, M. J., Stanish, W., Waite, H., Sullivan, M., & Tripp, D. A. (1998). Catastrophizing, pain, and disability in patients with soft-tissue injuries. *Pain, 77,* 253–260.

Sullivan, M. J., Thorn, B., Haythornthwaite, J., Keefe, F., Martin, M., Bradley, L., & Lefebvre, J. C. (2001). Theoretical perspectives on the relation between catastrophizing and pain. *Clinical Journal of Pain, 17,* 52–64.

Sutcher, H. (1997). Hypnosis as adjunctive therapy for multiple sclerosis: A progress report. *American Journal of Clinical Hypnosis, 39,* 283–290.

Sutcliffe, J. P. (1961). "Credulous" and "skeptical" views of hypnotic phenomena: Experiments in esthesia, hallucination, and delusion. *Journal of Abnormal and Social Psychology, 62,* 189–200.

Syrjala, K. L., Cummings, C., & Donaldson, G. W. (1992). Hypnosis or cognitive behavioral training for the reduction of pain and nausea during cancer treatment: A controlled clinical trial. *Pain, 48,* 137–146.

Taal, L. A., & Faber, A. W. (1997). The Burn Specific Pain Anxiety Scale: Introduction of a reliable and valid measure. *Burns, 23,* 147–150.

Tang, N. K., Wright, K. J., & Salkovskis, P. M. (2007). Prevalence and correlates of clinical insomnia co-occurring with chronic back pain. *Journal of Sleep Research, 16,* 85–95.

ter Kuile, M. M., Spinhoven, P., Linssen, A. C., Zitman, F. G., Van Dyck, R., & Rooijmans, H. G. (1994). Autogenic training and cognitive self-hypnosis for the treatment of recurrent headaches in three different subject groups. *Pain, 58,* 331–340.

Turk, D. C. (1978). Cognitive behavioral techniques in the management of pain. In J. P. Foreyt & C. P. Rathjen (Eds.), *Cognitive behavior therapy* (pp. 199–232). New York, NY: Plenum Press.

Turk, D. C. (1996). Biopsychosocial perspective on chronic pain. In R. J. Gatchel & D. C. Turk (Eds.), *Psychological approaches to pain management: A practitioner's handbook* (pp. 3–32). New York, NY: Guilford Press.

Turk, D. C., & Flor, H. (1999). Chronic pain: A biobehavioral perspective. In R. J. Gatchel & D. C. Turk (Eds.), *Psychosocial factors in pain: Critical perspectives* (pp. 18–34). New York, NY: Guilford Press.

Turk, D. C., & Gatchel, R. J. (1999). Psychosocial factors and pain: Revolution and evolution. In R. J. Gatchel & D. C. Turk (Eds.), *Psychosocial factors in pain: Critical perspectives* (pp. 481–493). New York, NY: Guilford Press.

Turk, D. C., Meichenbaum, D., & Genest, M. (1983). *Pain and behavioral medicine: A cognitive–behavioral perspective.* New York, NY: Guilford Press.

Turk, D. C., & Okifuji, A. (1998a). Interdisciplinary approach to pain management: Philosophy, operations, and efficacy. In M. A. Ashburn & L. J. Rice (Eds.), *The management of pain* (pp. 235–248). Baltimore, MD: Churchill-Livingstone.

Turk, D. C., & Okifuji, A. (1998b). Treatment of chronic pain patients: Clinical outcomes, cost-effectiveness, and cost-benefits of multidisciplinary pain centers. *Critical Reviews in Physical and Rehabilitation Medicine, 10,* 181–208.

Turner, J. A., & Chapman, C. R. (1982). Psychological interventions for chronic pain: A critical review: II. Operant conditioning, hypnosis, and cognitive–behavioral therapy. *Pain, 12,* 23–46.

Turner, J. A., Ersek, M., Herron, L., Haselkorn, J., Kent, D., Ciol, M. A., & Deyo, R. (1992). Patient outcomes after lumbar spinal fusions. *Journal of the American Medical Association, 268,* 907–911.

Turner, J. A., & Jensen, M. P. (1993). Efficacy of cognitive therapy for chronic low back pain. *Pain, 52*, 169–177.

Turner, J. A., & Romano, J. M. (2001). Cognitive–behavioral therapy for chronic pain. In J. D. Loeser, S. H. Butler, C. R. Chapman, & D. C. Turk (Eds.), *Bonica's management of pain* (3rd ed., pp. 1751–1758). Philadelphia, PA: Lippincott Williams & Wilkins.

Viswesvaran, C., & Schmidt, F. L. (1992). A meta-analytic comparison of the effectiveness of smoking cessation methods. *Journal of Applied Psychology, 77*, 554–561.

Vlaeyen, J. W., & Linton, S. J. (2000). Fear-avoidance and its consequences in chronic musculoskeletal pain: A state of the art. *Pain, 85*, 317–332.

Vlaeyen, J. W., Seelen, H. A., Peters, M., de Jong, P., Aretz, E., Beisiegel, E., & Weber, W. E. (1999). Fear of movement/(re)injury and muscular reactivity in chronic low back pain patients: An experimental investigation. *Pain, 82*, 297–304.

Wakeman, J. R., & Kaplan, J. Z. (1978). An experimental study of hypnosis in painful burns. *American Journal of Clinical Hypnosis, 21*, 3–12.

Walters, S. T., Vader, A. M., Harris, T. R., Field, C. A., & Jouriles, E. N. (2009). Dismantling motivational interviewing and feedback for college drinkers: A randomized clinical trial. *Journal of Consulting and Clinical Psychology, 77*, 64–73.

Wark, D. M. (1996). Teaching college students better learning skills using self-hypnosis. *American Journal of Clinical Hypnosis, 38*, 277–287.

Wark, D. M. (2006). Alert hypnosis: A review and case report. *American Journal of Clinical Hypnosis, 48*, 291–300.

Watkins, H. H., & Watkins, J. G. (1997). *Ego states: Theory and therapy:* New York, NY: Norton.

Watkins, J. G., & Barabasz, A. (2008). *Advanced hypnotherapy: Hypnodynamic techniques.* New York, NY: Routledge.

Weinstein, E. J., & Au, P. K. (1991). Use of hypnosis before and during angioplasty. *American Journal of Clinical Hypnosis, 34*, 29–37.

Weinstein, N. D., Rothman, A. J., & Sutton, S. R. (1998). Stage theories of health behavior: Conceptual and methodological issues. *Health Psychology, 17*, 290–299.

Weisenberg, M., Tepper, I., & Schwarzwald, J. (1995). Humor as a cognitive technique for increasing pain tolerance. *Pain, 63*, 207–212.

Weitzenhoffer, A. M., Hilgard, E. R. (1959). *Stanford Hypnotic Susceptibility Scale Forms A and B.* Palo Alto, CA: Consulting Psychologists Press.

Weitzenhoffer, A. M., & Hilgard, E. R. (1962). *Stanford Hypnotic Susceptibility Scale, Form C.* Palo Alto, CA: Consulting Psychologists Press.

Werch, C. E., & DiClemente, C. C. (1994). A multi-component stage model for matching drug prevention strategies and messages to youth stage of use. *Health Education Research, 9*, 37–46.

West, L. J., Niell, K. C., & Hardy, J. D. (1952). Effects of hypnotic suggestion on pain perception and galvanic skin response. *American Medical Association Archives of Neurology and Psychiatry, 68,* 549–569.

Whorwell, P. J., Prior, A., & Colgan, S. M. (1987). Hypnotherapy in severe irritable bowel syndrome: Further experience. *Gut, 28,* 423–425.

Whorwell, P. J., Prior, A., & Faragher, E. B. (1984). Controlled trial of hypnotherapy in the treatment of severe refractory irritable-bowel syndrome. *Lancet, 2,* 1232–1234.

Wiechman Askay, S. A., Bombardier, C. H., & Patterson, D. R. (2009). Effect of acute and chronic alcohol abuse on pain management in a trauma center. *Expert Review of Neurotherapeutics, 9,* 271–277.

Wiechman Askay, S. A., & Patterson, D. R. (2007). Hypnotic analgesia. *Expert Review of Neurotherapeutics, 7,* 1675–1683.

Wiechman Askay, S. A., Patterson, D. R., Jensen, M. P., & Sharar, S. R. (2007). A randomized controlled trial of hypnosis for burn wound care. *Rehabilitation Psychology, 52,* 247–253.

Williams, D. A. (1999). Acute pain (with special emphasis on painful medical procedures). In R. J. Gatchel & D. C. Turk (Eds.), *Psychosocial factors in pain: Critical perspectives* (pp. 151–163). New York, NY: Guilford Press.

Willoughby, F. W., & Edens, J. F. (1996). Construct validity and predictive utility of the Stages of Change Scale for alcoholics. *Journal of Substance Abuse, 8,* 275–291.

Wilson, K. G., Eriksson, M. Y., D'Eon, J. L., Mikail, S. F., & Emery, P. C. (2002). Major depression and insomnia in chronic pain. *Clinical Journal of Pain, 18,* 77–83.

Winocur, E., Gavish, A., Emodi-Perlman, A., Halachmi, M., & Eli, I. (2002). Hypnorelaxation as treatment for myofascial pain disorder: A comparative study. *Oral Surgery, Oral Medicine, Oral Pathology, Oral Radiology, Endodontics, 93,* 429–434.

Woodrow, K. M., Friedman, G. D., Siegelaub, A. B., & Collen, M. F. (1972). Pain tolerance: Differences according to age, sex and race. *Psychosomatic Medicine, 34,* 548–556.

Woody, E. Z., & Sadler, P. (2008). Dissociation theories of hypnosis. In M. R. Nash & A. J. Barnier (Eds.), *The Oxford handbook of hypnosis: Theory, research and practice* (pp. 81–110). New York, NY: Oxford University Press.

Woody, E. Z., & Szechtman, H. (2003). How can brain activity and hypnosis inform each other? *International Journal of Clinical and Experimental Hypnosis, 51,* 232–255.

Wright, B. R., & Drummond, P. D. (2000). Rapid induction analgesia for the alleviation of procedural pain during burn care. *Burns, 26,* 275–282.

Yaniv, I., & Meyer, D. E. (1987). Activation and metacognition of inaccessible stored information: Potential bases for incubation effects in problem solving. *Journal of Experimental Psychology: Learning, Memory, and Cognition, 13,* 187–205.

Yapko, M. (1992). *Hypnosis and the treatment of depressions*. New York, NY: Brunner/Mazel.

Zachariae, R., & Bjerring, P. (1994). Laser-induced pain-related brain potentials and sensory pain ratings in high and low hypnotizable subjects during hypnotic suggestions of relaxation, dissociated imagery, focused analgesia, and placebo. *International Journal of Clinical and Experimental Hypnosis, 42,* 56–80.

Zeig, J. K. (Ed.). (1985). *Ericksonian psychotherapy: Vol. 1: Structures.* New York, NY: Brunner/Mazel.

Zeig, J. K., & Lankton, S. R. (1988). *Developing Ericksonian therapy.* Bristol, PA: Brunner/Mazel.

Zeltzer, L., & LeBaron, S. (1982). Hypnosis and nonhypnotic techniques for reduction of pain and anxiety during painful procedures in children and adolescents with cancer. *Journal of Pediatrics, 101,* 1032–1035.

Zitman, F. G., Van Dyck, R., Spinhoven, P., & Linssen, A. C. (1992). Hypnosis and autogenic training in the treatment of tension headaches: A two-phase constructive design study with follow-up. *Journal of Psychosomatic Research, 36,* 219–228.

INDEX

ABOUT THE AUTHOR

David R. Patterson, PhD, ABPP, is a professor in the departments of rehabilitation medicine, surgery, and psychology at the University of Washington School of Medicine. Currently, he is head of the Division of Psychology for his home department and chair of the ethics committee at Harborview Medical Center. Dr. Patterson has been working as a clinical psychologist at Harborview Medical Center since 1983, particularly in the burn unit and the psychology consultation and liaison service he created. He holds diplomate degrees in the areas of psychological hypnosis and rehabilitation psychology. Dr. Patterson has been instrumental in running psychology intern and postdoctoral training programs for more than 20 years and has mentored hundreds of clinical and research students. His research has been funded by the National Institutes of Health since 1989, and he has published more than 150 articles and chapters in the areas of hypnosis, pain control, and adjustment to burn injuries and other types of trauma. His articles can be found in such journals as *Psychological Bulletin, Journal of Consulting and Clinical Psychology, Journal of Abnormal Psychology, Pain,* and the *New England Journal of Medicine.* As a long time soccer player, he enjoys coaching his sons in this sport and playing drums for the *Shrinking Heads* rock-and-roll band.